Cardiology Research and Clinical Developments

nova
Medicine & Health
New York

Cardiology Research and Clinical Developments

Perspectives in Aortic Valve Disease: Clinical and Morphological Characteristics, Diagnosis and Treatments
Giovanni Concistrè (Editor)
2020. ISBN: 978-1-53618-769-4 (Hardcover)
2020. ISBN: 978-1-53618-848-6 (eBook)

The Interventional Cardiology World: User's Manual of the Cath. Lab. for Students and Apprentices
Dario Buccheri, MD (Editor)
Bernardo Cortese (Editor)
Alessio La Manna, MD (Editor)
2020. ISBN: 978-1-53618-249-1 (Hardcover)
2020. ISBN: 978-1-53618-675-8 (eBook)

Nd:Yag Laser Treatment for Various Vascular Lesions
Ekrem Civas, Berna Aksoy and Hasan Mete Aksoy (Authors)
2011. ISBN: 978-1-61761-099-8 (Softcover)
2010. ISBN: 978-1-61761-646-4 (eBook)

Abdominal Aortic Aneurysms: New Approaches to Rupture Risk Assessment
Barry J. Doyle (Author)
David S. Molony (Author)
Michael T. Walsh (Author)
Timothy M. McGloughlin (Author)
2011. ISBN: 978-1-61668-312-2 (Softcover)
2011. ISBN: 978-1-61209-807-4 (eBook)

More information about this series can be found at
https://novapublishers.com/product-category/series/cardiology-research-and-clinical-developments/

Elian Facundo Giordanino
Editor

Heart Transplantation

Indications, Postoperative Management and Long-Term Outcomes

nova
Medicine & Health
New York

DOI: https://doi.org/10.52305/KNCI5528

Library of Congress Cataloging-in-Publication Data

Names: Giordanino, Elian Facundo, editor.
Title: Heart transplantation : indications, postoperative management and long-term outcomes / Elian Facundo Giordanino, MD (editor), Cardiologist, Heart Failure and Heart Transplantation, Favaloro Foundation University Hospital, BA Argentina.
Description: New York : Nova Science Publishers, [2022] | Series: Cardiology research and clinical developments | Includes bibliographical references and index. |
Identifiers: LCCN 2022021688 (print) | LCCN 2022021689 (ebook) | ISBN 9781685077594 (hardcover) | ISBN 9781685079413 (pdf)
Subjects: LCSH: Heart--Transplantation. | Heart--Transplantation--Complications. | Heart failure--Treatment.
Classification: LCC RD598.35.T7 H44 2022 (print) | LCC RD598.35.T7 (ebook) | DDC 617.4/120592--dc23/eng/20220609
LC record available at https://lccn.loc.gov/2022021688
LC ebook record available at https://lccn.loc.gov/2022021689

Published by Nova Science Publishers, Inc. † New York

To my teachers and colleagues at the Favaloro Foundation University Hospital, for being a group of professionals of excellence with whom I have the honor of having written this book and working side by side.

To my patients, who continue to teach me how to take care of them.

To Carolina, for her unconditional love and her tender companionship.

Contents

Preface

Heart failure is an increasingly prevalent syndrome worldwide with a high impact on quality of life and survival. Although there have been great advances in the treatment of this condition that effectively increase survival, mortality remains unacceptably high, exceeding 40% at 5 years, which worse than a large number of cancers. Furthermore, patients with advanced heart failure are a particular subgroup with higher hospitalizations and mortality, with a short-term survival that can be as low as 50% in the case of cardiogenic shock. Heart transplantation remains the gold standard treatment for these patients when other pharmacological and non-pharmacological interventions have failed, with a 1-year survival of approximately 90%. However, not all patients are suitable candidates for this procedure, and knowing the indications as well as the contraindications for heart transplantation is essential for appropriate patient selection.

Heart Transplantation: Indications, Postoperative Management and Long-Term Outcomes is a highly illustrated, didactic book that comprehensively describes the pretransplant assessment of the advanced heart failure patient, the perioperative management of heart transplantation, and the early and late complications of the heart transplant recipient. It also covers special situations in heart transplantation such as Chagas cardiomyopathy, congenital heart disease, hypertrophic/restrictive cardiomyopathy and pediatric heart transplantation.

Apart from the editor, this work has been reviewed by a distinguished group of specialists in the field of heart failure and heart transplantation. Drs. Absi, Bertolotti, Favaloro L., Favaloro R. and Renedo provided their expert review to improve the different chapters of this book.

The first part of the book is focused on the pretransplantation assessment. Dr. Ratto makes a precise introduction to the patient with heart failure and Drs. Cáneva, Ossés and Ahumada describe in detail the usefulness of cardiopulmonary exercise testing in heart transplant candidates. Patients with advanced heart failure being considered for heart transplantation often require complex monitoring and treatment. Dr. Sacatularo summarizes the hemodynamic assessment in the heart transplant candidate using the Swan-Ganz catheter, Drs. Cicolini and Giordanino briefly describe the main aspects of the intraortic balloon pump in heart transplantation, and Drs. Candioti and Giordanino present the challenging aspects of short-term mechanical circulatory support in heart transplant candidates. This gives place to the indications and contraindications for heart transplantation, which form the core of the book, didactically described by Dr. Giordanino. Finally, Moscoloni and Martinez offer an insightful look at psychosocial evaluation in heart transplantation.

The second part of the book centers on the perioperative management of heart transplantation. Dr. Absi comprehensively details the surgical techniques and Dr. Renedo describes the principal aspects of graft dysfunction and postoperative management of heart transplantation.

The third part concentrates on the follow-up care after heart transplantation. Drs. Salmo, Sánchez Luceros, Ganum, Moukarzel, Seijo Behety and Guevara highlight the value of echocardiography in heart transplant recipients, Drs. Giordanino, Padros and Vigliano explain the diagnosis and treatment of cardiac allograft rejection, and Dr. Giordanino briefly describes the diagnosis and follow-up of cardiac allograft vasculopathy. Infectious diseases in heart transplantation are thoroughly covered by Drs. Di Masi, Gago, Giorgio, Martínez Rios, Pujato and Villamandos. Last but not least, the challenges in nursing care and follow-up of the heart transplant patient are outlined by registered nurses Ibañez, Yakobas and Zacarias.

Finally, there are special situations in heart transplantation that deserve their own chapters. The singularities of pediatric heart transplantation are extensively reviewed by Dr. Trentadue and the increasingly common scenario of heart transplantation in Chagas cardiomyopathy is summarized by Drs. Vigliano and Favaloro L. In addition, the challenging aspects of heart transplantation in congenital heart disease are excellently described by Dr. Zeppa, while Drs. Fernández and Quiroga exhaustively detail the peculiarities of heart transplantation in familial hypertrophic/restrictive cardiomyopathy.

This book is intended for cardiology fellows in training, surgeons, cardiologists, internists, and other health professionals involved in the care of heart transplant patients. It includes the extensive experience of the exceptional health professionals of the Favaloro Foundation University Hospital in the management of this special population.

Elian Facundo Giordanino, MD

Part I: Pretransplantation Assessment

Chapter 1

Introduction to the Patient with Heart Failure

Roxana Daniela Ratto*
Heart Failure and Heart Transplantation, Favaloro Foundation University Hospital, Buenos Aires, Argentina

Abstract

Heart failure is one of the cardiovascular syndromes of greatest interest in recent years due to the increase in its prevalence with high rates of hospitalization and disability with enormous health costs. This increase is due to the aging of the population and the improvement in survival of other heart diseases and other non-cardiovascular diseases such as cancer. As patients get older, overcoming other diseases, they reach more advanced stages of heart failure. This chapter describes the different classifications, pathophysiology and pharmacological and non-pharmacological treatment of the patient with heart failure with reduced ejection fraction.

Keywords: heart failure, classification, medication therapy management

Introduction

Heart failure (HF) is a clinical syndrome consisting of symptoms (dyspnea, paroxysmal nocturnal dyspnea, fatigue and exercise intolerance, dry cough, ankle swelling) and/or signs (peripheral edema and fluid retention, elevated jugular venous pressure, pulmonary crackles, pleural effusion), caused by a

---

* Corresponding Author's E-mail: rratto@ffavaloro.org.

In: Heart Transplantation
Editor: Elian Facundo Giordanino
ISBN: 978-1-68507-759-4

structural and/or functional cardiac abnormality that results in elevated intracardiac pressures and/or inadequate cardiac output at rest and/or during exercise. This functional and cardiac abnormality is usually corroborated by elevated natriuretic peptide levels and/or objective evidence of pulmonary or systemic congestion [1].

Global prevalence of HF was 63.6 million in 2016 [2]. Multicenter, multinational studies have suggested that 1–2% of people have HF. However, some single-center, national studies have reported a higher prevalence of HF [3]. Despite the stable incidence, the prevalence of HF is increasing with a projected rise of 23%, from 2.4% (2012) to 3.0% (2030), due to the aging of the population and the increase in comorbidities leading to the development of the disease [3-5]. By 2030, more than 26% of HF patients will be 80 years of age or older [4].

In the THIN study (The Health Improvement Network), patients with HF have reduced 1-, 5-, and 10-year survival estimates compared with patients without HF. Data were collected over a period of more than 10 years to determine overall survival rates for patients; more than 54.000 patients were enrolled. Survival rates of patients with HF, aged 55–64, were reduced by more than 15% at each interval measured (1-, 5-, and 10-year). The difference between 10-year survival rates of patients with and without HF, aged 65–74, was over 30% [6].

Initial hospitalizations for HF appear to be declining, but readmissions remain high [7]. Acute events contribute to the progression of the disease; with each admission for decompensated HF, there is a short-term improvement, but the patient leaves the hospital with an additional decrease in cardiac function [8]. Patients with clinical worsening of HF are associated with a reduced quality of life. As functional class progresses, physical functioning, general perceptions of health, and vitality are significantly reduced. Role limitations are observed due to physical and emotional limitations [9].

Identifying the etiology of cardiac dysfunction is mandatory, since in some cases resolution of the underlying pathology is possible, determining an improvement in the prognosis of the disease [1].

Heart failure etiology is diverse and overlapping, causes include: *diseased myocardium* as previous ischemic events (myocardial infarction, coronary heart disease), toxic damage (substance abuse, heavy metals, medications, radiation), immune-mediated and inflammatory damage (infectious or noninfectious), infiltration (malignant or nonmalignant), metabolic disorders (diabetes/nutritional) and genetic abnormalities; *abnormal loading conditions* as hypertension, valve and myocardium structural defects, pericardial pathology, endomyocardial pathology, high output states (severe anemia, sepsis, thyrotoxicosis), volume overload (renal failure) and finally *arrhythmias*: tachyarrhythmias and bradyarrhythmias [10].

The etiology of HF varies by geography. In developed and Western-type countries, coronary artery disease and hypertension are predominant factors. The prevalence of ischemic heart disease by territory ranges from 4.6% (Sub-Saharan Africa) to 51.6% (Western high-income). In contrast, hypertension has a prevalence between 13.2% (Asia Pacific high income) and 35% (Central and Eastern Europe) and 33.5% (Sub-Saharan Africa) [1].

Terminology and Classification

The definition of HF considers different types of classifications according to the following parameters: functional class, ejection fraction, etiology, disease progression, genetic alterations, and severity profiles in patients with advanced HF (Table 1).

The importance of the points agreed upon in the latest European and American guidelines has been based on providing a simple but complete definition of clinically relevant HF that has prognostic and therapeutic validity. Subclassification provides clarity in its concept and allows it to be used by all physicians regardless of their specialty. Likewise, clinical research requires standardized definitions to identify HF cases and collect endpoints of interest, such as cardiovascular (CV) mortality, all-cause mortality, HF related hospitalizations, and improved quality of life [11].

Typically, in clinical practice, the ejection fraction is used to classify HF. This point becomes relevant when establishing pharmacological treatment since the pathophysiological mechanisms in patients with heart failure with reduced ejection fraction (HFrEF) probably differ from those with heart failure with preserved ejection fraction (HFpEF). This has led to large pharmacological research studies to define ejection fraction cutoff points to identify the different phenotypes of HF [1, 12-15].

Throughout the evolution of the disease there are changes of trajectory in the clinical state. The identification of each stage is essential for optimal pharmacological and non-pharmacological treatment, implementing risk mitigation strategies and conducting patient-centered discussions.

Table 1. Heart failure classifications

Etiology	Ejection Fraction	NYHA Functional Classification	Disease Progression	MOGES	INTERMACS Profiles for Advanced HF
Ischemic / Non-ischemic Valvular Hypertensive Infiltrative (amyloidosis) Peripartum Myocarditis Chemotherapy-induced	HFrEF: LVEF$\leq$40% HFmrEF: 41-49% HFpEF: $\geq$ 50% HFimpEF: $\leq$40% baseline, $\geq$10point increase and second measurement of LVEF >40%	 I II III IV	Stages A B C D	Morphofunctional phenotype Organ (s) involvement Genetic inheritance pattern Etiological annotation, including genetic defect or underlying disease/substrate, Functional status	Profiles 1 2 3 4 5 6 7
According to specific etiology	According to LVEF	According to severity of symptoms	According to presence of HF symptoms and signs and cardiac structural changes	According to nosologic system	According to symptoms, functional capacity and hemodynamic stability for patients who are considered for advanced HF therapies

HErEF, heart failure with reduced ejection fraction; HFmEF, heart failure with mildly reduced ejection fraction; HEpEF, heart failure with preserved ejection fraction; HFimpEF, heart failure with improved ejection fraction; LVEF, left ventricular ejection fraction; NYHA, New York Heart Association; HF, heart failure. (Data from McDonagh TA et al. ESC Scientific Document Group. 2021 ESC Guidelines for the diagnosis and treatment of acute and chronic heart failure. *Eur Heart J.* 2021 Sep 21;42(36):3599-3726 and Bozkurt B et al. Universal Definition and Classification of Heart Failure. *J Card Fail.* 2021 Feb 7:S1071-9164(21)00050-6.)

The different classifications according to the natural course of the disease include: *New onset/the novo HF* defined as newly diagnosed HF without previous history of HF. *Worsening HF,* characterized by worsening symptoms, signs, and functional capacity, requiring intensification of therapies or other advanced treatments with or without hospitalization. Otherwise, in the face of an improvement in signs, symptoms and functional capacity, the patient is considered to be in a stage of *improvement in HF*. It is important to note that in this new terminology the persistence of symptoms with limitation of functional capacity (previously defined as stable HF) is defined as *persistent HF* due to the chronicity of the process and the importance of continuing to optimize drugs with impact on morbidity and mortality. Finally, those patients who evolve with resolution of the symptoms and signs of HF and structural and functional heart disease are defined as *HF in remission*. At this point, it is important to understand that the continuity of pharmacological and non-pharmacological treatment will be necessary for most patients who have presented HF because there are few etiologies that justify the definitive suspension of treatment due to its prognosis and nature of complete remission [14, 16].

Pathophysiology

As previously mentioned, different etiologies contribute to the progression of HF. The main causes are cardiomyopathies, coronary artery disease, and comorbidities such as high blood pressure, diabetes, and dyslipemia. These lead to a reduction in cardiac output and subsequently to the activation of compensatory mechanisms such as overactivation of the sympathetic nervous system and the renin angiotensin aldosterone system (RAAS), which lead to an increase in blood pressure and heart rate, fluid and sodium retention and finally myocardial inflammation. These compensatory mechanisms, as a main initiative, improve cardiac output. However, in the long term, they play a very important role in the remodeling and deterioration of cardiac function [10, 17, 18].

There are several changes that occur in the heart as HF progresses, such as remodeling of the left ventricle. This process differs significantly between HFrEF and HFpEF. In HFrEF there is a thinning and weakening of the left ventricular wall due to dilation of the ventricle (eccentric remodeling) correlating with a decrease in systolic function and the pumping capacity of the heart, which increases the heart rate and reduces cardiac output [10, 18, 19].

Unlike HFrEF, the ventricular size of patients with HFpEF appears normal or slightly reduced, with increased thickness and stiffness of the left ventricle (concentric remodeling), leading to reduced efficiency of the heart muscle due to the altered diastolic function. It is important to note that cardiac pumping capacity is maintained at the expense of higher filling pressures [10, 19].

The interaction between various systems that contribute to HF is mediated by the activation of several pathways that focus on restoring hemodynamic homeostasis. There are circulating mediators which are implicated in different subtypes and severities of HF. Endothelin, tumor necrosis factor (TNF) and interleukins are examples of cytokines in response to renal activity in HF. Vasopressin regulates water and sodium reabsorption, which is subsequently responsible for renal contribution in decompensated HF. Atrial natriuretic peptide (ANP) and B-type natriuretic peptide (BNP) are released as a response to elevated central venous pressure [10, 20].

Evidence from both experimental and clinical trials indicates that inflammatory cytokines contribute to the pathogenesis of HF. In patients with HFrEF, elevated levels of TNF-α and interleukins 1, 6 and 8 are often observed. Simultaneously, patients with HFpEF also have elevated TNF-α and interleukins 1β and 6. There is strong evidence that these mediators contribute to cardiomyocyte apoptosis-mediated cardiac remodeling, cardiac hypertrophy, fibrosis, peripheral vascular abnormalities, and elevated metalloproteinase 9 activity. These inflammatory mediators mark the severity of the disease and the prognosis [21, 22].

Natriuretic peptides have a wide range of effects on the heart, kidneys, and central nervous system. Natriuretic peptides are secreted in response to elevated cardiac filling pressures. These peptides oppose the effect of the RAAS and mediate increases in natriuresis, diuresis, and vasodilation. Increased BNP is an indicator of ventricular dysfunction; therefore, it is considered an important endpoint for evaluating the treatment and prognosis of HF [20, 23].

Clinical Presentation Profiles

It is important to define the clinical profile in acute HF. During the physical examination, symptoms and signs of congestion and/or hypoperfusion are detected [21]. Congestion is characterized by peripheral and bilateral edema, jugular venous dilation, hepatomegaly, intestinal and lung congestion, ascites, hepatojugular reflux. Distinguishingly, the patient may refer orthopnea or paroxysmal nocturnal dyspnea. On the other hand, presence of hypoperfusion is characterized by cold sweated extremities, mental confusion, dizziness and oliguria. Based on these signs and symptoms, patients can be classified in four groups of clinical symptoms [10]. The most common group, *warm and wet,* indicates that the patient is well perfused and congestive. *Cold and wet* are signs that the patient is hypoperfused and congestive, determining a bad prognosis, with a risk of worse evolution. The group *cold and dry* indicates that the patient is hypoperfused without congestion, this is the least common combination in the healthcare practice. Finally, patients tend to have a better prognosis when they have good perfusion without congestion or are *warm and dry* [24].

Pharmacological Treatment of Heart Failure with Reduced Ejection Fraction

Disease modification strategies and symptom control are the main categories into which drug therapies for HF are divided.

Disease modification strategies aim to stabilize hemodynamics and provide neurohormonal control to improve symptoms, survival, and reduce hospitalization. These therapies include angiotensin-converting enzyme inhibitors (ACE-I), angiotensin receptor-neprilysin inhibitor (ARNI), beta-blockers, mineralocorticoid receptor antagonists (MRAs) and sodium-glucose co-transporter 2 inhibitors (SGLT2i) as the first line of treatment. Other medications should be considered in selected patients for specific situations: Angiotensin II type I receptor blockers (ARBs), *If*-channel inhibitor (ivabradine), combination of hydralazine and isosorbide dinitrate, digoxin, soluble guanylate cyclase receptor stimulator (vericiguat) and cardiac myosin activator (omecamtiv mecarbil) (Table 2) [1].

The individual profile of the patient according to the clinical presentation based on blood pressure, heart rate, kidney disease and/or hyperkalemia will be essential to start the disease-modifying treatment in early stages which is based on the four pharmacological groups previously mentioned. These drugs will be uptitrated according to the tolerance and response of the patient [25].

Table 2. Treatment of heart failure with reduced ejection fraction

<table>
<tr><td colspan="7">Pharmacological treatment</td></tr>
<tr><td colspan="7">To reduce mortality and hospitalization in all patients</td></tr>
<tr><td>ACE-I /ARNI
I-A</td><td colspan="2">BB
I-A</td><td colspan="2">MRA
I-A</td><td colspan="2">SGLT2i
I-A</td></tr>
<tr><td colspan="7">Volume overload</td></tr>
<tr><td colspan="7">DIURETICS
I-C</td></tr>
<tr><td colspan="7">Special situations</td></tr>
<tr><td>Heart rate > 70 bpm

Ivabradine
IIa-B*(With BB)
IIa-C**(Without BB)</td><td>Atrial fibrillation

Digoxin/PVI
IIb-B</td><td colspan="2">ACE-I/ARNI intolerance

ARB
I-B</td><td colspan="2">Black Race

Hydralazine/ISDN
IIa-B</td><td>Symptomatic patients NYHA class II-IV$^{\pm}$
Vericiguat
IIb-B</td></tr>
<tr><td colspan="7">Implantable devices</td></tr>
<tr><td colspan="2">LVEF ≤35% and QRS <130 ms
ICD</td><td colspan="5">SR and LVEF ≤35% and QRS ≥130 ms
CRT-D</td></tr>
<tr><td>Ischemic
I-A</td><td>Non ischemic
IIa-A</td><td colspan="3">QRS > 150 ms
I-A(LBBB)IIa-B(non-LBBB)</td><td colspan="2">QRS 130-149 ms
IIa-B(LBBB)</td></tr>
<tr><td colspan="7">If symptoms persist and devices are not indicated or are inappropriate consider other Class II therapies</td></tr>
</table>

* Symptomatic patients, LVEF ≤ 35%, SR at rest and heart rate > 70 b.p.m. Beta-blocker treatment (maximum tolerated dose), ACE-I/(or ARNI), and MRA ** Symptomatic patients, with LVEF ≤ 35%, SR at rest and heart rate > 70 b.p.m. who are unable to tolerate or have contraindications to a beta blocker. They must also receive an ACE-I (or ARNI) and an MRA. ± Despite optimal treatment with an ACE-I (or ARNI), a beta-blocker and an MRA. ACE-I, angiotensin-converting enzyme inhibitor; ARB, angiotensin receptor blocker; ARNI, angiotensin receptor-neprilysin inhibitor; BB, beta-blocker; b.p.m., beats per minute; CRT-D, cardiac resynchronization therapy with defibrillator; ICD, implantable cardioverter defibrillator; ISDN, isosorbide dinitrate; HFrEF, heart failure with reduced ejection fraction; LBBB, left bundle branch block; LVEF, left ventricular ejection fraction; MRA, mineralocorticoid receptor antagonist; ms, milliseconds; NYHA, New York Heart Association; PVI, pulmonary vein isolation; SGLT2i, sodium-glucose co-transporter 2 inhibitor; SR, sinus rhythm. (Data from McDonagh TA et al. ESC Scientific Document Group. 2021 ESC Guidelines for the diagnosis and treatment of acute and chronic heart failure. *Eur Heart J.* 2021 Sep 21;42(36):3599-3726.)

Beta-Blockers

The desired effect of beta-blockers includes rate control, blood pressure reduction and improved reverse remodeling. The mechanisms of action of beta blockers in HF include: antagonism of neuronal and cardiac β2 adrenergic receptor, reduced cardiac and adrenal protein-coupled receptor kinase 2 activity and reduced adrenergic nervous system activity.

Common adverse events include hypotension, dizziness, and bradycardia. Multiple studies have been carried out with proven efficacy reducing morbidity and mortality [26-28]. Beta-blockers are indicated in clinically stable patients with HFrEF, initially at a low dose, and increased to the maximum tolerated dose, in addition to other disease modifying drugs.

Angiotensin-Converting Enzyme Inhibitors

Angiotensin converting enzyme regulates the balance between the vasodilator and natriuretic properties of bradykinin and the vasoconstrictive and salt-retaining properties of angiotensin II. This peptide has a direct vasoconstrictive effect on vascular smooth muscle cells, while interacting with the sympathetic nervous system [29]. The consequent effects of angiotensin II production are sodium and fluid retention. By reducing its formation and bradykinin breakdown, ACE inhibitors limit vasoconstriction and improve hemodynamics [30]. They reduce mortality and morbidity and improve symptoms, which makes this pharmacological group one of the recommended treatments for patients with HF and they should be uptitrated to the maximum tolerated doses [31-33]. In those patients that cannot tolerate ACE-I due to serious side effects, ARBs can be used as a replacement [34, 35].

Mineralocorticoid Receptor Antagonists

Mineralocorticoid receptor antagonists inhibit the receptors for aldosterone and other steroid hormones with varying degrees of affinity, achieving beneficial effects on both the heart and the kidneys. These drugs manage to reduce endothelial dysfunction and vasoconstriction, myocardial and glomerular hypertrophy, and ventricular remodeling [36]. They also reduce kidney damage and subsequent proteinuria. One of these drugs, eplerenone, has greater selectivity for aldosterone blockade, producing fewer associated side effects [37].

This pharmacological group showed to reduce mortality, morbidity and improve symptoms [38, 39].

Angiotensin Receptor-Neprilysin Inhibitors

Sacubitril/valsartan is a combined drug that achieves both the inhibition of neprilysin (reducing the rate of degradation of bradykinin, ANP and BNP) and angiotensin II type I receptor (inhibiting the RAAS). The achieved effects include diuresis, natriuresis, myocardial relaxation and vasodilation with the consequent reduction of hypertrophy and ventricular remodeling [10, 40].

The benefits of this drug were demonstrated in the PARADIGM-trial, where it was compared to enalapril and showed a reduction in hospitalizations for worsening HF, CV mortality, and all-cause mortality in ambulatory patients with left ventricular ejection fraction (LVEF) $\leq 40\%$ [41]. Therefore, it is recommended that an ACE-I be replaced by sacubitril/valsartan in outpatients with HFrEF, who remain symptomatic despite optimal treatment and in naive patients as first line of treatment, according to different international guides [1, 42].

Sodium-Glucose Co-Transporter 2 Inhibitors

Sodium-glucose co-transporter 2 inhibitors drugs have shown a beneficial effect at the CV level through several potential mechanisms. The effect on natriuresis and diuresis decreases plasma volume and tissue sodium content, producing a decrease in interstitial edema, improving congestion and ventricular filling pressures with the consequent decrease in preload, afterload and wall stress, and in the activation of the sympathetic system [43]. In turn, there is an improvement in oxygen supply to the myocardium and in cellular metabolism, through a change of substrate that replaces free fatty acids and glucose with ketone bodies. This results in a more efficient production of *adenosine triphosphate* (ATP), reducing the consumption of oxygen at both myocardial and renal levels [44, 45]. The latter has an impact on the adequate production of erythropoietin, improving hematocrit and hemoglobin levels. Another of the postulated cardioprotective effects of these drugs is related to the inhibition of the sodium hydrogen exchanger 1 (NHE1) with the consequently decrease in intracellular calcium, thus reducing the toxic effect that this represents for the cardiomyocyte [46]. Based on the results of randomized studies that demonstrated a reduction in hospitalizations for HF, CV death and all-cause mortality as well as an improvement in quality of life, dapagliflozin or empagliflozin are recommended in addition to optimal medical therapy (OMT) with an ACE-I / ARNI, a beta-blocker and an MRAs, for HFrEF patients regardless of their diabetes status [47, 48].

Diuretics

Loop diuretics are recommended to reduce volume overload, producing symptomatic improvement and having a short-term impact on the clinical status of patients, improving exercise capacity and reducing hospitalizations. Daily weight control and self-monitoring of signs and symptoms allow patients to modify diuretic doses, achieving better management of congestion and self-care [1].

Angiotensin II Type I Receptor Blockers

Angiotensin II type I receptor blockers are recommended for those patients who cannot tolerate ARNI or ACE-I. ARBs have a favorable effect on the treatment of HFrEF by antagonizing vasoconstriction, aldosterone release, and hypertrophic response. Studies carried out with this group of drugs showed a benefit in reducing CV death and hospitalizations for HF [34], but not in reducing all-cause mortality [35].

I_f-Channel Inhibitors

Ivabradine is a therapeutic option in patients who are in sinus rhythm (SR) with heart rate (HR) ≥70 beats per minute (bpm), under maximum tolerated dose of beta blockers or who present contraindications for their use. Ivabradine reduces the HR by inhibiting the I_f channel of the sinus node. The SHIFT trial demonstrated a reduction in the combined end point of CV mortality and hospitalization for HF in patients with symptomatic HFrEF with LVEF ≤35%, who have been hospitalized for HF in the last 12 months and were in SR and HR ≥ 70 bpm under OMT [49].

Hydralazine and Isosorbide Dinitrate

The combination of hydralazine/isosorbide dinitrate is indicated in patients with contraindications for ARNI, ACE-I or ARBs and for those who continue to be symptomatic despite OMT. This benefit has been proved mainly in black-race patients with HFrEF, in addition to conventional therapy [1, 10, 50].

Digoxin

The use of digoxin is recommended in patients with SR and symptomatic HFrEF despite OMT [1]. In patients with atrial fibrillation, its use is suggested for HR control, between 70 and 90 bpm. Clinical trials showed a reduction in hospitalizations for HF or for any cause [51, 52].

Soluble Guanylate Cyclase Receptor Stimulator

Vericiguat, an oral soluble guanylate cyclase receptor stimulator, may be considered for the treatment of patients with worsening heart failure despite OMT to reduce hospitalizations for HF, based on the results of the VICTORIA trial [53].

Cardiac Myosin Activator

Omecamtiv mecarbil is a cardiac myosin activator that was evaluated in the GALACTIC-HF trial and showed a modest reduction in the combined endpoint of first HF event or CV death in patients with worsening heart failure despite OMT [54].

Implantable Devices in Heart Failure

In an individualized group of patients, the need to implement non-pharmacological therapies must be defined, since one of the forms of death in patients with HF is due to sudden death, especially in those with milder symptoms [55-57]. It is important when making the decision to consider short and long-term prognostic factors, such as the etiology of the heart disease (size of the scar, fibrosis), fragility, progression of dementia, comorbidities and adequacy of the OMT. The most frequent causes of death in this setting are due to electrical disturbances (ventricular arrhythmia, bradycardia, and asystole) or acute vascular events. In these cases, implantable cardioverter defibrillators (ICDs) are effective in protecting against arrhythmic events. Pharmacological antiarrhythmic treatment manages to reduce the rate of tachyarrhythmia and sudden death, but not overall mortality [1].

In the case of cardiac resynchronization therapy (CRT), the evidenced benefit marks a reduction in morbidity and mortality [58]. There are specific criteria for the indication of CRT. It is important to evaluate the clinical and echocardiographic response to resynchronization therapy in the follow-up since reverse remodeling is one of the most important therapeutic mechanisms and is often accompanied by an improvement in morbidity, mortality and quality of life. There are some specific parameters that help select the appropriate patients for this therapy, such as QRS width and morphology (left bundle branch block), sinus rhythm, female gender, non-ischemic etiology, and functional class [59, 60].

When evaluating the indication for ICDs and CRT, it is of utmost importance to first consider the prescription of OMT in patients with HFrEF, since these drugs can also produce reverse remodeling and improvement in LVEF that may avoid the need for these devices [61].

Conclusion

Heart failure is a complex syndrome that requires a multidisciplinary approach and pharmacological as well as non-pharmacological treatments. Medical care for patients with heart failure has improved in recent years and, consequently, so have their outcomes. However, when patients remain symptomatic despite optical medical therapy, a referral to a specialized heart failure clinic with availability of heart transplantation should always be considered.

References

[1] McDonagh TA, Metra M, Adamo M, Gardner RS, Baumbach A, Böhm M, Burri H, Butler J, Čelutkienė J, Chioncel O, Cleland JGF, Coats AJS, Crespo-Leiro MG,

Farmakis D, Gilard M, Heymans S, Hoes AW, Jaarsma T, Jankowska EA, Lainscak M, Lam CSP, Lyon AR, McMurray JJV, Mebazaa A, Mindham R, Muneretto C, Francesco Piepoli M, Price S, Rosano GMC, Ruschitzka F, Kathrine Skibelund A; ESC Scientific Document Group. 2021 ESC Guidelines for the diagnosis and treatment of acute and chronic heart failure. *Eur Heart J.* 2021 Sep 21;42(36):3599-3726.

[2] GBD 2016 Disease and Injury Incidence and Prevalence Collaborators. Global, regional, and national incidence, prevalence, and years lived with disability for 328 diseases and injuries for 195 countries, 1990-2016: a systematic analysis for the Global Burden of Disease Study 2016. *Lancet.* 2017 Sep 16;390(10100):1211-1259.

[3] Ponikowski P, Anker SD, AlHabib KF, Cowie MR, Force TL, Hu S, Jaarsma T, Krum H, Rastogi V, Rohde LE, Samal UC, Shimokawa H, Budi Siswanto B, Sliwa K, Filippatos G. Heart failure: preventing disease and death worldwide. *ESC Heart Fail.* 2014 Sep;1(1):4-25.

[4] Heidenreich PA, Albert NM, Allen LA, Bluemke DA, Butler J, Fonarow GC, Ikonomidis JS, Khavjou O, Konstam MA, Maddox TM, Nichol G, Pham M, Piña IL, Trogdon JG; American Heart Association Advocacy Coordinating Committee; Council on Arteriosclerosis, Thrombosis and Vascular Biology; Council on Cardiovascular Radiology and Intervention; Council on Clinical Cardiology; Council on Epidemiology and Prevention; Stroke Council. Forecasting the impact of heart failure in the United States: a policy statement from the American Heart Association. *Circ Heart Fail.* 2013 May;6(3):606-19.

[5] Conrad N, Judge A, Tran J, Mohseni H, Hedgecott D, Crespillo AP, Allison M, Hemingway H, Cleland JG, McMurray JJV, Rahimi K. Temporal trends and patterns in heart failure incidence: A population-based study of 4 million individuals. *Lancet.* 2018 Feb 10;391(10120):572-580.

[6] Taylor CJ, Ryan R, Nichols L, Gale N, Hobbs FR, Marshall T. Survival following a diagnosis of heart failure in primary care. *Fam Pract.* 2017 Apr 1;34(2):161-168.

[7] Roger VL. Epidemiology of heart failure. *Circ Res.* 2013 Aug 30;113(6):646-59.

[8] Gheorghiade M, De Luca L, Fonarow GC, Filippatos G, Metra M, Francis GS. Pathophysiologic targets in the early phase of acute heart failure syndromes. *Am J Cardiol.* 2005 Sep 19;96(6A):11G-17G.

[9] Juenger J, Schellberg D, Kraemer S, Haunstetter A, Zugck C, Herzog W, Haass M. Health related quality of life in patients with congestive heart failure: comparison with other chronic diseases and relation to functional variables. *Heart.* 2002 Mar;87(3):235-41.

[10] Ponikowski P, Voors AA, Anker SD, Bueno H, Cleland JGF, Coats AJS, Falk V, González-Juanatey JR, Harjola VP, Jankowska EA, Jessup M, Linde C, Nihoyannopoulos P, Parissis JT, Pieske B, Riley JP, Rosano GMC, Ruilope LM, Ruschitzka F, Rutten FH, van der Meer P; ESC Scientific Document Group. 2016 ESC Guidelines for the diagnosis and treatment of acute and chronic heart failure: The Task Force for the diagnosis and treatment of acute and chronic heart failure of the European Society of Cardiology (ESC)Developed with the special contribution

of the Heart Failure Association (HFA) of the ESC. *Eur Heart J.* 2016 Jul 14;37(27):2129-2200.

[11] Hicks KA, Mahaffey KW, Mehran R, Nissen SE, Wiviott SD, Dunn B, Solomon SD, Marler JR, Teerlink JR, Farb A, Morrow DA, Targum SL, Sila CA, Hai MTT, Jaff MR, Joffe HV, Cutlip DE, Desai AS, Lewis EF, Gibson CM, Landray MJ, Lincoff AM, White CJ, Brooks SS, Rosenfield K, Domanski MJ, Lansky AJ, McMurray JJV, Tcheng JE, Steinhubl SR, Burton P, Mauri L, O'Connor CM, Pfeffer MA, Hung HMJ, Stockbridge NL, Chaitman BR, Temple RJ; Standardized Data Collection for Cardiovascular Trials Initiative (SCTI). 2017 Cardiovascular and Stroke Endpoint Definitions for Clinical Trials. *Circulation.* 2018 Feb 27;137(9):961-972.

[12] Bozkurt B. Reasons for Lack of Improvement in Treatment With Evidence-Based Therapies in Heart Failure. *J Am Coll Cardiol.* 2019 May 21;73(19):2384-2387.

[13] Greene SJ, Fonarow GC, DeVore AD, Sharma PP, Vaduganathan M, Albert NM, Duffy CI, Hill CL, McCague K, Patterson JH, Spertus JA, Thomas L, Williams FB, Hernandez AF, Butler J. Titration of Medical Therapy for Heart Failure With Reduced Ejection Fraction. *J Am Coll Cardiol.* 2019 May 21;73(19):2365-2383.

[14] Bozkurt B, Coats A, Tsutsui H. Universal Definition and Classification of Heart Failure. *J Card Fail.* 2021 Feb 7:S1071-9164(21)00050-6.

[15] Khatibzadeh S, Farzadfar F, Oliver J, Ezzati M, Moran A. Worldwide risk factors for heart failure: a systematic review and pooled analysis. *Int J Cardiol.* 2013 Sep 30;168(2):1186-94.

[16] Halliday BP, Wassall R, Lota AS, Khalique Z, Gregson J, Newsome S, Jackson R, Rahneva T, Wage R, Smith G, Venneri L, Tayal U, Auger D, Midwinter W, Whiffin N, Rajani R, Dungu JN, Pantazis A, Cook SA, Ware JS, Baksi AJ, Pennell DJ, Rosen SD, Cowie MR, Cleland JGF, Prasad SK. Withdrawal of pharmacological treatment for heart failure in patients with recovered dilated cardiomyopathy (TRED-HF): an open-label, pilot, randomised trial. *Lancet.* 2019 Jan 5;393(10166):61-73.

[17] Hartupee J, Mann DL. Neurohormonal activation in heart failure with reduced ejection fraction. *Nat Rev Cardiol.* 2017 Jan;14(1):30-38.

[18] Jessup M, Brozena S. Heart failure. *N Engl J Med.* 2003 May 15;348(20):2007-18.

[19] Wright DFB, Anakin MG, Duffull SB. Clinical decision-making: An essential skill for 21st century pharmacy practice. *Res Social Adm Pharm.* 2019 May;15(5):600-606.

[20] Jönsson S, Agic MB, Narfström F, Melville JM, Hultström M. Renal neurohormonal regulation in heart failure decompensation. *Am J Physiol Regul Integr Comp Physiol*. 2014 Sep 1;307(5):R493-7.

[21] Gullestad L, Ueland T, Vinge LE, Finsen A, Yndestad A, Aukrust P. Inflammatory cytokines in heart failure: mediators and markers. *Cardiology.* 2012;122(1):23-35.

[22] Shou X, Lin J, Xie C, Wang Y, Sun C. Plasma IL-37 Elevated in Patients with Chronic Heart Failure and Predicted Major Adverse Cardiac Events: A 1-Year Follow-Up Study. *Dis Markers*. 2017;2017:9134079.

[23] Rodeheffer RJ. Measuring plasma B-type natriuretic peptide in heart failure: good to go in 2004? J Am Coll Cardiol. 2004 Aug 18;44(4):740-9.

[24] Nohria A, Tsang SW, Fang JC, Lewis EF, Jarcho JA, Mudge GH, Stevenson LW. Clinical assessment identifies hemodynamic profiles that predict outcomes in patients admitted with heart failure. *J Am Coll Cardiol.* 2003 May 21;41(10):1797-804.

[25] Rosano GMC, Moura B, Metra M, Böhm M, Bauersachs J, Ben Gal T, Adamopoulos S, Abdelhamid M, Bistola V, Čelutkienė J, Chioncel O, Farmakis D, Ferrari R, Filippatos G, Hill L, Jankowska EA, Jaarsma T, Jhund P, Lainscak M, Lopatin Y, Lund LH, Milicic D, Mullens W, Pinto F, Ponikowski P, Savarese G, Thum T, Volterrani M, Anker SD, Seferovic PM, Coats AJS. Patient profiling in heart failure for tailoring medical therapy. A consensus document of the Heart Failure Association of the European Society of Cardiology. *Eur J Heart Fail.* 2021 Jun;23(6):872-881.

[26] Effect of metoprolol CR/XL in chronic heart failure: Metoprolol CR/XL Randomised Intervention Trial in Congestive Heart Failure (MERIT-HF). *Lancet.* 1999 Jun 12;353(9169):2001-7.

[27] The Cardiac Insufficiency Bisoprolol Study II (CIBIS-II): a randomised trial. *Lancet.* 1999 Jan 2;353(9146):9-13.

[28] Fowler MB. Effects of beta blockers on symptoms and functional capacity in heart failure. *Am J Cardiol.* 1997 Dec 4;80(11A):55L-58L.

[29] Brown NJ, Vaughan DE. Angiotensin-converting enzyme inhibitors. *Circulation.* 1998 Apr 14;97(14):1411-20.

[30] Perkovic V, Jardine M, Vijapurkar U, Meininger G. Renal effects of canagliflozin in type 2 diabetes mellitus. *Curr Med Res Opin.* 2015 Dec;31(12):2219-31.

[31] Enalapril for congestive heart failure. *N Engl J Med.* 1987 Nov 19;317(21):1349-51.

[32] Garg R, Yusuf S. Overview of randomized trials of angiotensin-converting enzyme inhibitors on mortality and morbidity in patients with heart failure. Collaborative Group on ACE Inhibitor Trials. JAMA. 1995 May 10;273(18): 1450-6. *Erratum in: JAMA* 1995 Aug 9;274(6):462.

[33] SOLVD Investigators, Yusuf S, Pitt B, Davis CE, Hood WB, Cohn JN. Effect of enalapril on survival in patients with reduced left ventricular ejection fractions and congestive heart failure. *N Engl J Med.* 1991 Aug 1;325(5):293-302.

[34] Granger CB, McMurray JJ, Yusuf S, Held P, Michelson EL, Olofsson B, Ostergren J, Pfeffer MA, Swedberg K; CHARM Investigators and Committees. Effects of candesartan in patients with chronic heart failure and reduced left-ventricular systolic function intolerant to angiotensin-converting-enzyme inhibitors: the CHARM-Alternative trial. *Lancet.* 2003 Sep 6;362(9386):772-6.

[35] Cohn JN, Tognoni G; Valsartan Heart Failure Trial Investigators. A randomized trial of the angiotensin-receptor blocker valsartan in chronic heart failure. *N Engl J Med.* 2001 Dec 6;345(23):1667-75.

[36] Bauersachs J, Jaisser F, Toto R. Mineralocorticoid receptor activation and mineralocorticoid receptor antagonist treatment in cardiac and renal diseases. *Hypertension.* 2015 Feb;65(2):257-63.

[37] Manolis AA, Manolis TA, Melita H, Manolis AS. Eplerenone Versus Spironolactone in Resistant Hypertension: an Efficacy and/or Cost or Just a Men's Issue? *Curr Hypertens Rep.* 2019 Mar 2;21(3):22.

[38] Pitt B, Zannad F, Remme WJ, Cody R, Castaigne A, Perez A, Palensky J, Wittes J. The effect of spironolactone on morbidity and mortality in patients with severe heart failure. Randomized Aldactone Evaluation Study Investigators. *N Engl J Med.* 1999 Sep 2;341(10):709-17.

[39] Zannad F, McMurray JJ, Krum H, van Veldhuisen DJ, Swedberg K, Shi H, Vincent J, Pocock SJ, Pitt B; EMPHASIS-HF Study Group. Eplerenone in patients with systolic heart failure and mild symptoms. *N Engl J Med.* 2011 Jan 6;364(1):11-21.

[40] Yandrapalli S, Andries G, Biswas M, Khera S. Profile of sacubitril/valsartan in the treatment of heart failure: patient selection and perspectives. *Vasc Health Risk Manag.* 2017 Oct 5;13:369-382.

[41] McMurray JJ, Packer M, Desai AS, Gong J, Lefkowitz MP, Rizkala AR, Rouleau JL, Shi VC, Solomon SD, Swedberg K, Zile MR; PARADIGM-HF Investigators and Committees. Angiotensin-neprilysin inhibition versus enalapril in heart failure. *N Engl J Med.* 2014 Sep 11;371(11):993-1004.

[42] Writing Committee, Maddox TM, Januzzi JL Jr, Allen LA, Breathett K, Butler J, Davis LL, Fonarow GC, Ibrahim NE, Lindenfeld J, Masoudi FA, Motiwala SR, Oliveros E, Patterson JH, Walsh MN, Wasserman A, Yancy CW, Youmans QR. 2021 Update to the 2017 ACC Expert Consensus Decision Pathway for Optimization of Heart Failure Treatment: Answers to 10 Pivotal Issues About Heart Failure With Reduced Ejection Fraction: A Report of the American College of Cardiology Solution Set Oversight Committee. *J Am Coll Cardiol.* 2021 Feb 16;77(6):772-810. doi: 10.1016/j.jacc.2020.11.022. Epub 2021 Jan 11. PMID: 33446410.

[43] Heerspink HJL, Kosiborod M, Inzucchi SE, Cherney DZI. Renoprotective effects of sodium-glucose cotransporter-2 inhibitors. *Kidney Int.* 2018 Jul;94(1):26-39. doi: 10.1016/j.kint.2017.12.027. Epub 2018 May 5. PMID: 29735306.

[44] Tamargo J. Sodium-glucose Cotransporter 2 Inhibitors in Heart Failure: Potential Mechanisms of Action, Adverse Effects and Future Developments. *Eur Cardiol.* 2019 Apr;14(1):23-32.

[45] Verma S, Garg A, Yan AT, Gupta AK, Al-Omran M, Sabongui A, Teoh H, Mazer CD, Connelly KA. Effect of Empagliflozin on Left Ventricular Mass and Diastolic Function in Individuals With Diabetes: An Important Clue to the EMPA-REG OUTCOME Trial? *Diabetes Care.* 2016 Dec;39(12):e212-e213. doi: 10.2337/dc16-1312. Epub 2016 Sep 27. PMID: 27679584.

[46] Favaloro LE, Ratto RD, Musso C. Heart Failure And Diabetes: Perspective Of A Dangerous Association. *Curr Hypertens Rev.* 2021 Apr 5.

[47] McMurray JJV, DeMets DL, Inzucchi SE, Køber L, Kosiborod MN, Langkilde AM, Martinez FA, Bengtsson O, Ponikowski P, Sabatine MS, Sjöstrand M, Solomon SD; DAPA-HF Committees and Investigators. A trial to evaluate the effect of the sodium-glucose co-transporter 2 inhibitor dapagliflozin on morbidity and mortality

in patients with heart failure and reduced left ventricular ejection fraction (DAPA-HF). *Eur J Heart Fail.* 2019 May;21(5):665-675.

[48] Packer M, Anker SD, Butler J, Filippatos G, Pocock SJ, Carson P, Januzzi J, Verma S, Tsutsui H, Brueckmann M, Jamal W, Kimura K, Schnee J, Zeller C, Cotton D, Bocchi E, Böhm M, Choi DJ, Chopra V, Chuquiure E, Giannetti N, Janssens S, Zhang J, Gonzalez Juanatey JR, Kaul S, Brunner-La Rocca HP, Merkely B, Nicholls SJ, Perrone S, Pina I, Ponikowski P, Sattar N, Senni M, Seronde MF, Spinar J, Squire I, Taddei S, Wanner C, Zannad F; EMPEROR-Reduced Trial Investigators. Cardiovascular and Renal Outcomes with Empagliflozin in Heart Failure. *N Engl J Med.* 2020 Oct 8;383(15):1413-1424.

[49] Swedberg K, Komajda M, Böhm M, Borer JS, Ford I, Dubost-Brama A, Lerebours G, Tavazzi L; SHIFT Investigators. Ivabradine and outcomes in chronic heart failure (SHIFT): a randomised placebo-controlled study. *Lancet.* 2010 Sep 11;376(9744):875-85.

[50] Taylor AL, Ziesche S, Yancy C, Carson P, D'Agostino R Jr, Ferdinand K, Taylor M, Adams K, Sabolinski M, Worcel M, Cohn JN; African-American Heart Failure Trial Investigators. Combination of isosorbide dinitrate and hydralazine in blacks with heart failure. *N Engl J Med.* 2004 Nov 11;351(20):2049-57.

[51] Ouyang AJ, Lv YN, Zhong HL, Wen JH, Wei XH, Peng HW, Zhou J, Liu LL. Meta-analysis of digoxin use and risk of mortality in patients with atrial fibrillation. *Am J Cardiol.* 2015 Apr 1;115(7):901-6.

[52] Ziff OJ, Lane DA, Samra M, Griffith M, Kirchhof P, Lip GY, Steeds RP, Townend J, Kotecha D. Safety and efficacy of digoxin: systematic review and meta-analysis of observational and controlled trial data. *BMJ.* 2015 Aug 30;351:h4451.

[53] Armstrong PW, Pieske B, Anstrom KJ, Ezekowitz J, Hernandez AF, Butler J, Lam CSP, Ponikowski P, Voors AA, Jia G, McNulty SE, Patel MJ, Roessig L, Koglin J, O'Connor CM; VICTORIA Study Group. Vericiguat in Patients with Heart Failure and Reduced Ejection Fraction. *N Engl J Med.* 2020 May 14;382(20):1883-1893.

[54] Teerlink JR, Diaz R, Felker GM, McMurray JJV, Metra M, Solomon SD, Adams KF, Anand I, Arias-Mendoza A, Biering-Sørensen T, Böhm M, Bonderman D, Cleland JGF, Corbalan R, Crespo-Leiro MG, Dahlström U, Echeverria LE, Fang JC, Filippatos G, Fonseca C, Goncalvesova E, Goudev AR, Howlett JG, Lanfear DE, Li J, Lund M, Macdonald P, Mareev V, Momomura SI, O'Meara E, Parkhomenko A, Ponikowski P, Ramires FJA, Serpytis P, Sliwa K, Spinar J, Suter TM, Tomcsanyi J, Vandekerckhove H, Vinereanu D, Voors AA, Yilmaz MB, Zannad F, Sharpsten L, Legg JC, Varin C, Honarpour N, Abbasi SA, Malik FI, Kurtz CE; GALACTIC-HF Investigators. Cardiac Myosin Activation with Omecamtiv Mecarbil in Systolic Heart Failure. *N Engl J Med.* 2021 Jan 14;384(2):105-116.

[55] Shen L, Jhund PS, Petrie MC, Claggett BL, Barlera S, Cleland JGF, Dargie HJ, Granger CB, Kjekshus J, Køber L, Latini R, Maggioni AP, Packer M, Pitt B, Solomon SD, Swedberg K, Tavazzi L, Wikstrand J, Zannad F, Zile MR, McMurray JJV. Declining Risk of Sudden Death in Heart Failure. *N Engl J Med.* 2017 Jul 6;377(1):41-51.

[56] Barisani JM, Fernandez A, Fairman E, Diez M, Thierer J, Christen A, Porcile R, Trainini J, Kotowicz V, Comignani P, Nul D, Hirschson Prado A, Avellana P, Falconi M, Perez de Arenaza D. Consensus Statement on Acute and Advanced Heart Failure. *Rev argent Cardiol.* 2010 May-June;78(3):264-280.

[57] Ezekowitz JA, O'Meara E, McDonald MA, Abrams H, Chan M, Ducharme A, Giannetti N, Grzeslo A, Hamilton PG, Heckman GA, Howlett JG, Koshman SL, Lepage S, McKelvie RS, Moe GW, Rajda M, Swiggum E, Virani SA, Zieroth S, Al-Hesayen A, Cohen-Solal A, D'Astous M, De S, Estrella-Holder E, Fremes S, Green L, Haddad H, Harkness K, Hernandez AF, Kouz S, LeBlanc MH, Masoudi FA, Ross HJ, Roussin A, Sussex B. 2017 Comprehensive Update of the Canadian Cardiovascular Society Guidelines for the Management of Heart Failure. *Can J Cardiol.* 2017 Nov;33(11):1342-1433.

[58] Cleland JG, Abraham WT, Linde C, Gold MR, Young JB, Claude Daubert J, Sherfesee L, Wells GA, Tang AS. An individual patient meta-analysis of five randomized trials assessing the effects of cardiac resynchronization therapy on morbidity and mortality in patients with symptomatic heart failure. *Eur Heart J.* 2013 Dec;34(46):3547-56.

[59] Cleland JG, Mareev Y, Linde C. Reflections on EchoCRT: sound guidance on QRS duration and morphology for CRT? *Eur Heart J.* 2015 Aug 7;36(30):1948-51.

[60] Zusterzeel R, Selzman KA, Sanders WE, Caños DA, O'Callaghan KM, Carpenter JL, Piña IL, Strauss DG. Cardiac resynchronization therapy in women: US Food and Drug Administration meta-analysis of patient-level data. *JAMA Intern Med.* 2014 Aug;174(8):1340-8.

[61] Woods B, Hawkins N, Mealing S, Sutton A, Abraham WT, Beshai JF, Klein H, Sculpher M, Plummer CJ, Cowie MR. Individual patient data network meta-analysis of mortality effects of implantable cardiac devices. *Heart.* 2015 Nov;101(22):1800-6.

Chapter 2

Cardiopulmonary Exercise Testing in Heart Transplant Candidates

Jorge Osvaldo Cáneva[1,*], Juan Manuel Ossés[1] and Rosalía Ahumada[1]

[1]Exercise Physiopathology Laboratory, Pneumonology Section, Department of Medicine, Favaloro Foundation University Hospital, Buenos Aires, Argentina

Abstract

End-stage heart failure is a complex syndrome of multiple etiologies and heart transplantation is the gold standard treatment. However, identifying those patients that will benefit from heart transplantation might be challenging, especially in an outpatient setting. Cardiopulmonary exercise testing is an invaluable tool for the proper evaluation of patients with heart failure and for the selection of candidates for heart transplantation. Furthermore, it allows for a comprehensive assessment of a patient's respiratory, cardiovascular and musculoskeletal response to maximal exercise. Understanding its components and interpreting its results is essential for the adequate management of heart failure patients.

Keywords: heart transplantation, heart failure, exercise test

---

* Corresponding Author's E-mail: jcaneva@ffavaloro.org.

In: Heart Transplantation
Editor: Elian Facundo Giordanino
ISBN: 978-1-68507-759-4

Introduction

Cardiopulmonary exercise testing (CPET) is the "gold standard" test to assess a subject's physical capacity, primarily aerobic. Additionally, the anaerobic complement may be recognized [1]. This test identifies and defines the respiratory, cardiovascular and/or musculoskeletal limitations, and the coupling between all of them, that limit physical activity. This is achieved by evaluating the behavior of a series of primary variables, such as maximum oxygen consumption (VO_2max), carbon dioxide production (VCO_2), maximum ventilation achieved (VE), anaerobic threshold (AT) and heart rate (HR).

There are also equally important secondary variables that enrich the pathophysiological knowledge of a certain clinical condition for which this procedure is performed. Interpretation of CPET results has diagnostic, prognostic and therapeutic implications [2].

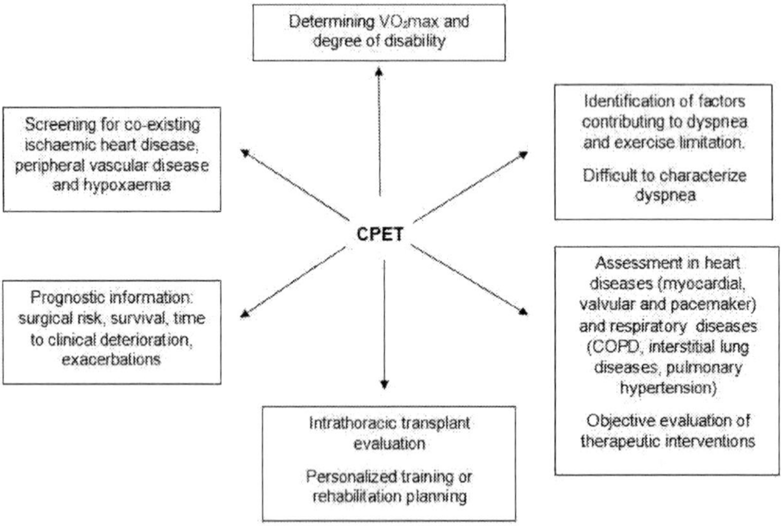

Figure 1. Clinical utility of cardiopulmonary exercise testing. COPD, Chronic obstructive pulmonary disease; CPET, cardiopulmonary exercise testing; VO_2max maximum oxygen consumption (Data from Laveneziana P et al. The clinical value of cardiopulmonary exercise testing in the modern era. *Eur Respir Rev*. 2021 Jan 6;30(159):200187).

This test is indicated in different medical situations, such as heart failure, pulmonary hypertension, respiratory diseases, pacemaker regulation, evaluation for heart, lung and heart-lung transplantation, cardiovascular and respiratory rehabilitation programs, surgical risk assessment, sports fitness assessment and in situations of dyspnea of unknown origin, difficult diagnosis or in cases which dyspnea is of multifactorial cause in order to determine the contribution of different systems to maximal exercise limitation (Figure 1) [3, 4].

Determinants of Physiological Responses to Exercise in Normal Subjects

CPET should be seen as an adjunct to a prior comprehensive medical evaluation comprising clinical history, physical examination, and appropriate complementary tests. The latter vary according to the specific condition and may include laboratory tests, electrocardiography, chest imaging, arterial blood gases and acid-base status, resting pulmonary function and/or echocardiography, among others. Therefore, there is a key interpretative feature of CPET that, if ignored, can be a major source of frustration for the ordering physician: the test must always be interpreted in light of the likelihood of abnormality [5].

Indeed, many patients referred for CPET have undergone extensive additional studies, such that it is the referring physicians' task to integrate the pathophysiological dysfunction patterns obtained by this test with their diagnostic plan and/or prognostic assessment. Patients referred for CPET usually have multiple comorbidities in addition to polypharmacy, obesity and extreme sedentary lifestyle. Therefore, an individual with a single mechanism of exercise intolerance has become extremely rare in the CPET laboratory [5].

Exercise intolerance, or the inability to maintain muscle exertion, is a central feature of many cardiopulmonary diseases. Conceptually, this depends on the restrictions and limitations of the mitochondrial electron transport chain. This ultimately expresses an operational failure within the normally coordinated interaction between skeletal muscle energy and the cardiovascular and respiratory systems in response to exertion. The aim of CPET is to establish the underlying contributions of these systems to exercise intolerance, using pre-designed exercise test formats. Thus, there are intensity- and time-related response profiles to either incremental (ramped) or constant-load exercise performed up to the limit of tolerance; it is for this reason that CPET is also referred to as symptom-limited CPET at maximal exertion [6].

A rapidly incremental test (following a continuous "ramp" or stepwise 1-2 minutes increments in workload) is the most commonly used protocol in the clinical setting. In addition to standard metabolic, cardiovascular, gas exchange and ventilatory variables, measurements of symptom intensity (Borg dyspnea and leg strain indices) and exercise breathing capacity are required [7].

There are logical sequences for collecting the information provided by the test, a procedure that is very useful, particularly for the assessment of subjects with multiple potential causes of exercise intolerance. Numerical cut-off values of normality based on age and gender are available for key variables that may influence decision making [8-10]. Therefore, the results obtained in this test should be presented in numerical (tabular report) and graphical format. Normality is established if the results follow an expected behavioral profile and the values read in a report are not outside the proposed cut-off values according to the age group. Thus, a CPET can be maximal or submaximal: maximal when it meets those normal values and submaximal when the key variables are outside the expected range or in the presence of large chronotropic, ventilatory and mechanical reserves when all other responses are considered normal in a subject with a low symptom load at the end of exercise [11].

Equipment and Report

CPET relies on a number of devices and sensors which must function properly to ensure the validity of all the assessments. It is important to choose an appropriate test methodology for a given clinical population, as well as to choose the appropriate ergometer to be used in any particular population. The accuracy of clinical judgment when considering CPET results is only guaranteed if the user is confident in the accuracy of the measurements made [12].

The aim of CPET protocols is to impose substantial stress on all organ systems involved in exercise response to test their functional reserve and to observe the pattern of this response in order to draw clinical conclusions. For this reason, exercise testing generally involves large muscle groups, usually the muscles of the lower extremities. An important requirement is that the exercise stimulus be quantifiable in terms of the rate of external work performed.

Simpler tests, such as the 6-minute walk test, can provide measures of exercise performance and, in some cases, exercise tolerance. However, it should be noted that they are submaximal tests, which limits clinical judgment compared to data provided by a CPET [13]. In contrast, incremental CPET protocols allow a series of exercise intensities to be imposed for a relatively short period during which physiological responses to exertion are continuously recorded. Nevertheless, the accuracy and reliability of these measurements depend on strict adherence to some key technical aspects [12].

Two types of exercise equipment are commonly used for this test: the bicycle ergometer, also called cycloergometer, and the treadmill. In the case of cycloergometers, an ergometer with an electromagnetic brake is preferred since ergometers with friction brakes often do not provide sufficiently accurate load settings [14]. On the other hand, it is still debated whether treadmill exercise can be used effectively in CPET. Since walking is a more familiar activity than cycling for most subjects, more muscle mass is used during treadmill exercise; hence, this leads to greater stress on the organ systems that mediate the exercise response, such that VO_2max is 5-10% higher on a treadmill than on a cycloergometer [15-18].

Several incremental treadmill protocols are popular, but their use in CPET has been slow to gain ground in clinical diagnostic testing or clinical trials [19-21].

With a focus on patients with heart disease, and specifically those with end-stage heart disease, CPET is applied to those who require evaluation as potential heart transplant candidates [22].

Regarding the correct presentation of the CPET results for a consistent final interpretation, there are different ways of preparing a report. Regardless of the form of the report, it is convenient and advisable that, in addition to expressing the parameters with the obtained values and the reference values individually, they should also be grouped into different domains, such as:

Working parameters
Work capacity.
AT.

Respiratory parameters
Respiratory reserve at maximum effort.

Respiratory rate at rest and at maximum effort.
Tidal volume/forced vital capacity ratio (TV/FVC) at rest and at maximal effort.
Pulse oximetry saturation at rest and at maximal effort.
Arterial blood gases at rest and at maximal effort (if available).

Ventilation/perfusion ratio (V/Q) parameters
Alveolar-arterial oxygen gradient or difference ($P(A\text{-}a)O_2$) at rest and at maximal effort.
Dead space (Vd/Vt) at rest and at maximum effort.
Arterial carbon dioxide (CO_2)-end-expiratory CO_2 gradient ($P(a\text{-}ET)CO_2$) or difference at rest and at maximal effort.
Ventilatory efficiency at rest and at maximal effort: respiratory minute ventilation/CO_2 production ratio (VE/VCO_2).

Cardiac parameters
Cardiac reserve at maximal effort.
Oxygen/heart rate (O_2/HR) at rest and at maximal effort.
Blood pressure behavior at rest and at maximal effort.

Usefulness in Heart Failure and Selection of Patients for Heart Transplantation

CPET makes a variety of contributions to the understanding of dyspnea and exercise limitation in chronic heart failure [23].

Numerous studies have shown that both invasive and noninvasive measurements of resting cardiac function are poor predictors of symptoms, exercise capacity, prognosis and the need for heart transplantation. Weber et al. compared resting cardiac function with exercise capacity in patients with heart failure and found that variables such as cardiac index, left ventricular ejection fraction, pulmonary capillary wedge pressure and heart size on chest radiography correlated poorly with VO_2max. Pulmonary capillary wedge pressure, both at rest and during exercise, does not correlate significantly with VO_2max; however, the authors established the correlation between functional capacity measured as VO_2max during CPET with the cardiac index, which gave rise to the "Weber Classification" (Table 1) [24].

Table 1. Weber's functional classification by cardiopulmonary exercise test

Class	Severity	VO_2max (ml/kg/min)	AT (ml/kg/min)	Maximal CI (L/min/m^2)
A	None to mild	>20	>14	>8
B	Mild to moderate	16-20	11-14	6-8
C	Moderate to severe	10-15	8-11	4-6
D	Severe	<10	<8	<4

AT, anaerobic threshold; CI, cardiac index; VO_2max: maximum oxygen consumption. (Data from Weber KT et al. Oxygen utilization and ventilation during exercise in patients with chronic cardiac failure. *Circulation.* 1982 Jun; 65(6):1213-23).

Van den Broek et al. reported that 88% of patients in New York Heart Association (NYHA) functional class II were in Weber classes A and B, as opposed to 73% of patients in NYHA functional class III, who were in Weber class C and D [25]. Similarly, Matsumura et al. and Itoh et al. demonstrated that VO_2max and AT correlated with symptom severity as measured by the NYHA class. AT was 90% ± 15%, 77% ± 14% and 60% ± 12% of the predicted values for NYHA Class I, Class II and Class III, respectively. On the other hand, AT correlates weakly with left ventricular ejection fraction, measured by echocardiography or angiography [26, 27].

Szlachik et al. found that patients with a VO_2max less than 10 ml/kg/min had a 1-year mortality of 77%, and if VO_2max was between 10 and 18 ml/kg/min the 1-year mortality was only 14% [28].

In a study led by Rickenbacher, 116 consecutive patients with severe but stable congestive heart failure, referred for heart transplantation, were evaluated under strict medical control and management. This working group demonstrated a very good prognosis, with a survival of 98% at one year and 84% at four years. Mean VO_2max was 17.4 ± 4.3 ml/kg/min. The authors concluded that stability of symptoms and a relatively high VO_2max identifies patients with a favorable prognosis despite a low resting ejection fraction [29].

The importance of CPET in risk stratification of patients with heart failure has been well established in several studies, allowing prioritization for heart transplantation. A prospective study by Mancini et al. included 114 patients with chronic heart failure referred for transplantation who were divided into three groups, the first with a VO_2max >14 ml/kg/min considered too well for transplantation, the second group with a VO_2max <14 ml/kg/min who were accepted for transplantation and finally a third group with a VO_2max <14 ml/kg/min who were not accepted for surgery due to non-cardiac reasons. The 1-year survival for patients with a VO_2max > 14 ml/kg/min was 94%, with only 70% survival for those with a VO_2max < 14 ml/kg/min who were ineligible for heart transplantation [30].

Osada et al. evaluated 154 of 500 congestive heart failure patients referred for heart transplantation with a $VO_2max \leq 14$ ml/kg/min, finding that the 3-year survival rate was reduced from 83 to 55% in those patients with an inability to achieve a systemic blood pressure of 120 mm Hg [31].

Stevenson et al. presented data from 68 heart transplant candidates (VO_2max < 14 ml/kg/min) who repeated the CPET within 6 ± 5 months after the initial assessment. The purpose of repeating this test was to determine the possibility of excluding patients from the transplant waiting list after a period of medical therapy. All patients were strictly treated with diuretics and ventricular afterload reduction and complied with a supervised muscle rehabilitation plan. Thirty patients had no improvement, but 38 had an increase of more than 2 ml/kg/min in VO_2max. Of the latter 7 reported no clinical improvement, but the remaining 31 improved clinically. The increase in VO_2max of the clinically improved patients was also associated with an increase in AT, oxygen pulse, HR reserve and a decrease in resting HR. All 31 patients were excluded from the waiting list with a survival rate of 100% [32]. Myers et al. reported the results of 644 patients with chronic heart failure over a 10-year period. They found that VO_2max outperformed cardiac catheterization data and the usual clinical variables used to assess and predict outcomes in patients with chronic heart failure. The authors concluded that direct measurement of VO_2max should be performed when clinical or surgical decisions are needed in patients referred for evaluation of their heart failure and/or eventual heart transplantation [33].

Although many studies establish the predicted VO_2max value based on body weight and ignore other variables such as age and gender, Stelken et al. compared the sensitivity of the percent predicted VO_2max using weight, age and gender in 181 outpatients in functional class II-III. The results showed that both VO_2max, percent VO_2max and AT were significantly different between survivors and non-survivors compared at 12 and 24 months. A total of 89 patients with a percent predicted VO_2max less than 50% had a 1-year and 2-year survival of 74% and 43%, respectively, compared with 98% and 90% of 92 patients with a percent predicted VO_2max greater than 50% [34].

For more than three decades, transplant cardiologists have accepted VO_2max as a more sensitive predictor of prognosis than classical heart failure prognostic factors, such as left ventricular ejection fraction, functional class

IV and neurohumoral markers. Growing experience has confirmed the prognostic value of VO_2max in the evaluation of patients for heart transplantation [30-35]. At the Bethesda Conference (1993), the indications for heart transplantation were developed and are shown in Table 2. A low VO_2max, having reached anaerobic metabolism, was considered a primary criterion for heart transplantation [36].

Table 2. Bethesda conference: indications for heart transplantation

Accepted indications for transplantation
VO_2max less than 10 ml/kg/min, reaching anaerobic metabolism. Severe ischemia, limiting activities of daily living and not amenable to surgical or hemodynamic revascularization. Recurrent ventricular arrhythmia refractory to all accepted therapeutic measures.
Probable indications for cardiac transplantation
VO_2max less than 14 ml/kg/min, with significant limitations in activities of daily living Recurrent unstable ischemia not amenable to surgical or hemodynamic revascularization Inadequate fluid balance and/or renal function, with adequate adherence to therapeutic regimens, including diuretics and saline restriction.
Inadequate indications for transplantation
Ejection fraction less than 20% Heart failure with symptoms in functional class III or IV. History of ventricular arrhythmias VO_2max greater than 15 ml/kg/min

VO_2max, maximum oxygen consumption. (Data from Mudge GH et al. Task Force 3: Recipient guidelines/prioritization. *J Am Coll Cardiol*. 1993 Jul; 22(1):21-31).

Finally, it is worth mentioning that VO_2max may be underestimated due to poor patient effort or early termination of exercise by the examiner. Gitt et al. studied submaximal AT and VE criteria versus the slope of VCO_2 below the ventilatory compensation point compared with VO_2max as a measure of heart failure severity and survival [37].

AT reflects sustainable VO_2max and is an objective parameter of cardiopulmonary exercise capacity. It can be derived from submaximal exercise and therefore does not require maximal patient effort. Another measure of submaximal CPET that has been found to have prognostic value in survival is the slope of VE/VCO_2 below the ventilatory compensation point [38-39]. Gitt et al. compared VO_2max and submaximal parameters as predictors of survival at 6 and 24 months in 223 patients. In this study, the risk of mortality was high in patients with VO_2max less than 14ml/kg/min, AT less than 11ml/kg/min and VE/VCO_2 slope below the compensation point of plus 35. The combination of AT and VE/VCO_2 were the best predictors of early mortality (within 6 months) in patients with left ventricular failure. Sun et al. using the previously discussed threshold values confirmed an increase in mortality and frequency of hospitalizations within the first 6 months of follow-up [40].

Conclusion

CPET is currently considered a central and irreplaceable tool in the evaluation of patients with advanced heart failure and candidates for heart transplantation, with diagnostic, prognostic and therapeutic implications.

References

[1] Guazzi M, Adams V, Conraads V, Halle M, Mezzani A, Vanhees L, Arena R, Fletcher GF, Forman DE, Kitzman DW, Lavie CJ, Myers J. European Association for Cardiovascular Prevention & Rehabilitation; American Heart Association. EACPR/AHA Scientific Statement. Clinical recommendations for cardiopulmonary exercise testing data assessment in specific patient populations. *Circulation,* 2012 Oct 30; 126(18):2261-74.

[2] Mezzani A. Cardiopulmonary Exercise Testing: Basics of Methodology and Measurements. *Ann Am Thorac Soc,* 2017 Jul; 14(Supplement_1):S3-S11.

[3] Corrà U, Agostoni PG, Anker SD, Coats AJS, Crespo Leiro MG, de Boer RA, Harjola VP, Hill L, Lainscak M, Lund LH, Metra M, Ponikowski P, Riley J, Seferović PM, Piepoli MF. Role of cardiopulmonary exercise testing in clinical stratification in heart failure. A position paper from the Committee on Exercise Physiology and Training of the Heart Failure Association of the European Society of Cardiology. *Eur J Heart Fail,* 2018 Jan; 20(1):3-15.

[4] Laveneziana P, Weatherald J. Pulmonary Vascular Disease and Cardiopulmonary Exercise Testing. *Front Physiol,* 2020 Aug 5; 11:964.

[5] ERS Task Force, Palange P, Ward SA, Carlsen KH, Casaburi R, Gallagher CG, Gosselink R, O'Donnell DE, Puente-Maestu L, Schols AM, Singh S, Whipp BJ. Recommendations on the use of exercise testing in clinical practice. *Eur Respir J,* 2007 Jan; 29(1):185-209.

[6] Ward SA. Determinants of the physiological systems responses to muscular exercise in healthy subjects, In: Palange P, Laveneziana P, Neder JA, Ward SA. Clinical

Exercise Testing (ERS Monograph). Sheffield: *European Respiratory Society,* 2018, 1–33.

[7] Karlsson J, Saltin B. Lactate, ATP, and CP in working muscles during exhaustive exercise in man. *J Appl Physiol*, 1970 Nov; 29(5):596-602.

[8] Jones NL, McCartney N, Graham T, Spriet LL, Kowalchuk JM, Heigenhauser GJ, Sutton JR. Muscle performance and metabolism in maximal isokinetic cycling at slow and fast speeds. *J Appl Physiol,* (1985). 1985 Jul; 59(1):132-6.

[9] Schiaffino S, Reggiani C. Fiber types in mammalian skeletal muscles. *Physiol Rev,* 2011 Oct; 91(4):1447-531.

[10] Clanton TL, Hogan MC, Gladden LB. Regulation of cellular gas exchange, oxygen sensing, and metabolic control. *Compr Physiol,* 2013 Jul; 3(3):1135-90.

[11] Neder JA, Berton DC, Rocha A, Arbex FF, Alencar MC, Degani-Costa LH, Ferreira EM, Ramos R. Abnormal patterns of response to incremental CPET, In: Palange P, Laveneziana P, Neder JA, Ward SA. Clinical Exercise Testing (ERS Monograph). Sheffield: *European Respiratory Society,* 2018, 34–58.

[12] Porszasz J, Stringer W, Casaburi R. Equipment, measurements and quality control, In: Palange P, Laveneziana P, Neder JA, Ward SA. Clinical Exercise Testing (ERS Monograph). Sheffield: *European Respiratory Society,* 2018, 59–81.

[13] Ries AL. The role of exercise testing in pulmonary diagnosis. *Clin Chest Med,* 1987 Mar; 8(1):81-9.

[14] Hellerstein HK. Specifications for exercise testing equipment. American Heart Association subcommittee on rehabilitation target activity group. *Circulation,* 1979 Apr; 59(4):849A-854A.

[15] Hermansen L, Saltin B. Oxygen uptake during maximal treadmill and bicycle exercise. *J Appl Physiol,* 1969 Jan; 26(1):31-7.

[16] Koyal SN, Whipp BJ, Huntsman D, Bray GA, Wasserman K. Ventilatory responses to the metabolic acidosis of treadmill and cycle ergometry. *J Appl Physiol,* 1976 Jun; 40(6):864-7.

[17] McArdle WD, Katch FI, Pechar GS. Comparison of continuous and discontinuous treadmill and bicycle tests for max Vo2. *Med Sci Sports,* 1973 Fall; 5(3):156-60.

[18] McKay GA, Banister EW. A comparison of maximum oxygen uptake determination by bicycle ergometry at various pedaling frequencies and by treadmill running at various speeds. *Eur J Appl Physiol Occup Physiol,* 1976 Aug 12; 35(3):191-200.

[19] Bruce RA. Exercise testing of patients with coronary heart disease. Principles and normal standards for evaluation. *Ann Clin Res,* 1971 Dec; 3(6):323-32.

[20] Buchfuhrer MJ, Hansen JE, Robinson TE, Sue DY, Wasserman K, Whipp BJ. Optimizing the exercise protocol for cardiopulmonary assessment. *J Appl Physiol Respir Environ Exerc Physiol,* 1983 Nov; 55(5):1558-64.

[21] Patterson JA, Naughton J, Pietras RJ, Gunnar RM. Treadmill exercise in assessment of the functional capacity of patients with cardiac disease. *Am J Cardiol,* 1972 Nov; 30(7):757-62.

[22] Khush KK, Cherikh WS, Chambers DC, Goldfarb S, Hayes D Jr, Kucheryavaya AY, Levvey BJ, Meiser B, Rossano JW, Stehlik J. International Society for Heart and Lung Transplantation. The International Thoracic Organ Transplant Registry of

the International Society for Heart and Lung Transplantation: Thirty-fifth Adult Heart Transplantation Report-2018; Focus Theme: Multiorgan Transplantation. *J Heart Lung Transplant,* 2018 Oct; 37(10):1155-1168.

[23] Sullivan MJ, Hawthorne MH. Exercise intolerance in patients with chronic heart failure. *Prog Cardiovasc Dis,* 1995 Jul-Aug; 38(1):1-22.

[24] Weber KT, Kinasewitz GT, Janicki JS, Fishman AP. Oxygen utilization and ventilation during exercise in patients with chronic cardiac failure. *Circulation,* 1982 Jun; 65(6):1213-23.

[25] van den Broek SA, van Veldhuisen DJ, de Graeff PA, Landsman ML, Hillege H, Lie KI. Comparison between New York Heart Association classification and peak oxygen consumption in the assessment of functional status and prognosis in patients with mild to moderate chronic congestive heart failure secondary to either ischemic or idiopathic dilated cardiomyopathy. *Am J Cardiol,* 1992 Aug 1; 70(3):359-63.

[26] Matsumura N, Nishijima H, Kojima S, Hashimoto F, Minami M, Yasuda H. Determination of anaerobic threshold for assessment of functional state in patients with chronic heart failure. *Circulation,* 1983 Aug; 68(2):360-7.

[27] Itoh H, Taniguchi K, Koike A, Doi M. Evaluation of severity of heart failure using ventilatory gas analysis. *Circulation,* 1990 Jan; 81(1 Suppl):II31-7. PMID: 2295150.

[28] Szlachcic J, Massie BM, Kramer BL, Topic N, Tubau J. Correlates and prognostic implication of exercise capacity in chronic congestive heart failure. *Am J Cardiol,* 1985 Apr 1; 55(8):1037-42.

[29] Rickenbacher PR, Trindade PT, Haywood GA, Vagelos RH, Schroeder JS, Willson K, Prikazsky L, Fowler MB. Transplant candidates with severe left ventricular dysfunction managed with medical treatment: characteristics and survival. *J Am Coll Cardiol,* 1996 Apr; 27(5):1192-7.

[30] Mancini DM, Eisen H, Kussmaul W, Mull R, Edmunds LH Jr, Wilson JR. Value of peak exercise oxygen consumption for optimal timing of cardiac transplantation in ambulatory patients with heart failure. *Circulation,* 1991 Mar; 83(3):778-86.

[31] Osada N, Chaitman BR, Miller LW, Yip D, Cishek MB, Wolford TL, Donohue TJ. Cardiopulmonary exercise testing identifies low risk patients with heart failure and severely impaired exercise capacity considered for heart transplantation. *J Am Coll Cardiol,* 1998 Mar 1; 31(3):577-82.

[32] Stevenson LW, Steimle AE, Fonarow G, Kermani M, Kermani D, Hamilton MA, Moriguchi JD, Walden J, Tillisch JH, Drinkwater DC, Laks H. Improvement in exercise capacity of candidates awaiting heart transplantation. *J Am Coll Cardiol,* 1995 Jan; 25(1):163-70.

[33] Myers J, Christle JW, Tun A, Yilmaz B, Moneghetti KJ, Yuen E, Soofi M, Ashley E. Cardiopulmonary Exercise Testing, Impedance Cardiography, and Reclassification of Risk in Patients Referred for Heart Failure Evaluation. *J Card Fail,* 2019 Dec; 25(12):961-968.

[34] Stelken AM, Younis LT, Jennison SH, Miller DD, Miller LW, Shaw LJ, Kargl D, Chaitman BR. Prognostic value of cardiopulmonary exercise testing using percent achieved of predicted peak oxygen uptake for patients with ischemic and dilated cardiomyopathy. *J Am Coll Cardiol,* 1996 Feb; 27(2):345-52.

[35] Likoff MJ, Chandler SL, Kay HR. Clinical determinants of mortality in chronic congestive heart failure secondary to idiopathic dilated or to ischemic cardiomyopathy. *Am J Cardiol,* 1987 Mar 1; 59(6):634-8.

[36] Mudge GH, Goldstein S, Addonizio LJ, Caplan A, Mancini D, Levine TB, Ritsch ME Jr, Stevenson LW. 24th Bethesda conference: Cardiac transplantation. Task Force 3: Recipient guidelines/prioritization. *J Am Coll Cardiol,* 1993 Jul; 22(1):21-31.

[37] Gitt AK, Wasserman K, Kilkowski C, Kleemann T, Kilkowski A, Bangert M, Schneider S, Schwarz A, Senges J. Exercise anaerobic threshold and ventilatory efficiency identify heart failure patients for high risk of early death. *Circulation,* 2002 Dec 10; 106(24):3079-84.

[38] Chua TP, Ponikowski P, Harrington D, Anker SD, Webb-Peploe K, Clark AL, Poole-Wilson PA, Coats AJ. Clinical correlates and prognostic significance of the ventilatory response to exercise in chronic heart failure. *J Am Coll Cardiol,* 1997 Jun; 29(7):1585-90.

[39] Kleber FX, Vietzke G, Wernecke KD, Bauer U, Opitz C, Wensel R, Sperfeld A, Gläser S. Impairment of ventilatory efficiency in heart failure: Prognostic impact. *Circulation,* 2000 Jun 20; 101(24):2803-9.

[40] Sun XG, Hansen JE, Beshai JF, Wasserman K. Oscillatory breathing and exercise gas exchange abnormalities prognosticate early mortality and morbidity in heart failure. *J Am Coll Cardiol*, 2010 Apr 27; 55(17):1814-23.

Chapter 3

Invasive Hemodynamic Assessment in the Heart Transplant Candidate: Swan-Ganz Catheter

Cristhian Emmanuel Scatularo*
Heart Failure and Heart Transplantation, Favaloro Foundation University Hospital, Buenos Aires, Argentina

Abstract

The Swan-Ganz catheter (SGC) is a tool available in most intensive care units for the management of hemodynamically complex patients, especially with advanced heart failure (HF). Although it allows the identification of different hemodynamic patterns and orienting the appropriate therapy accordingly, it must always be evaluated which patients will benefit from it and how to interpret the information it provides.

There is still great controversy about the true usefulness of the SGC and the reliability of the data derived from it, as the cardiac function, vascular resistance or tissue oxygenation. These data must be interpreted with caution, knowing their possible limitations. Unfortunately, several studies show insufficient knowledge of the proper use and interpretation of the SGC.

This chapter aims to provide information on the catheter implantation technique, the main hemodynamic patterns and how to interpret them to guide the therapy of patients with advanced heart failure.

Keywords: Swan-Ganz catheterization, heart failure, heart transplantation

---

* Corresponding Author's E-mail: emmanuelscatularo@gmail.com.

In: Heart Transplantation
Editor: Elian Facundo Giordanino
ISBN: 978-1-68507-759-4

Introduction

Structural Characteristics

The Swan-Ganz catheter (SGC) is a central venous access created by Swan and Ganz in 1970 that evaluates the hemodynamic status of a patient through the direct measurement of different hemodynamic variables in the right heart chambers and the pulmonary artery [1].

It is a catheter made of different materials (the most frequently used is polyvinyl chloride), with a length between 60 and 110 cm and gauges between 4 to 8 French. It has thin marks every 10 cm and thick marks every 50 cm to determine the location of the catheter tip during its insertion. Additionally, it has lumens through which it is possible to measure intracavitary pressures, instill solutions or implant a temporary pacemaker. There are catheters with 2, 4, 5 or even 7 lumens, although the most frequently used is the 4-lumen catheter (Figure 1). Those with the highest number of lumens allow for a greater number of simultaneous applications, such as the implantation of a temporary pacemaker, measurement of continuous cardiac output (CO) or continuous venous oxygen saturation [2-4].

The proximal lumen is at 30 cm from the tip, which will be located approximately in the right atrium (RA). At the tip is the distal lumen and a balloon (proximal to the tip) that can be inflated from the outside (inflation volume between 0.7 to 1.5 ml of air) and allows occluding a subsegmental branch of the pulmonary artery and to measure the pulmonary capillary pressure (PCP) (Figure 1). The thermistor (transducer that registers changes in temperature), located in the external surface of the catheter 4 cm from its end, allows the calculation of CO by thermodilution [1, 3-5].

The SGC should be placed in a similar way to a central line, so that the proximal lumen is located in the RA and the distal in one of the branches of the pulmonary artery (with the deflated balloon). The proximal lumen allows to measure the pressure in the RA or central venous pressure (CVP), and to administrate electrolyte solutions and drugs [6, 7]. The distal lumen allows to measure the systolic, diastolic and mean pressures of the pulmonary artery (sPAP, dPAP, mPAP, respectively). When the balloon is inflated, it occludes a subsegmental branch of the pulmonary artery and the PCP can be measured. (Figure 2) CO can be measured by injecting a bolus of saline into the proximal lumen or by continuous measurement through a thermal filament in more complex catheters [1, 8-10].

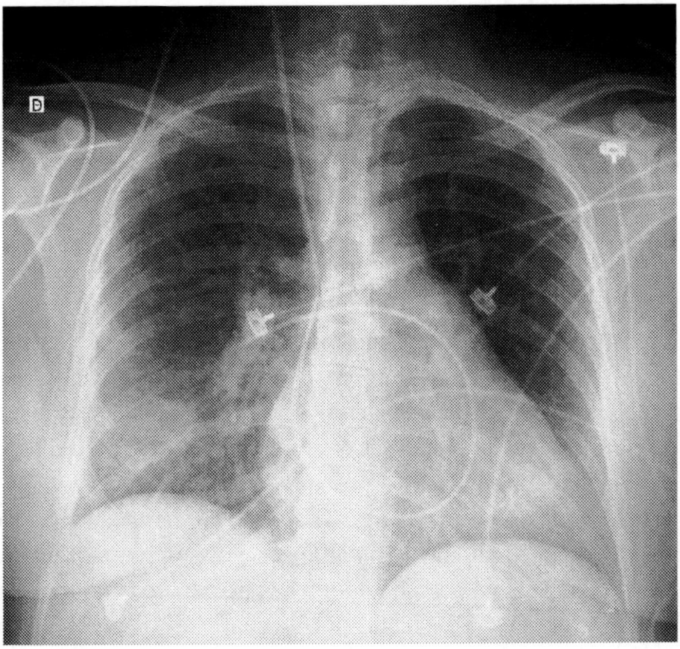

Figure 1. Swan-Ganz Catheter on chest radiography. Tip of the catheter located at the right pulmonary artery.

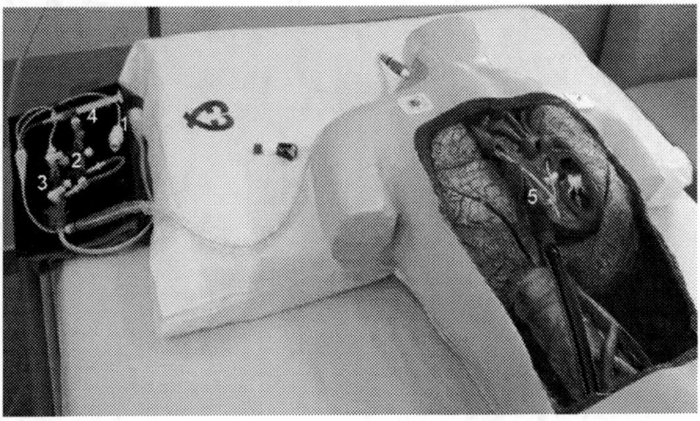

Figure 2. Placement of the Swan-Ganz catheter. 1. Thermistor lumen port. 2. Proximal lumen port. 3. Distal lumen port. 4. Balloon inflation lumen port. 5. Swan-Ganz catheter inside the heart. (Simulation manikins courtesy of Licensed Practical Nurse Ricardo Rosero, ricardorosero40@gmail.com.)

Implant Technique

During its insertion, when the tip of the catheter is in the RA a curve with three positive waves will be observed: wave "a" (atrial contraction), wave "c" (closure of the tricuspid valve due to contraction of the right ventricle) and wave "v" (passive atrial filling) [4, 5]. Once in the RA, the balloon must be inflated and the catheter advanced until it reaches the right ventricle (RV), and a wide curve with a sharp rise and fall will be observed. Then, it should be advanced towards the pulmonary artery, and a lower amplitude curve will appear, with a diastolic pressure greater than the diastolic ventricular pressure and a dicrotic notch in its descending branch (produced by the closure of the pulmonary valve). If SGC is advanced with the inflated balloon until it occludes the corresponding pulmonary subsegmental branch, a curve will appear again with the "a", "c" and "v" waves corresponding to the PCP, which reflects the left atrial (LA) pressure [7]. Once the PCP has been obtained, the balloon must be deflated passively, obtaining the appropriate location of the catheter (Figure 3). The balloon should always be deflated while it is in the pulmonary artery and the PCP should not be continuously recorded (inflate less than 15 seconds) to reduce the risk of pulmonary infarction. Once the SGC is correctly placed, the CVP and PAP can be recorded continuously [2, 5].

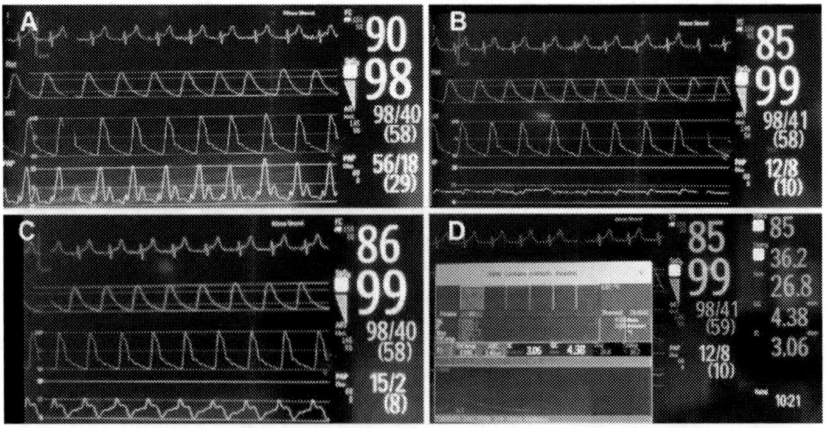

Figure 3. Curves and measurements of the Swan-Ganz catheter. A. Pulmonary artery pressure B. Wedge pressure C. Right atrial pressure D. Cardiac output.

The correct placement of the catheter must be confirmed by the following checklist [2]:

- The action of inflating and deflating the balloon should make the PCP and PAP curves appear, respectively.
- The morphology of the PCP curve must be that of an atrial pressure curve, with its two characteristic waves "a" and "v".
- The mean value of the PCP should be equal to or lower than the dPAP, except if there is a "v" wave of mitral regurgitation or if the patient has severe pulmonary hypertension.
- Perform chest X-ray to control the adequate position of the catheter (below the left atrium) and rule out possible complications secondary to the puncture.

Common Problems with Implantation

- SGC does not advance towards the RV: inflating the balloon with sterile saline solution and placing the patient in the left lateral decubitus position can be useful for the balloon to fall into the RV by gravity [5-7].
- SGC does not show the PCP despite its complete introduction: the cause could be non-uniform inflation of the balloon. dPAP can be assumed as the PCP value, except in the case of severe pulmonary hypertension [5-7].
- SGC shows a line without curves during PCP measurement: this may be due to over inflation of the balloon or catheter located too distal. The catheter should be withdrawn with the balloon deflated until the curve of the pulmonary artery is obtained and advance again with the balloon inflated.

Indications

The SGC has two fundamental objectives: to assess the hemodynamic status of a patient, especially in complex cases where multiple variables are involved, and to guide therapy based on the hemodynamic patterns found. SGC implantation is recommended in the following situations [1, 2, 10].

General Conditions

- Cardiogenic shock with poor response to standard doses of inotropic/vasopressor support or intra-aortic balloon pump.
- Diagnosis and characterization of pulmonary hypertension (PH), and evaluation of the efficacy of its treatment.
- Evaluation of a candidate for heart transplantation.
- Vasoplegic shock with associated ventricular dysfunction.

Pre- and Intraoperative Conditions (Cardiovascular Surgery)

- Reduced ventricular function (ejection fraction <40%)
- Pulmonary hypertension (mPAP > 25 mmHg)
- Isolated or combined heart transplant.

Hemodynamic Variables

The main hemodynamic parameters that can be obtained through the SGC are described below. Their expression in relation to body surface area is used to minimize differences between individuals, and when this is the case the term index is added. The direct measurements using the SGC are CVP, PCP, mPAP and CO. The rest of the variables are derived from formulas that include these direct measurements and others such as heart rate (HR) and body surface area (Table 1) [9-11].

Table 1. Hemodynamic variables obtained or calculated through the Swan-Ganz catheter

Hemodynamic variables	Formula	Normal value
Measured Hemodynamic variables		
CVP	Central Venous Pressure	1 – 7 mmHg
PCP	Pulmonary Capillary Pressure	4 – 12 mmHg
CO	Cardiac Output	4 – 8 L/min

Hemodynamic variables	Formula	Normal value
MAP	Mean Arterial Pressure	70 – 105 mmHg
HR	Heart Rate	60 – 100 beats/min
mPAP	Mean Pulmonary Artery Pressure	9 – 20 mmHg
sPAP	Systolic Pulmonary Artery Pressure	15 – 30 mmHg
dPAP	Diastolic Pulmonary Artery Pressure	4 – 12 mmHg
Calculated hemodynamic variables		
CI	CO/BSA	2.8 – 4.2 L/min/m2
SV	CO/HR	40 - 70 ml/beat
SVi	CO/(HR x BSA)	36 - 49 ml/beat/m2
LVSWi	(MAP - PCP) x SVi x 0.0136	40 - 56 g-m/m2/beat
RVSWi	(mPAP - CVP) x SVi x 0.0136	7 - 10 g-m/m2/beat
SVR	(MAP - CVP) x 80/CO	700 – 1600 din-s/cm5
PVR	(mPAP - PCP) x 80/CO	150 - 200 din-s/cm5
TGP	mPAP – PCP	< 12 mmHg
PDG	dPAP – PCP	< 7 mmHg

BSA, body surface area; CI, cardiac index; CO, cardiac output; CVP, central venous pressure; HR, heart rate; LVSWi, left ventricular systolic work index; MAP, mean arterial pressure; dPAP, diastolic pulmonary artery pressure; mPAP, mean pulmonary artery pressure; sPAP, systolic pulmonary artery pressure; PDG, pulmonary diastolic gradient; PCP, pulmonary capillary pressure; PVR, pulmonary vascular resistance; RVSWi, right ventricular systolic work index; SV, systolic volume or stroke volume; SVI, SV index; SVR, systemic vascular resistance; TPG, transpulmonary gradient. (Data from Bonow R et al. Braunwald's Heart Disease a textbook of cardiovascular medicine. 10ed. Philadelphia, United States of America: 2015; Elsevier; 364-391, and Carrasco Rueda JM et al. Invasive hemodynamic monitoring by Swan-Ganz pulmonary artery catheter: concepts and utility. *Arch Peru Cardiol Cir Cardiovasc.* 2021 Oct 4;2(3):175-86).

Central Venous Pressure

It is the pressure located in the RA and registered from the proximal lumen of the SGC. The maximum pressure should be used in patients on spontaneous ventilation and the minimum when on mechanical ventilation.

Pulmonary Capillary Pressure or Wedge Pressure

It is the pressure registered through the distal lumen of the catheter with the inflated balloon until it has occluded a pulmonary subsegmental branch. Under these conditions, the value obtained reflects the LA pressure. Since the LA pressure is usually equal to the left ventricular end-diastolic pressure, the PCP estimates the left ventricle (LV) preload, except if the catheter is not located below the LA (pulmonary zone 3), if there is severe aortic insufficiency, or in the presence of a less compliant LV and early closure of the mitral valve (in cases of severe hypertrophy or restrictive cardiomyopathy). Its normal value ranges between 4 – 12 mmHg [5].

Cardiac Output and Cardiac Index

The thermistor records changes in blood temperature at the distal lumen of the SGC and calculates the CO applying the thermodilution principle. The thermodilution principle is based on the fact that the speed of blood flow is inversely proportional to the change in temperature of a liquid injected into the blood. In order to measure CO, 10 cc of physiological saline solution with a different temperature from blood (ice-cold or room temperature) must be injected through the proximal lumen during 2 to 4 seconds. The change of the temperature's velocity at the thermistor is related to the speed of the blood flow and therefore to the CO. In a high CO patient, the recorded curve has a rapid rise and fall, and the opposite is true for those of low CO (area under the curve is inversely proportional to the blood flow in the pulmonary artery). It is recommended to perform three measurements to avoid possible errors, discarding the measurements with a difference of more than 10% between them.

When the CO is adjusted by the body surface area the cardiac index (CI) is obtained (normal value is 2.8 – 4.2 L/min/m2) and is the most reliable parameter to comparatively measure the blood flow.

In severe tricuspid regurgitation there may be falsely low CO values due to regurgitation of the injected fluid. In cases of intracardiac shunts from right to left, falsely elevated CO can be obtained since part of the injected fluid goes into the left chambers and not through the pulmonary artery (abbreviated curve similar to that of elevated CO). In left to right shunt, since the blood is at higher temperature than the injected solution and equal to that of the right ventricle blood, the CO measurement is usually not affected [5, 6].

Oxygen Consumption and Cardiac Index by Fick's Formula

Oxygen Consumption (VO_2) reflects the amount of oxygen extracted by the tissues of the systemic circulation. It is usually constant, except in pre-mortem patients, and its normal value ranges between 110 - 160 ml/min/m2. VO_2 is a function of CI and the difference in oxygen concentration between arterial (CaO_2) and venous (CvO_2) blood, according to Fick's formula [VO_2 = CI x (CaO_2 - CvO_2)], and therefore [VO_2 = CI x 1.34 x Hemoglobin x (arterial oxygen saturation - venous oxygen saturation)]. Assuming that VO_2 is constant, the CI can be calculated as: CI = VO_2/(CaO_2 - CvO_2) (CI by Fick's formula). For Fick's formula calculation, arterial blood and mixed venous blood (from the pulmonary artery) must be drawn, which represents the oxygen content in blood after it was removed by all body tissues. Venous oxygen saturation varies directly with the CI, hemoglobin, and arterial oxygen saturation [9-11].

Systolic Volume or Stroke Volume and Systolic Volume Index

It refers to the volume ejected in each cardiac beat. The formula for its calculation is CO/HR. Its normal value ranges between 40 - 70 ml/beat. The systolic volume index is the systolic volume adjusted by the body surface area and its normal value is 36 - 49 ml/beat/m2.

Left Ventricular Systolic Work Index

Left ventricular systolic work Index (LVSWi) reflects the work done by the LV in order to eject blood, and it depends on the mean arterial pressure (MAP), the PCP and the systolic volume index (SVi). It is calculated with the formula: LVSWi = (MAP - PCP) x SVi x 0.0136 and its normal value ranges between 40 and 56 g-m/m2/beat [5].

Right Ventricular Systolic Work Index

Right ventricular systolic work index (RVSWi) reflects the work required to eject the systolic volume through the pulmonary circulation, and is dependent on mPAP, CVP, and stroke volume index. The formula for its calculation is: RVSWi = (mPAP - CVP) x SVi x 0.0136. Its normal value ranges between 7 and 10 g-m/m2/beat [5].

Systemic Vascular Resistance

Systemic vascular resistance (SVR) represents peripheral vascular resistance. It is calculated as the pressure gradient from the aorta to the RA and is inversely related to CO. The formula for its calculation is: SVR = (MAP - CVP) x 80/CO. Its normal value ranges between 700 – 1600 din-s/cm5 [5].

Pulmonary Vascular Resistance

Pulmonary vascular resistance (PVR) is the resistance of the pulmonary vasculature, is directly proportional to gradient between mPAP and PCP, and inversely proportional to CO. It is calculated as PVR = (mPAP - PCP) x 80/CO. Normal value of PVR ranges between 150 - 200 din-s/cm5 [5].

Transpulmonary Gradient and Pulmonary Diastolic Gradient

Transpulmonary gradient (TPG) results from the difference in pressure between the pulmonary capillaries, represented by the PCP, and the mPAP. The formula for its calculation is TPG = mPAP – PCP. In patients with pulmonary hypertension (PH), which is usually the case in most patients with advanced HF, if it is less than or equal to 12 mmHg it is called passive PH, which will probably not respond to specific vasodilator treatment in pulmonary vasoreactivity tests as it is mainly driven by the passive congestion of the failing heart [9-11]. The opposite occurs if the TPG is greater than 12 mmHg, in which case it is called reactive PH.

Pulmonary diastolic gradient (PDG) orients towards the origin of the PH and is calculated according to the following formula PDG = dPAP – PCP. Its normal value is less than or equal to 7 mmHg. Values greater than 7 mmHg indicate PH of real vascular origin caused by an alteration at the pulmonary vascular level. Therefore, it is a fundamental measurement to be carried out in the evaluation of the heart transplant candidate [5, 9-11].

Hemodynamic Patterns in Advanced Heart Failure

The variables measured and calculated using the SGC allow us to evaluate the hemodynamic status of a patient which must be analyzed in conjunction with both clinical findings and complimentary studies such as echocardiography [12-15]. It must be considered that in most real-life patients the following hemodynamic patterns are not found in isolation, but rather are combined. Therefore, it is necessary to have a thorough understanding of the SGC findings and their correlation with other parameters to reach an adequate diagnosis and treatment (Table 2).

Table 2. Hemodynamic patterns detected through Swan-Ganz catheter in advanced heart failure patients

	Hemodynamic patterns				
	CI	**CVP**	**PCP**	**SVR**	**PVR**
Hypovolemia	Low	Low	Low	Normal or high	Normal or high
Pulmonary congestion	Normal	Normal or high	High	Normal or high	Normal or high
Cardiogenic shock	Low	Normal or high	High	High	Normal or high
Primary failure of the RV	Low	High	Low	Normal or high	Normal or low
Vasoplegia	Normal or high	Low	Low	Low	Normal or low

CI, cardiac index; CVP, central venous pressure; PCP, pulmonary capillary pressure; PVR, pulmonary vascular resistance; SVR, systemic vascular resistance. (Data from Gonzalez-Hermosillo JA et al. Hemodynamic profiles related to circulatory shock in cardiac care units. Arch Cardiol Mex. 2020;90(1):47-54 and Carrasco Rueda JM et al. Invasive hemodynamic monitoring by Swan-Ganz pulmonary artery catheter: concepts and utility. *Arch Peru Cardiol Cir Cardiovasc*. 2021 Oct 4;2(3):175-86).

Hypovolemia

In patients with advanced heart failure under high doses of diuretics (especially in the elderly) or in patients hospitalized for heart failure with very abrupt pharmacological water depletion, relative hypovolemia (decreased intravascular volume) is frequent. This determines a systemic hypoperfusion, affecting mainly the renal function and mental status. In these cases, the SGC can determine the presence of a CI < 2.2 L/min/m2 and low filling pressures (PVC and PCP), which are quickly corrected with controlled fluid inputs. In hypovolemia, systemic vascular resistance is usually normal or elevated [12].

Pulmonary Congestion

Due to the increase in pulmonary capillary pressure in heart failure patients, it can be observed an extravasation of fluids from the pulmonary vasculature towards the interstitium and alveoli of the lungs, which leads to a progressive deterioration in gas exchange and consequently in hypoxia. Most patients with simple pulmonary congestion or acute pulmonary edema have a PCP > 18 mmHg, but with CI > 2.2 L/min/m2. In pulmonary congestion, systemic and pulmonary vascular resistances are usually normal or elevated [13, 14].

Cardiogenic Shock

It is defined as the state of severe hypoperfusion resulting from a primary cardiac dysfunction, presenting a systolic blood pressure <90 mmHg, a mean arterial pressure <65 mmHg for thirty minutes or the need to use vasopressors to achieve these values despite adequate preload. Additionally, pulmonary congestion or high filling pressures in the left ventricle and signs of organ hypoperfusion (altered mental status, cold skin, oliguria, increased serum lactate) are also present. The characteristic pattern in the SGC measurement is the presence of a CI ≤ 2.2 L/min/m2 and PCP > 18 mmHg, with high systemic and pulmonary vascular resistance. LVSWi is decreased and is one of the most reliable parameters in these cases to assess LV ejection, since it is adjusted to HR and preload [7, 12-14].

Primary Failure of the Right Ventricle

In the case of cardiogenic shock secondary to RV failure, as occurs in the setting of RV acute myocardial infarction, systemic hypoperfusion occurs in the context of insufficient preload of the LV. The decrease in RV ejection generates a retrograde increase in right atrial pressure, and a fall in sPAP, mPAP and PCP. In the SGC measurement, we can observe a CI < 2.2 L/min/m2, lower PCP than CVP (inversion of preload pressures) or high CVP. Other calculations that aid the diagnosis of RV failure are the presence of low RVSWi or CVP/PCP > 0.54 [8, 10-12].

In some cases, when a patient with primary RV failure also presents hypovolemia, low and equal filling pressures, or even slightly higher PCP than CVP can be observed. In these situations, a preload test with saline solution corrects the hypovolemia and unmasks the underlying RV failure, showing an elevation of the CVP but not the PCP, with inversion of filling pressures.

Vasoplegia

Although it is not a typical pattern of a patient with advanced HF it can be observed as a consequence of a recent infarction, a concomitant infectious process, existence of systemic inflammatory comorbidities such as chronic kidney disease or concomitant treatment with vasodilators. In these scenarios, systemic vascular resistance might be decreased due to vasodilatation leading to a reduction in LV afterload which favors a high CO. The characteristic pattern in the SGC measurement is the presence of a CI > 2.2 L/min/m2, low PCP and CVP, with low systemic and pulmonary vascular resistance. An increase in differential pressures (systolic minus diastolic) can also be observed due to a low dPAP and low diastolic blood pressure [9-12].

Complications

The SGC implantation is an invasive procedure, and its complications, although infrequent, can be serious.

It is essential to know them in order to prevent them, to early diagnose them, and to treat them properly. Its principal complications are described below [1-8].

Related to Puncture

- Pneumothorax
- Hematoma.
- Air embolism
- Nerve injuries
- Arteriovenous fistula

Related to Insertion

- Arrhythmias: The most frequent (90%) is ventricular tachycardia when crossing the RV, especially in an ischemic RV. This resolves when the catheter is repositioned or removed, so no additional treatment is required. There is also a minimum risk of right bundle branch block, which can be serious if the patient has a previous left bundle branch blocks as it can lead to a complete atrioventricular block.
- Injury to cardiac structures.

Related to Use

- Pulmonary infarction due to distal migration of the catheter. It can also occur as a consequence of excessive balloon inflation time with the formation of a thrombus around the end of the catheter, which can also lead to thromboembolism (Incidence 1.3%).
- Rupture of the pulmonary artery is a rare complication (0.06-0.2%) but very serious (50% mortality). Predisposing factors are excessive balloon inflation, age, hypothermia and pulmonary arterial hypertension. It should be suspected when hemoptysis is present, sometimes with a cataclysmic clinical course.
- Catheter infection: Bacterial colonization can be present in up to 10% of catheters, although sepsis occurs in only 2% of cases [8]. The risk of infection increases significantly if the SGC remains for more than 72 hours. The risk of endocarditis due to SGC is low.
- Endocardial lesions such as parietal thrombi or subendocardial hemorrhages. Its most frequent localization is the pulmonary valve, followed by the tricuspid, the right atrium, the RV and the main pulmonary artery. They occur as a consequence of removal of the catheter with the balloon inflated, especially if it has been inserted with the balloon deflated.
- Balloon rupture: It generates air embolism.

Contraindications

Contraindications for SGC implantation should always be ruled out to avoid complications [1-8].

Absolute Contraindications

- Tricuspid or pulmonary valve stenosis
- Tricuspid prosthesis
- Right intracavitary masses
- Tetralogy of Fallot
- Latex allergy

Relative Contraindications

- Severe arrhythmias
- Coagulopathy
- Newly placed permanent pacemakers (<4-6 weeks)

Current Evidence

The evidence about the diagnostic and therapeutic benefits of the SGC in patients with advanced HF is controversial and heterogeneous, making it difficult to define whether its application in real practice provides a real benefit beyond clinical findings and Doppler ultrasound [15-17]. Although the SGC is used to guide therapeutic decisions in cardiogenic shock, the evidence supporting its optimal use is insufficient [18-22].

In the Evaluation Study of Congestive Heart Failure and Pulmonary Artery Catheterization Effectiveness (ESCAPE) trial, a randomized multicentric controlled trial, 433 HF patients were assigned to receive therapy guided by clinical assessment and a SGC or clinical assessment alone. The objective in both groups was resolution of clinical congestion. In patients with a SGC additional targets of a PCP of 15 mmHg and a CVP of 8 mmHg were pursued. The primary end point was days alive out of hospital during the first 6 months. This trial did not demonstrate a superiority of SGC over conventional guided therapy: both strategies led to a marked improvement in signs and symptoms by treating volume overload. Furthermore, the SGC group had a higher rate of adverse events, without impact on mortality or hospitalizations [23].

In a multicenter study by Reshad Garan et al., 1414 patients with cardiogenic shock were retrospectively analyzed, 53.6% were in advanced cardiogenic shock and 84% of those patients with advanced stages of shock required mechanical circulatory support devices. Of this cohort, 598 patients (42%) had complete hemodynamic data by SGC. The SGC-guided therapy reduced mortality in the group where complete hemodynamic data were obtained in comparison to the group that did not present a complete set of data ($p < 0.001$), a benefit that was persistent in all stages of shock. The non-use of SGC in the management of cardiogenic shock in this study was associated with higher in-hospital mortality (adjusted odds ratio 1.57; 95% CI: 1.06 to 2.33) [24].

Even though some studies have observed benefits in reducing mortality, the available evidence is controversial, heterogeneous, and sometimes contradictory. In general, the usefulness of invasive monitoring with SGC is based on its correct use and interpretation, making it a valuable tool in some settings where it provides key information that allows for a more hemodynamically tailored therapy [18-24].

Conclusion

Although the SGC has allowed for an extraordinary advance in the monitoring and diagnosis of the critically ill patient, its usefulness is being reassessed, since it is closely related to the correct measurement and interpretation of the data it provides. Therefore, the adequate interpretation of the information provided by the physical examination, the SGC and other non-invasive methods such as the echocardiogram is essential when establishing the correct diagnosis of the hemodynamic status of a patient and its proper treatment.

References

[1] Asereny DJ, Farrando S, Vera Y. Capitulo 4: Cateter de Swan Ganz. In: *Manual de Unidad Coronaria de CONAREC.* [*Chapter 4: Swan-Ganz catheter, In CONAREC Handbook of Coronary Unit*] Argentina: Marketing & Research; 2020, 48-66.

[2] McGee WT, Headley JM, Frazier JA, Lichtentha PR. Swan-Ganz catheters - Advanced and standard technology. In: McGee WT, Headley JM, Frazier JA, Lichtentha PR. *Edwards Critical Care Education: Quick guide to cardiopulmonary care.* United States of América: Editorial Edwards Lifesciences; 2014; 120-180.

[3] Lauga A, D'Ortencio A. Monitoreo de las presiones de la arteria pulmonar: Catéter de Swan-Ganz Parte I. [*Monitoring of pulmonary artery pressures. Swan-Ganz catheter Part I*] *Rev Insuf Cardiac* 2007;2(1):5-11.

[4] Gidwani UK, Mohanty B, Chatterjee K. The pulmonary artery catheter: a critical reappraisal. *Cardiol Clin.* 2013 Nov;31(4):545-565.

[5] Elefteriades, JA. Chapter 5. In: Elefteriades, JA. House Officer Guide to ICU Care. *Fundamentals of management of the heart and lungs.* United States of America: 1994. Raven Press.

[6] Jimenez Perez R, Allona Dueñas A, Diaz Fernandez C, Lopez Gonzalez G. Cateterismo cardiaco izquierdo y derecho. In: Argibay Pytlik V, Gomez Fernandez M, Jimenez Perez R, Santos Velez S, Serrano Poyato C. *Manual de Enfermeria en Cardiologia Intervencionista Hemodinamica. Protocolos unificados.* [*Left and right heart catheterization*, In *Nursing Manual in Hemodynamic Interventional Cardiology. Unified protocols*] 1st ed, Madrid, España: Graficas Diumaro;2007, 117-125.

[7] Carrasco Rueda JM, Gabino Gonzalez GA, Sánchez Cachi JL, Pariona Canchiz RP, Valdivia Gómez AF, Aguirre Zurita ON. Invasive hemodynamic monitoring by Swan-Ganz pulmonary artery catheter: concepts and utility. *Arch Peru Cardiol Cir Cardiovasc.* 2021 Oct 4;2(3):175-86.

[8] Valdivieso LR, Mendiz OA. Hemodinamia y diagnostico cardiovascular por cateter. In: Mautner B. *Cardiologia basada en la evidencia y la experiencia de la Fundacion Favaloro.* [*Hemodynamics and cardiovascular diagnosis by catheter, In Cardiology based on evidence and on the experience of the Favaloro Foundation*] Argentina: Mediterraneo; 2009; 291-313.

[9] Lauga A, D'Ortencio A. Monitoreo de las presiones de la arteria pulmonar: Catéter de Swan-Ganz Parte I. [*Monitoring of pulmonary artery pressures. Swan-Ganz catheter Part I*] *Rev Insuf Cardiac* 2007;2(2):48-54.

[10] Davidson CJ, Bonow R. Cardiac Catheterization. In: Bonow R, Mann D, Zipes D, Libby P. *Braunwald's Heart Disease a textbook of cardiovascular medicine.* 10ed. Philadelphia, United States of America: 2015; Elsevier; 364-391.

[11] Martino E, Martin Napoli V, Moles G. Capitulo 5: Monitoreo hemodinamico en Unidad Coronaria. In: Manual de Unidad Coronaria de CONAREC. [*Chapter 5: Hemodynamic monitoring in the Coronary Unit, In CONAREC Handbook of Coronary Unit*] Argentina: Marketing & Research; 2020,67-85.

[12] Gonzalez-Hermosillo JA, Palma-Carbajal R, Rojas-Velasco G, Cabrera-Jardines R, Gonzalez-Galvan LM, Manzur-Sandoval D, Jimenez-Rodriguez GM, Ortiz-Solis WA. Hemodynamic profiles related to circulatory shock in cardiac care units. *Arch Cardiol Mex.* 2020;90(1):47-54.

[13] VanDyck TJ, Pinsky MR. Hemodynamic monitoring in cardiogenic shock. *Curr Opin Crit Care.* 2021 Aug 1;27(4):454-459.

[14] Vallabhajosyula S, Shankar A, Patlolla SH, Prasad A, Bell MR, Jentzer JC, Arora S, Vallabhajosyula S, Gersh BJ, Jaffe AS, Holmes DR Jr, Dunlay SM, Barsness GW. Pulmonary artery catheter use in acute myocardial infarction-cardiogenic shock. *ESC Heart Fail.* 2020 Jun;7(3):1234-1245.

[15] Oh JK, Seward JB, Khandheria BK, Gersh BJ, McGregor CG, Freeman WK, Sinak LJ, Tajik AJ. Transesophageal echocardiography in critically ill patients. *Am J Cardiol.* 1990 Dec 15;66(20):1492-5.

[16] Pearson AC. Noninvasive evaluation of the hemodynamically unstable patient: the advantages of seeing clearly. *Mayo Clin Proc.* 1995 Oct;70(10):1012-4.

[17] Ashes C, Roscoe A. Transesophageal echocardiography in thoracic anesthesia: pulmonary hypertension and right ventricular function. *Curr Opin Anaesthesiol.* 2015 Feb;28(1):38-44.

[18] Fang JC, Jones TL. Can a Pulmonary Artery Catheter Improve Outcomes in Cardiogenic Shock? *JACC Heart Fail.* 2020 Nov;8(11):914-916.

[19] Saxena A, Garan AR, Kapur NK, O'Neill WW, Lindenfeld J, Pinney SP, Uriel N, Burkhoff D, Kern M. Value of Hemodynamic Monitoring in Patients With Cardiogenic Shock Undergoing Mechanical Circulatory Support. *Circulation.* 2020 Apr 7;141(14):1184-1197.

[20] Sionis A, Rivas-Lasarte M, Mebazaa A, Tarvasmäki T, Sans-Roselló J, Tolppanen H, Varpula M, Jurkko R, Banaszewski M, Silva-Cardoso J, Carubelli V, Lindholm MG, Parissis J, Spinar J, Lassus J, Harjola VP, Masip J. Current Use and Impact on 30-Day Mortality of Pulmonary Artery Catheter in Cardiogenic Shock Patients: Results From the CardShock Study. *J Intensive Care Med.* 2020 Dec;35(12):1426-1433.

[21] Zorzi MF, Cancelli E, Rusca M, Kirsch M, Yerly P, Liaudet L. The prognostic value of pulmonary artery compliance in cardiogenic shock. *Pulm Circ.* 2019 Sep 19;9(3):2045894019877161.

[22] Hernandez GA, Lemor A, Blumer V, Rueda CA, Zalawadiya S, Stevenson LW, Lindenfeld J. Trends in Utilization and Outcomes of Pulmonary Artery Catheterization in Heart Failure With and Without Cardiogenic Shock. *J Card Fail.* 2019 May;25(5):364-371.

[23] Binanay C, Califf RM, Hasselblad V, O'Connor CM, Shah MR, Sopko G, Stevenson LW, Francis GS, Leier CV, Miller LW. Evaluation study of congestive heart failure and pulmonary artery catheterization effectiveness: the ESCAPE trial. *JAMA.* 2005 Oct 5;294(13):1625-33.

[24] Garan AR, Kanwar M, Thayer KL, Whitehead E, Zweck E, Hernandez-Montfort J, Mahr C, Haywood JL, Harwani NM, Wencker D, Sinha SS, Vorovich E, Abraham J, O'Neill W, Burkhoff D, Kapur NK. Complete Hemodynamic Profiling With Pulmonary Artery Catheters in Cardiogenic Shock Is Associated With Lower In-Hospital Mortality. *JACC Heart Fail.* 2020 Nov;8(11):903-913.

Chapter 4

Intraaortic Balloon Pump in Heart Transplantation

Alejandro Cicolini[1,*] and Elian Facundo Giordanino[2]
[1]Cardiovascular Intensive Care Unit, Favaloro Foundation University Hospital, Buenos Aires, Argentina
[2]Heart Failure and Heart Transplantation, Favaloro Foundation University Hospital, Buenos Aires, Argentina

Abstract

The intraaortic balloon pump is the most widely used mechanical circulatory support device. Knowing its complications and its proper setting is essential to achieve good results. Heart transplant patients are a special population that may require hemodynamic support before transplantation, due to their underlying disease, but also afterwards, due to early graft dysfunction. This chapter describes the main aspects of intraaortic balloon pump in heart transplantation.

Keywords: intra-aortic balloon pumping, heart transplantation, cardiogenic shock

Introduction

The intraaortic balloon pump (IABP) is one of the oldest and most common forms of mechanical circulatory support, mainly due to its simplicity and accessibility.

---

* Corresponding Author's E-mail: aciccoli@ffavaloro.org.

In: Heart Transplantation
Editor: Elian Facundo Giordanino
ISBN: 978-1-68507-759-4

The physiologic principles of counterpulsation consist of diastolic augmentation of aortic pressure and systolic reduction of left ventricular afterload. In patients with myocardial ischemia, these result in hemodynamic benefits through increased coronary perfusion pressure and improved myocardial oxygen balance [1, 2]. The counterpulsation effect is accomplished by displacing a volume of blood of approximately 30 to 50 mL by alternately inflating and deflating a balloon positioned in the proximal segment of the descending aorta (Figure 1). It can be inserted peripherally, including at the bedside, and is widely available in most centers. However, it provides only partial support which can be insufficient in some cases of severe cardiogenic shock [1, 3].

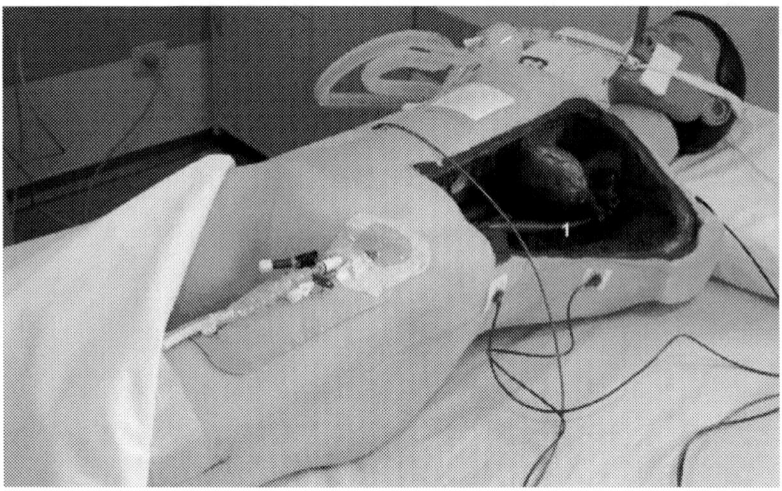

Figure 1. Positioning of an intra-aortic balloon pump. 1. Intraaortic balloon pump in the descending aorta. (Simulation manikins courtesy of Licensed Practical Nurse Ricardo Rosero, ricardorosero40@gmail.com.)

Components and Physiology

The IABP consists primarily of a two-lumen catheter and a mobile console. The two-lumen catheter is flexible, with one lumen for pressure monitoring and a second for the periodic delivery and removal of helium gas to a closed balloon that results in the displacement of blood through the aorta. The other essential part is the mobile console that contains the helium transfer system as well as a computer to control the inflation and deflation cycles (Figure 2) [1].

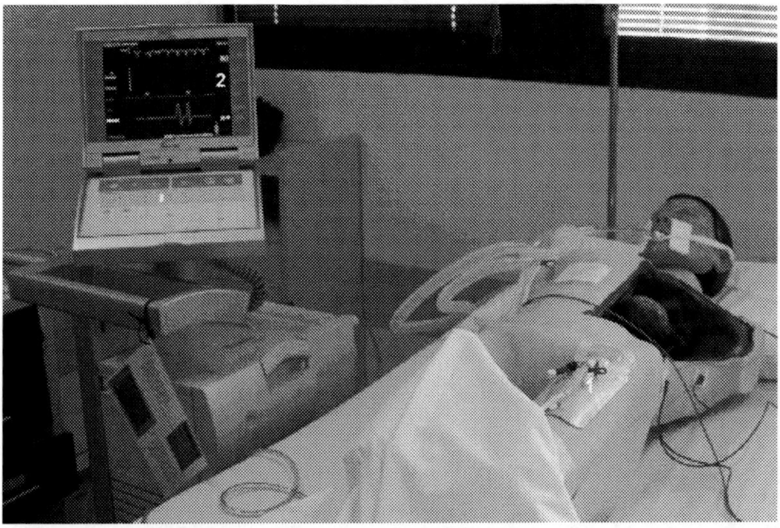

Figure 2. Components of the intra-aortic balloon pump. 1. Two-lumen catheter placed in the femoral artery. 2. Mobile console. (Simulation manikins courtesy of Licensed Practical Nurse Ricardo Rosero, ricardorosero40@gmail.com).

The IABP can be placed peripherally, with the most common and easiest insertion site being the femoral artery, but it can also be placed in the subclavian artery in selected patient to allow mobilization. Disadvantages of femoral insertion include:

- Supine position requirement (no ambulation)
- Leg ischemia
- High infection rate
- Requires femoral/iliac arteries without severe peripheral arterial disease

Subclavian artery insertion allows ambulation and has been described for patients with severe peripheral vascular disease or in those who need long-term support, such as patients waiting for heart transplantation. Nevertheless, this approach carries procedural demands as correct positioning may require fluoroscopic assistance, is associated with driveline kinking and has the potential risk of embolic stroke. In order to prevent some of these complications, the subclavian artery approach can be avoided in patients with low body mass index.

Once the catheter is inserted into the descending aorta, it should be placed 1–2 cm below the left subclavian artery (to avoid upper extremity or cerebral ischemia) and above the renal arteries (to avoid renal ischemia). On chest radiography, the tip of the IABP should be between the second and third intercostal space (Figure 3) [4]. In the case of subclavian/axillary insertion, the balloon lies in the reverse of its usual orientation, with the tip of the catheter in the distal descending aorta. Optimal positioning can be achieved through radiography, fluoroscopy or transesophageal echocardiography [1].

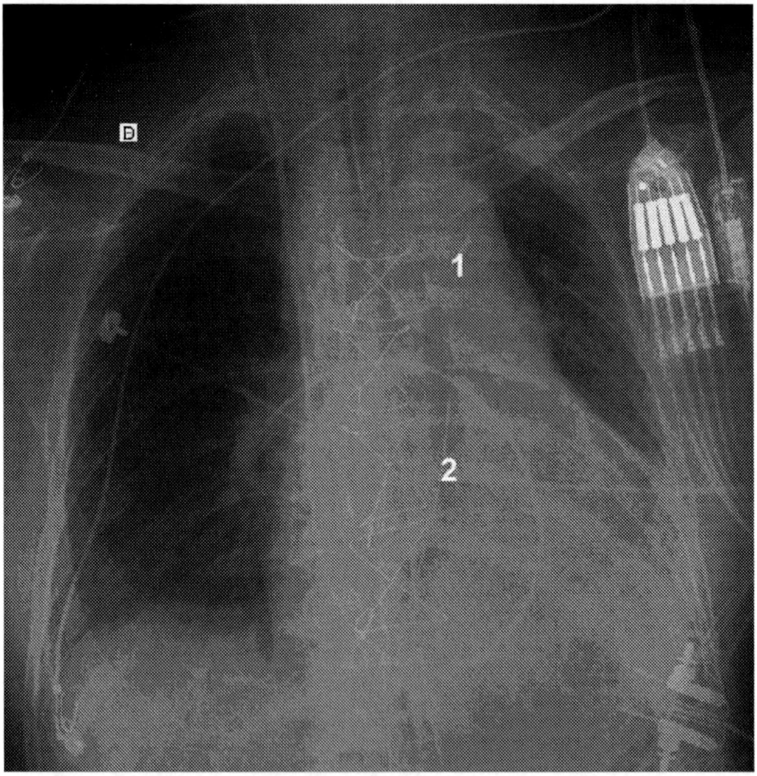

Figure 3. Radiographic imaging of an intra-aortic balloon pump. 1. Tip of the intraaortic balloon pump. 2. Inflated balloon.

The IABP provides hemodynamic support by diastolic augmentation of aortic pressure and left ventricular afterload reduction; during diastole, the balloon inflates, increasing coronary perfusion, whereas during systole, the balloon rapidly deflates, creating a temporary vacuum that reduces afterload and improves left ventricular unloading. In order to achieve the optimal effect of the IABP, inflation and deflation must be correctly timed to the cardiac cycle. Therefore, counterpulsation should be synchronized with either electrocardiogram or pressure trigger. In optimal inflation-deflation timing, balloon inflation occurs after aortic valve closure, at the onset of diastole, and deflation occurs just before the aortic valve opens, during isovolumetric contraction [1].

In the case of electrocardiographic triggering, in a properly timed waveform, the inflation is triggered during T wave – P wave interval and deflation triggered during R wave – T wave interval. In case of atrial fibrillation, the computer can analyze the QRS complex to time deflation with an R wave, whether positively or negatively deflected. Additionally, when patients have 100% ventricular pacing, pacer triggering mode determines augmentation based on the ventricular pacing spike. With pressure triggering, the identification of the dicrotic notch and systolic upstroke in the arterial waveform triggers inflation and deflation, respectively.

One inflation per cardiac cycle (1:1) provides maximum hemodynamic support, while a reduced assist ratio (1:2 or 1:3) may be used during tachycardia, arrhythmia, or for weaning prior to device removal. Augmentation may be decreased in cases of tachycardia, atrial fibrillation, increased aortic compliance, decreased systemic vascular resistance, or extremely low or high stroke volume.

It should be noted that IABP provides only partial support, with an increase of approximately 0.5 to 1 l/min in cardiac output [1, 2].

Complications and Contraindications

Complications related to the IABP include [1]:

- Vascular injury (5%–10% incidence).
- Incorrect balloon size, positioning, and/or timing, resulting in limb or organ ischemia, vascular injury, and/or reduced hemodynamic benefits.
- Infection
- Bleeding, hemolysis and thrombocytopenia
- Thrombosis, pseudoaneurysm, aneurysm, dissection, compartment syndrome

In order to decrease the risk of vascular trauma or dissection, the use of smaller diameter and/or "sheathless" catheters without an introducer can be considered. On the contrary, the use of large catheters, prolonged support, peripheral arterial disease, diabetes, female gender, older age or smoking history increase the risk of injury. In addition, the risk of thrombosis can be reduced by implementing systemic anticoagulation, especially in cases where support for more than one day is planned, there are previous risk factors for thrombosis, or when the patient is in weaning mode (1:2 or 1:3).

The main contraindications for the use of the IABP are [1, 5]:

- Moderate to severe aortic valve regurgitation
- Aortic aneurysm or dissection
- Active bleeding or contraindications to anticoagulation
- Severe thrombocytopenia

Triggering and Timing

Correct synchronization with cardiac cycle is essential to achieve the best results when using an IABP. It is recommended to assess proper timing by evaluating the arterial pressure waveform from the central lumen. When timing is correct, there is a diastolic augmentation of aortic pressure and the assisted end-diastolic pressure is lower than the end-diastolic pressure of the unassisted beat. Therefore, peak-assisted systolic pressure is lower than the peak systolic pressure of the unassisted beat (Figure 4) [1].

There are four errors of timing: early inflation, late inflation, early deflation and late deflation. In early inflation, IABP inflates before aortic valve closure, leading to increased afterload and reduced left ventricular ejection. Late IABP inflation reduces the time of diastolic augmentation, therefore the effectiveness of this device is reduced. Early deflation, before aortic valve opening, also reduces the effectiveness of the IABP secondary to an early decrease in diastolic augmentation, with no afterload reduction. Finally, late IABP deflation increases end-diastolic pressure and afterload during the early phase of left ventricular ejection (Figure 5) [1, 2].

Early inflation and late deflation are the most harmful errors in timing as they both increase afterload by being inflated during systole, which increases myocardial oxygen demand.

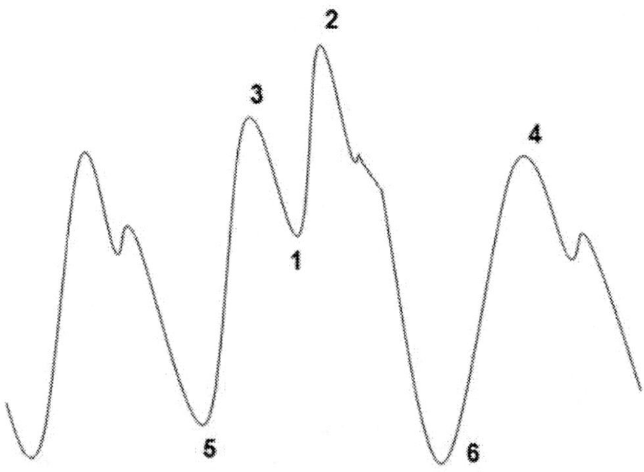

Figure 4. Correct timing. 1. Dicrotic notch. 2. Diastolic augmentation. 3. Peak unassisted systolic pressure. 4. Peak-assisted systolic pressure. 5. Unassisted end-diastolic pressure. 6. Assisted end-diastolic pressure.

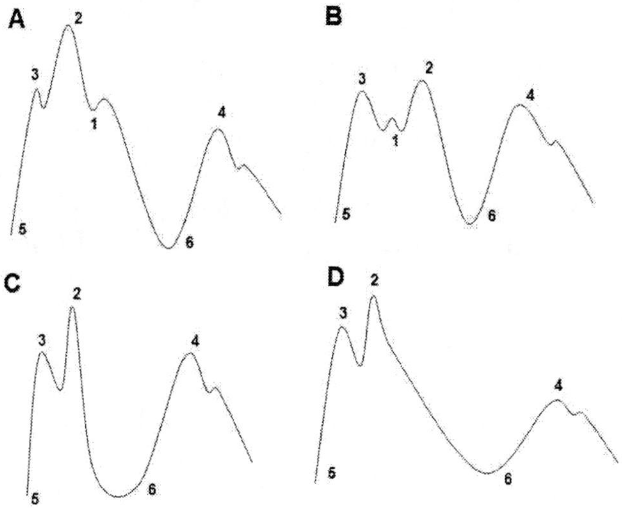

Figure 5. Errors of timing. A. Early inflation. B. Late inflation. C. Early deflation. D. Late deflation. 1. Dicrotic notch. 2. Diastolic augmentation. 3. Peak unassisted systolic pressure. 4. Peak-assisted systolic pressure. 5. Unassisted end-diastolic pressure. 6. Assisted end-diastolic pressure.

Current Evidence on the Use of Intraaortic Balloon Pump

Several studies have tried to assess the usefulness of IABP in different settings. The majority of these studies were focused on patients with myocardial infarction [6, 7]. Subsequently, some studies evaluated the use of IABP in the setting of low cardiac output following cardiac surgery with positive results [1, 8].

In recent years, there have been two mayor randomized controlled trials investigating the use of IABP in the setting of cardiogenic shock: the IABP-SHOCK and the IABP-SHOCK II trials. The IABP-SHOCK trial was a single-center study that included 45 patients with acute myocardial infarction and cardiogenic shock undergoing percutaneous coronary intervention. In this study, IABP did not improve hemodynamics or multiorgan failure scores [9]. Afterwards, the IABP-SHOCK II trial included 598 patients with cardiogenic shock secondary to myocardial infarction in multiple centers. Patients were assigned either to IABP (300 patients) or no IABP (298 patients), underwent early revascularization (percutaneous or surgical) and received optimal medical therapy. There were no differences in 30-day, 1-year, or 6-year mortality [10, 11].

Although these results do not support the routine use of IABP in patients with cardiogenic shock secondary to myocardial infarction undergoing early revascularization, it is difficult to draw definitive conclusions as there was a lack of standardization in revascularization therapy, since percutaneous coronary intervention or coronary artery bypass surgery were performed at the discretion of the treating physician. Despite these results, IABP continues to be the most widely used mechanical circulatory support device [12].

Current guidelines make different recommendations regarding the use of IABP. The 2013 AHA guidelines for the management of ST-elevation myocardial infarction recommend the use of IABP in patients with cardiogenic shock unresponsive to pharmacologic therapy (Class IIa) and also prior to surgical treatment for mechanical complications, such as ventricular rupture [13]. The 2014 AHA guidelines for the management of non–ST-elevation myocardial infarction recommend IABP in patients with refractory cardiogenic shock [14]. In contrast, European guidelines do not recommend routine use in cardiogenic shock complicating acute ST-elevation myocardial infarction (Class III), although it may be considered in selected patients. They do recommend its use in patients with non–ST-elevation myocardial infarction with hemodynamic instability secondary to mechanical complications (Class IIa) [15, 16].

Cardiogenic shock secondary to acutely decompensated chronic heart failure is different from that secondary to myocardial infarction. The use of IABP in the latter has been extensively studied as described above. However, studies on the use of IABP in the setting of acute-on-chronic heart failure are scarce, and are mostly small or observational reports. Gul et al., retrospectively analyzed 193 patients with IABP due to cardiogenic shock secondary to myocardial infarction (69.4%) and secondary to other causes (30.6%) and found that mortality was lower in patients who received an IABP within the first hour of diagnosis of cardiogenic shock, highlighting the importance of prompt utilization of these devices [17]. A randomized controlled trial by den Uil et al., that included 32 patients with acute decompensated heart failure compared IABP with inotropic therapy in this setting. They found that improvement in mixed venous saturation at 3 hours was achieved more frequently in the IABP group, as well as a reduction in 30-day mortality (23% vs. 44%) [18].

Despite these studies and guideline recommendations, the evidence for or against the use of IABP in cardiogenic shock is conflicting, and no universal statements can be made. Therefore, the use of IABP should be decided on an individual basis and according to the experience and availability of each center [19].

Intraaortic Balloon Pump in Heart Transplantation

Heart transplantation is the gold standard treatment for advanced heart failure (See Chapter 6). However, these patients are often critically ill and may require pharmacological and non-pharmacological support in order to achieve transplantation. The IABP can be useful in these situations to provide hemodynamic stabilization as a bridge to heart transplantation. However, candidates may remain on the waiting list for extended periods before undergoing transplantation, and an IABP in the femoral artery may prevent patients from ambulating for long periods of time, resulting in deterioration of the physical condition. In order to overcome this problem, a subclavian/axillary approach may be used to allow mobilization. Nishida et al., described their experience with 133 patients bridged to heart transplantation with axillary IABP with a median duration of 21 days. They reported that 98.5% of patients were able to mobilize during the waiting period, and 122 patients (91.7%) were successfully bridged to heart transplantation, with a 5-year survival after transplantation of 83.6% [20]. Additionally, the United Network for Organ Sharing (UNOS) recently changed its allocation policies, prioritizing patients bridged with an IABP. After this change, the number of patients bridged with IABP increased significantly compared to the previous period. Furthermore, patients requiring IABP support were more likely to survive to transplant when compared to patients before the policy change (76.4 vs. 89.8%, $P < 0.001$), probably in part due to shorter waitlist times (15 v. 35 days, $P < 0.001$) [21].

Finally, the use of IABP is not only useful in the pretransplant setting, but also after heart transplantation, when the patient may also require hemodynamic support. In fact, one of the most common early complications after transplantation is primary graft dysfunction (See Chapter 9). When this occurs, inotropic support may be insufficient to stabilize the patient, and mechanical circulatory support can be necessary to compensate for the hemodynamic condition, while waiting for the graft to recover. When IABP is required, primary graft dysfunction is classified as moderate, whereas if other types of mechanical circulatory support are needed it is classified as severe [22].

Conclusion

The IABP is the most common used mechanical circulatory support device. Although it provides only partial support, it can be quickly placed at the bedside and it is widely available. When used appropriately, it can be useful both in the pretransplant setting to allow bridge to transplantation and after heart transplantation for the treatment of early graft dysfunction. Therefore, despite conflictive evidence, its ease of use and wide availability make the IABP an useful tool in heart transplantation.

References

[1] González L S, Chaney M A. Intraaortic Balloon Pump Counterpulsation, Part I: History, Technical Aspects, Physiologic Effects, Contraindications, Medical Applications/Outcomes. *Anesth. Analg.* 2020 Sep;131(3):776-791.

[2] Parissis H, Graham V, Lampridis S, Lau M, Hooks G, Mhandu P C. IABP: history-evolution-pathophysiology-indications: what we need to know. *J. Cardiothorac. Surg.* 2016 Aug 4;11(1):122.

[3] Huu A L, Shum-Tim D. Intra-aortic balloon pump: current evidence & future perspectives. *Future Cardiol.* 2018 Jul;14(4):319-328.

[4] Rodriguez Lima D R, Duran E J, Rojas Díaz E L, Pinilla Rojas D I, Mercado Díaz MA, Bustos Martínez YF. Ultrasound-guided insertion of intra-aortic balloon counterpulsation in intensive care: description of the technique. *Ultrasound J.* 2020 Apr 21;12(1):23.

[5] MacKay E J, Patel P A, Gutsche J T, Weiss S J, Augoustides J G. Contemporary Clinical Niche for Intra-Aortic Balloon Counterpulsation in Perioperative Cardiovascular Practice: An Evidence-Based Review for the Cardiovascular Anesthesiologist. *J. Cardiothorac. Vasc. Anesth.* 2017 Feb;31(1):309-320.

[6] O'Rourke M F, Norris R M, Campbell T J, Chang V P, Sammel N L. Randomized controlled trial of intraaortic balloon counterpulsation in early myocardial infarction with acute heart failure. *Am. J. Cardiol.* 1981 Apr;47(4):815-20.

[7] Subramanian V A, Goldstein J E, Sos T A, McCabe J C, Hoover E A, Gay W A Jr. Preliminary clinical experience with percutaneous intraaortic balloon pumping. *Circulation.* 1980 Aug;62(2 Pt 2):I123-9.

[8] McEnany M T, Kay H R, Buckley M J, Daggett W M, Erdmann A J, Mundth E D, Rao R S, DeToeuf J, Austen W G. Clinical experience with intraaortic balloon pump support in 728 patients. *Circulation.* 1978 Sep;58(3 Pt 2):I124-32.

[9] Prondzinsky R, Lemm H, Swyter M, Wegener N, Unverzagt S, Carter J M, Russ M, Schlitt A, Buerke U, Christoph A, Schmidt H, Winkler M, Thiery J, Werdan K, Buerke M. Intra-aortic balloon counterpulsation in patients with acute myocardial infarction complicated by cardiogenic shock: the prospective, randomized IABP SHOCK Trial for attenuation of multiorgan dysfunction syndrome. *Crit. Care Med.* 2010 Jan;38(1):152-60.

[10] Thiele H, Zeymer U, Neumann F J, Ferenc M, Olbrich H G, Hausleiter J, Richardt G, Hennersdorf M, Empen K, Fuernau G, Desch S, Eitel I, Hambrecht R, Fuhrmann J, Böhm M, Ebelt H, Schneider S, Schuler G, Werdan K; IABP-SHOCK II Trial Investigators. Intraaortic balloon support for myocardial infarction with cardiogenic shock. *N. Engl. J. Med.* 2012 Oct 4;367(14):1287-96.

[11] Thiele H, Zeymer U, Thelemann N, Neumann F J, Hausleiter J, Abdel-Wahab M, Meyer-Saraei R, Fuernau G, Eitel I, Hambrecht R, Böhm M, Werdan K, Felix S B, Hennersdorf M, Schneider S, Ouarrak T, Desch S, de Waha-Thiele S; IABPSHOCK II Trial (Intraaortic Balloon Pump in Cardiogenic Shock II) Investigators. Intraaortic Balloon Pump in Cardiogenic Shock Complicating Acute Myocardial Infarction: Long-Term 6-Year Outcome of the Randomized IABP-SHOCK II Trial. *Circulation.* 2018 Nov 11.

[12] Shah M, Patnaik S, Patel B, Ram P, Garg L, Agarwal M, Agrawal S, Arora S, Patel N, Wald J, Jorde U.P. Trends in mechanical circulatory support use and hospital mortality among patients with acute myocardial infarction and non-infarction related cardiogenic shock in the United States. *Clin. Res. Cardiol.* 2018 Apr;107(4):287-303.

[13] O'Gara P T, Kushner F G, Ascheim D D, Casey D E Jr, Chung M K, de Lemos J A, Ettinger S M, Fang J C, Fesmire F M, Franklin B A, Granger C B, Krumholz H M,

Linderbaum J A, Morrow D A, Newby L K, Ornato J P, Ou N, Radford M J, Tamis-Holland J E, Tommaso C L, Tracy C M, Woo Y J, Zhao D X, Anderson J L, Jacobs A K, Halperin J L, Albert N M, Brindis R G, Creager M A, DeMets D, Guyton R A, Hochman J S, Kovacs R J, Kushner F G, Ohman E M, Stevenson W G, Yancy C W; American College of Cardiology Foundation/American Heart Association Task Force on Practice Guidelines. 2013 ACCF/AHA guideline for the management of ST-elevation myocardial infarction: a report of the American College of Cardiology Foundation/American Heart Association Task Force on Practice Guidelines. *Circulation.* 2013 Jan 29;127(4):e362-425.

[14] Amsterdam E A, Wenger N K, Brindis R G, Casey D E Jr, Ganiats T G, Holmes D R Jr, Jaffe A S, Jneid H, Kelly R F, Kontos M C, Levine G N, Liebson P R, Mukherjee D, Peterson E D, Sabatine M S, Smalling R W, Zieman S J. 2014 AHA/ACC Guideline for the Management of Patients with Non-ST-Elevation Acute Coronary Syndromes: a report of the American College of Cardiology/American Heart Association Task Force on Practice Guidelines. *J. Am. Coll. Cardiol.* 2014 Dec 23;64(24):e139-e228.

[15] Roffi M, Patrono C, Collet J P, Mueller C, Valgimigli M, Andreotti F, Bax J J, Borger M A, Brotons C, Chew D P, Gencer B, Hasenfuss G, Kjeldsen K, Lancellotti P, Landmesser U, Mehilli J, Mukherjee D, Storey R F, Windecker S; ESC Scientific Document Group. 2015 ESC Guidelines for the management of acute coronary syndromes in patients presenting without persistent ST-segment elevation: Task Force for the Management of Acute Coronary Syndromes in Patients Presenting without Persistent ST-Segment Elevation of the European Society of Cardiology (ESC). *Eur. Heart J.* 2016 Jan 14;37(3):267-315.

[16] Ibanez B, James S, Agewall S, Antunes M J, Bucciarelli-Ducci C, Bueno H, Caforio ALP, Crea F, Goudevenos J A, Halvorsen S, Hindricks G, Kastrati A, Lenzen M J, Prescott E, Roffi M, Valgimigli M, Varenhorst C, Vranckx P, Widimský P; ESC Scientific Document Group. 2017 ESC Guidelines for the management of acute myocardial infarction in patients presenting with ST-segment elevation: The Task Force for the management of acute myocardial infarction in patients presenting with ST-segment elevation of the European Society of Cardiology (ESC). *Eur. Heart J.* 2018 Jan 7;39(2):119-177.

[17] Gul B, Bellumkonda L. Usefulness of Intra-aortic Balloon Pump in Patients With Cardiogenic Shock. *Am. J. Cardiol.* 2019 Mar 1;123(5):750-756.

[18] den Uil C A, Van Mieghem N M, B Bastos M, Jewbali L S, Lenzen M J, Engstrom A E, Bunge J J H, Brugts J J, Manintveld O C, Daemen J, Wilschut J M, Zijlstra F, Constantinescu A A. Primary intra-aortic balloon support versus inotropes for decompensated heart failure and low output: a randomised trial. *EuroIntervention.* 2019 Sep 20;15(7):586-593.

[19] Morici N, Marini C, Sacco A, Tavazzi G, Saia F, Palazzini M, Oliva F, Ferrari G M, Colombo P C, Kapur N K, Garan A R, Pappalardo F. Intra-aortic Balloon Pump for Acute-on-Chronic Heart Failure Complicated by Cardiogenic Shock. *J. Card. Fail.* 2021 Nov 11:S1071-9164(21)00468-1.

[20] Nishida H, Koda Y, Kalantari S, Nguyen A, Chung B, Grinstein J, Kim G, Sarswat N, Smith B, Song T, Onsager D, Jeevanandam V, Ota T. Outcomes of Ambulatory

Axillary Intraaortic Balloon Pump as a Bridge to Heart Transplantation. *Ann. Thorac. Surg.* 2021 Apr;111(4):1264-1270.

[21] Huckaby L V, Seese L M, Mathier M A, Hickey G W, Kilic A. Intra-Aortic Balloon Pump Bridging to Heart Transplantation: Impact of the 2018 Allocation Change. *Circ. Heart Fail.* 2020 Aug;13(8):e006971.

[22] Kobashigawa J, Zuckermann A, Macdonald P, Leprince P, Esmailian F, Luu M, Mancini D, Patel J, Razi R, Reichenspurner H, Russell S, Segovia J, Smedira N, Stehlik J, Wagner F; Consensus Conference participants. Report from a consensus conference on primary graft dysfunction after cardiac transplantation. *J. Heart Lung Transplant.* 2014 Apr;33(4):327-40.

Chapter 5

Short-Term Mechanical Circulatory Support in Heart Transplant Candidates

Mariano Martin Candioti Lehmann*
and Elian Facundo Giordanino
Heart Failure and Heart Transplantation, Favaloro Foundation University Hospital, Buenos Aires, Argentina

Abstract

Heart transplant candidates may be critically ill despite pharmacological support while awaiting transplantation. In this situation, short-term mechanical circulatory support devices can be useful to compensate the hemodynamic status allowing bridge to transplantation. Furthermore, advanced heart failure patients may also require these devices as a bridge to recovery or another, more durable, device. There are different short-term mechanical circulatory support devices, each with its own advantages and disadvantages. Therefore, understanding their particular characteristics is essential to use these technologies appropriately.

Keywords: heart transplantation, heart-assist devices, extracorporeal membrane oxygenation

Introduction

One of the main objectives of every heart transplant team is to give patients the best chance to save or improve their lives and this is achieved through an

* Corresponding Author's E-mail: mcandiot@ffavaloro.org.

In: Heart Transplantation
Editor: Elian Facundo Giordanino
ISBN: 978-1-68507-759-4

adequate match between donor and recipient, among other factors. Selecting the right time for heart transplantation and achieving proper recipient conditioning are other key components to success. However, in a critically ill population, as is often the case with heart transplant candidates, these goals are sometimes difficult to achieve with medical therapy alone.

Although medical therapy was the last resort for this group of patients until two decades ago, today mechanical circulatory support devices (MCS) are a feasible option with increasing use and an acceptable safety profile. This offers the possibility of a complementary role for these two therapies for the treatment and stabilization of heart transplant candidates.

Currently, these technologies are being used earlier and earlier to avoid the use of maximum pharmacological support and its deleterious effects. Their goal is to minimize the probability of organ dysfunction in the setting of advanced heart failure by bridging patients in the best conditions possible to heart transplantation, long term support or decision, according to the clinical scenario [1, 2].

In this chapter, the different options regarding MCS will be discussed, with an emphasis on short-term MCS such as extracorporeal membrane oxygenation (ECMO), centrifugal pumps and Impella. Intra-aortic balloon pump is discussed in Chapter 4. Although there are some general principles when choosing an MCS, the ideal device for each situation is an area of ongoing debate.

Patient Selection

Choosing the right time and the right patient for short-term MCS placement is one of the most challenging aspects of this type of technology. Placing a MCS very early exposes the patient to the serious complications associated with its use, without offering a real benefit over usual inotropic support. On the other hand, using these devices too late may cause multiple organ failure secondary to shock to settle in, reaching a point of no return. Similarly, using these technologies in patients with multiple comorbidities may stabilize the hemodynamic situation but they will still not be suitable candidates for heart transplantation or destination therapy with left ventricular assist devices (LVADs). Furthermore, these patients will not have a chance of recovery and mechanical support would eventually be declared futile.

In order to overcome the challenges of patient selection, multiple classifications have been used [3, 4]. These classifications stratify patients based on their prognosis, allowing physicians to identify those patients who could benefit the most. Nevertheless, these classifications are only another tool in clinical decision making, and individual patient selection should always be the preferred strategy.

INTERMACS

One of the most widely used classifications in MCS candidates is the one developed by the Interagency Registry for Mechanically Assisted Circulatory Support (INTERMACS) database. This database was started in June 2006 by the National Heart, Lung and Blood Institute and was originally intended to register patients who received durable MCS approved by the Food and Drug Administration [4].

There are seven patient profiles/status, which also correlate with the New York Heart Association (NYHA) Functional Classification (Table 1).

- Critical cardiogenic shock.
- Progressive decline.
- Stable but inotrope dependent.
- Recurrent advanced Heart Failure.
- Exertion Intolerant.
- Exertion Limited
- Advanced NYHA class III

The usefulness of this classification has been evaluated in several studies and the database continues to provide meaningful data in the field. The 2020 annual report analyzed 25,551 patients with a ventricular assist device between 2010 and 2019, comparing two different eras (2010-2014 and 2015-2019). The usage of temporary MCS, including ECMO and intra-aortic balloon pump before durable LVAD showed an increase in the last era (36.8% vs. 26.0%; $p < 0.0001$). The 2-year survival has improved in 2015-2019 compared with 2010-2014 (73.1% vs.69.1%, $p <0.0001$). Nevertheless, serious adverse events remain common, with major bleeding and infection being the most frequent [5].

Table 1. INTERMACS Profiles

INTERMACS Profile	Description	NYHA class
1.	Life-threatening hypotension despite rapidly escalating inotropic support, critical organ hypoperfusion, often with worsening acidosis and/or lactate levels.	IV
2.	Declining function despite intravenous inotropic support, may be manifest by worsening renal function, nutritional depletion, inability to restore volume balance. Also describes declining status in patients unable to tolerate inotropic therapy.	IV
3.	Stable blood pressure, organ function, nutrition, and symptoms on continuous intravenous inotropic support/temporary circulatory support device, but demonstrating repeated failure to wean from support due to recurrent symptomatic hypotension or renal dysfunction.	IV
4.	Stabilized close to normal volume status but experiences daily symptoms of congestion at rest or during daily activities. Doses of diuretics generally fluctuate at very high levels.	IV
5.	Comfortable at rest and with daily activities but unable to engage in any other activity, living predominantly within the house. Comfortable at rest without congestive symptoms, but may have underlying refractory elevated volume status, often with renal dysfunction.	IV
6.	No evidence of fluid overload, comfortable at rest, and with daily activities and minor activities outside the home but fatigues after the first few minutes of any meaningful activity.	IIIb
7.	No current or recent episodes of unstable fluid balance, living comfortably with meaningful activity limited to mild physical exertion.	III

INTERMACS, Interagency Registry for Mechanically Assisted Circulatory Support; NYHA, New York Heart Association. (Data from Stevenson LW et al. INTERMACS profiles of advanced heart failure: the current picture. *J Heart Lung Transplant*. 2009 Jun; 28(6):535-41)

SCAI

The Society for Cardiovascular Angiography and Interventions (SCAI) classification was recently developed in order to categorize acute cardiogenic shock in different stages in order to identify subset of patients with different prognoses and therefore potentially different therapeutic approaches [3]. Patients with cardiogenic shock are a diverse population ranging from those at risk from progressing to actual shock to those with hemodynamic instability and severe multi-organ dysfunction. Inevitably, these different groups of patients have distinct characteristics and outcomes, and the therapies needed to improve their clinical status should also be different. The SCAI classification addresses this problem by dividing patients with cardiogenic shock into different progressive stages and has shown to be able to identify subsets of patients with different prognoses [6, 7].

The stages that are used in this classification are:

- A: "At risk" for cardiogenic shock. Patients who have no signs or symptoms of cardiogenic shock but are at risk of developing it
- B: "Beginning" shock. Patients who have relative hypotension or tachycardia without hypoperfusion.
- C: "Classic" cardiogenic shock. Patients with relative hypotension and with hypoperfusion that requires inotropes, vasopressors or mechanical support (including ECMO) apart from volume resuscitation in order to restore perfusion.
- D: "Deteriorating". Patients similar to category C but that are getting worse, failing to respond to initial interventions.
- E: "Extremis". Patients on cardiac arrest, supported by multiple interventions

As previously mentioned, there are different studies that evaluated the utility of this classification, but most have a retrospective design. However, there is a prospective single center study that used the SCAI classification in a real-world setting. This study showed that 30-day survival was 100%, 65.4%, 44.2% and 60% for patients with initial SCAI shock stage B, C, D, and E respectively ($p = 0.0004$), providing evidence of the usefulness of this classification in clinical practice [7]. However, it has some limitations, mainly the small sample size ($n = 166$) and short follow-up, which may explain why stage E patients seemed to have a better survival than stage D patients.

Regardless of the aid of these classifications in identifying groups of patients with different prognoses within the spectrum of cardiogenic shock, the decision of the best therapeutic approach should be made on an individual basis and to do this, it is paramount to understand the basic principles of the different short-term MCS.

Extracorporeal Membrane Oxygenation

ECMO was used for the first time in 1975 by Dr. Robert H. Barlett in a newborn that was dying from meconium aspiration pneumonia, and since then it has become one of the most complete, versatile and widely used MCS in the world [8].

ECMO Physiology

ECMO devices are designed to be able to supply the function of both the failing heart and lungs, providing circulatory and respiratory support. Thus, the two main functions of this device are as a pump, to provide circulatory support, and as an oxygenator, to provide respiratory support, depending mainly on the configuration of the ECMO circuit.

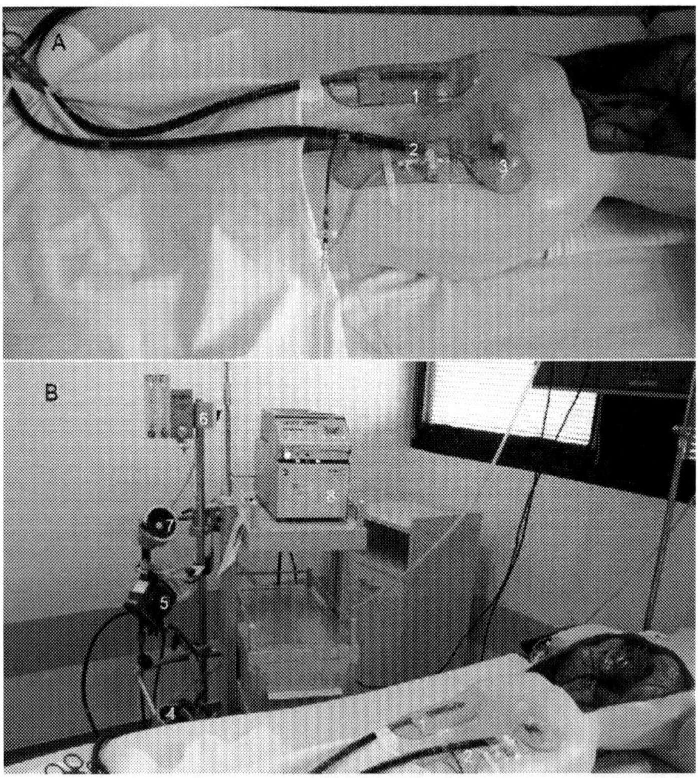

Figure 1. Veno-arterial Extracorporeal Membrane Oxygenation. **A.** Peripheral cannulation. **B.** Basic Components. 1. Inflow (venous) cannula. 2. Outlfow (arterial) cannula. 3. Distal perfusion cannula. 4. Pump. 5. Membrane oxygenator. 6. Gas blender. 7. Manual back-up pump. 8. Main console (Simulation manikins courtesy of Licensed Practical Nurse Ricardo Rosero, ricardorosero40@gmail.com.).

Regarding the pump function, initially ECMO devices used roller pumps, but currently these have mostly been replaced by centrifugal pumps. The purpose of the pump is to allow the circulation of the blood from the patient (via the inflow cannula) to the membrane oxygenator and heater, and finally return it back to the patient (via the outflow cannula). Depending on the ECMO configuration (veno-venous or veno-arterial), this process may provide circulatory support with a flow rate of up to 7-10 liters/minute depending on the cannulation strategy, replacing the function of the heart [8].

Regarding the oxygenator functionality, the main objective is to replace the failing lungs, providing respiratory support. In order to do this, ECMO devices have a membrane oxygenator that receives the deoxygenated blood drawn from the patient and adds oxygen while removing carbon dioxide. The membrane oxygenator mimics the function of the alveoli by providing an interface between air and blood to allow gas exchange (Figure 1). There are three phases in artificial oxygenators: gas phase, membrane phase and blood phase. Pressure gradients between the blood phase and the gas phase drive oxygen across the membrane and into the blood, whereas carbon dioxide is driven out of the blood and into the gas phase. Additionally, in order to maintain blood temperature and avoid hypothermia and other deleterious effects, thermo-regulated water passes through the oxygenator [9].

Configuration and Cannulation Strategy

There are several types of configurations and cannulation strategies in ECMO, according to the different clinical scenarios. Configurations are named according to the compartment from which blood is drawn (inflow cannula) and returned (outflow cannula). Thus, when blood is drawn from the venous compartment and returned to the arterial compartment, the ECMO configuration is referred as veno-arterial. Three main configurations will be considered in this chapter: veno-venous and arterio-venous, for respiratory support, and veno-arterial for cardiac support [10].

Veno-venous and arterio-venous are used when respiratory support is needed, the former in the case of refractory hypoxemia and the latter in the case of refractory hypercapnia. Veno-arterial configuration is used when circulatory support is also required.

Cannulation alternatives are central or peripheral, according to the access site of the inflow and outflow cannulas. For central cannulation, a sternotomy, clamshell incision or a thoracotomy are required in order to have access to the aorta, right and left atria and the pulmonary artery. Generally, inflow cannula is placed in the right atrium and outflow cannula in the ascending aorta, with the possibility of placing a vent usually in the right superior pulmonary vein that allows decompression of the left ventricle. This approach is used for instance in the setting of post-cardiotomy cardiogenic shock, as the cardiopulmonary bypass circuit can be replaced by an ECMO circuit on site. In the case of cardiogenic shock due to acute myocardial infarction, acute myocarditis or acute decompensation in a patient with chronic cardiomyopathy or acute respiratory failure despite mechanical ventilation, among others, an urgent cannulation is generally required, even bedside [11]. In this setting, peripheral cannulation is used via Seldinger technique. The inflow cannula can be placed through the femoral vein and into the inferior vena cava and the outflow cannula can be placed in the right Internal jugular vein or contralateral femoral vein, in case of veno-venous configuration, or in the femoral artery or subclavian artery in case or veno-arterial support. In case of arterio-venous configuration the inflow cannula is placed in the artery whereas the outflow cannula is placed in the vein.

Each cannulation strategy has its advantages and disadvantages. Peripheral ECMO allows rapid support, without surgery, even in the context of cardiac arrest. However, this configuration increases the afterload of the failing ventricle with consequent risk of pulmonary edema, and can also cause ischemia of the limb due to the arterial cannula. Central ECMO allows adequate unload of the left ventricle and a more physiological direction of the arterial flow but requires a surgical approach with higher rates of bleeding and infection [10-12].

ECMO in Different Scenarios

Short-term MCS can be a life-saving measure for critically ill patients. The term "short" makes reference to the intended duration of these devices. Therefore, an exit strategy should always be considered in order to be able to wean patients from MCS and transition them to a more durable strategy, including recovery. This is referred as a bridge strategy. There are different bridge strategies according to the clinical scenario: bridge to decision, bridge to bridge, bridge to candidacy, bridge to transplantation and bridge to recovery (Table 2) [12].

Table 2. Bridge strategies in mechanical circulatory support

BRIDGE TO DECISION/BRIDGE TO BRIDGE	Support in patients with cardiogenic shock until hemodynamics and end-organ perfusion are stabilized, contraindications for long-term MCS are excluded and additional therapeutic options including LVAD or heart transplant can be evaluated.
BRIDGE TO CANDIDACY	Support to improve end-organ function and to make an ineligible patient eligible for heart transplantation.
BRIDGE TO RECOVERY	Support to keep a patient alive until cardiac function recovers sufficiently to be weaned from MCS.
BRIDGE TO TRANSPLANTATION	Support to keep a patient alive until a donor organ becomes available

(Data from McDonagh TA et al. 2021 ESC Guidelines for the diagnosis and treatment of acute and chronic heart failure. *Eur Heart J.* 2021 Sep 21;42(36):3599-3726.)

Complications

ECMO is an invasive strategy that requires anticoagulation to avoid thrombosis of the circuit, and several complications can arise, especially with long runs.

Cheng et al. reported in a meta-analysis of 1866 patients the following rates of complications: acute kidney injury (55.6%), renal replacement therapy (46.0%), major bleeding (40.8%), rethoracotomy for bleeding or tamponade in postcardiotomy patients (41.9%), significant infection (30.4%), lower limb ischemia (16.9%), fasciotomy or compartment syndrome (10.3%), lower extremity amputation (4.7%), stroke (5.9%) and neurologic complications (13.3%) [13].

Some measures can be taken in order to decrease the rate of complications. Regarding bleeding, it is important to ensure proper fixation of the cannulas in peripheral ECMO as well as to maintain strict anticoagulation levels. Limb ischemia is another well-known complication of peripheral cannulation. In order to prevent it, a smaller, distal perfusion cannula can be placed in the femoral artery distal to the insertion point of the arterial cannula, providing flow to the limb (Figure 1A). Left ventricular thrombi can also appear when peripheral ECMO is used, which increases afterload and may close aortic valve. In order to avoid this, in addition of adequate anticoagulation levels, different strategies can be evaluated, for instance reducing afterload with another device such as Impella or intra-aortic balloon pump, increasing contractility with inotropes or decreasing ECMO flow if tolerated.

There are no formal contraindications to ECMO therapy apart from a pre-existing condition that is incompatible with recovery. Relative contraindications include uncontrollable bleeding or severe peripheral arterial disease that does not allow cannulation.

ECMO as Bridge to Heart Transplantation

The role of ECMO as a bridge to heart transplantation has been evaluated in different studies [14]. In general, ECMO is an effective therapy to obtain a rapid hemodynamic stabilization and allows bridge to heart transplantation in a critically ill population that would otherwise have practically no chance of survival. However, mortality and complications on ECMO remain high and careful patient selection is important at time of decision [15].

In a prospective analysis published by our center, 37 patients were supported with either ECMO or centrifugal pumps, and 30 patients (81.1%) underwent heart transplantation. Mortality at 30 days after transplantation was 23.3%, similar with both MCS, with no further deaths at median follow-up of 44.2 months [16].

Veno-arterial ECMO as bridge to transplantation is progressively used in the United States after the change of the heart allocation policies, leading to a more frequent use of this MCS before heart transplantation. This, together with the advances in the critical care of ECMO patients, makes it an increasingly viable option for these critical patients [15].

Centrifugal Pumps

In addition to ECMO, there are other short-term MCS that can be used to provide hemodynamic stabilization in advanced heart failure, which are centrifugal pumps. These devices use continuous centrifugal flow generated by a magnetically levitated pump that is implanted centrally in the chest, usually by a median sternotomy, and can provide left, right or biventricular support. These pumps can generate a flow rate of up to 10 liters per minute and a membrane oxygenator can be implanted halfway in the circuit to provide respiratory support if needed [17].

The main characteristics of these devices are their electromagnetic suspended impeller and totally bearingless technology, which minimizes friction, hemolysis, heat generation and platelet consumption. There are different possible configurations for these pumps depending on the hemodynamic support that is needed. For left support, the inflow cannula is inserted into the left ventricular apex or left atrium and the outflow cannula is placed in the ascending aorta. For right support, blood is extracted from the right atrium via the inflow cannula and is returned to the pulmonary artery via the outflow cannula (Figure 2).

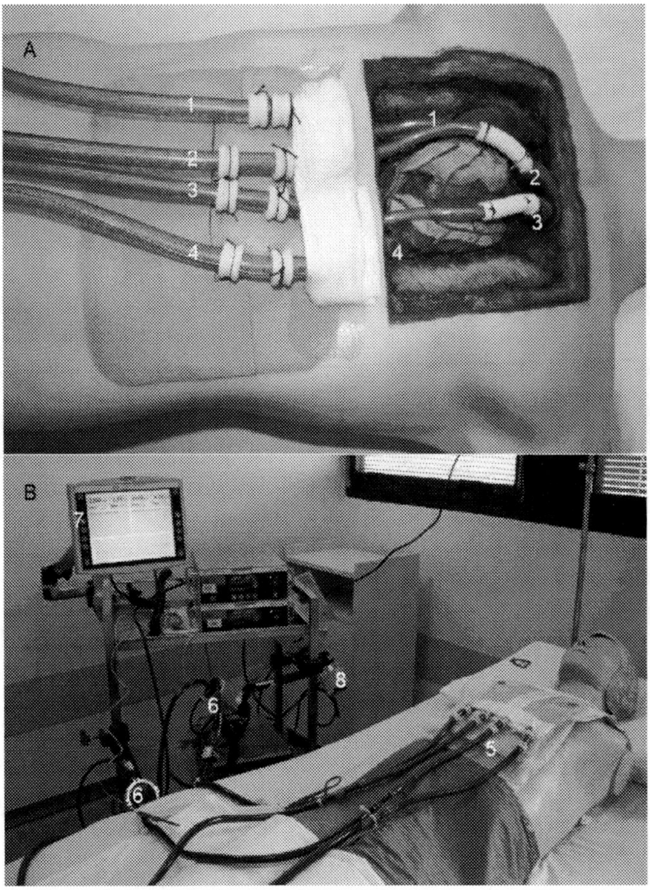

Figure 2. Biventricular support with centrifugal pump. **A.** Central cannulation. **B.** Basic Components. 1. Right inflow cannula in right atrium. 2. Left outlfow cannula in aorta. 3. Right outflow cannula in pulmonary artery. 4. Left inflow cannula in left ventricular apex. 5. Cannula exteriorization sites. 6. Right and left centrifugal pumps. 7. Main console. 8. Back-up pump (Simulation manikins courtesy of Licensed Practical Nurse Ricardo Rosero, ricardorosero40@gmail.com.).

There are several studies that analyzed the feasibility of centrifugal pumps to support patients with cardiogenic shock, including as a bridge to heart transplantation [18, 19]. A meta-analysis of 53 observational studies found a survival of 82% in precardiotomy cardiogenic shock (mean duration of support 25 days), 63% in postcardiac surgery cardiogenic shock (mean duration of support 10.9 days) and 62% in shock due to post-transplant graft rejection or failure (mean duration of support 8.8 days) [18]. As mentioned above, our institution published one of the largest single-center prospective studies with ECMO and centrifugal pumps as bridge to heart transplantation describing both pre- and post-transplant outcomes. Both strategies allowed for successful bridge to transplantation in more than 80% of patients, with a 30-days survival of 76.7% after heart transplantation [16].

One of the advantages of centrifugal pumps is the possibility to provide longer circulatory support than other short-term MCS. One study reported a mean duration of support of 38.7 days in a cohort of patients, and cases of more than 300 days of continuous operation have been described [20, 21]. Another advantage is the potential early mobilization due to its central cannulation approach [17].

Regarding some of their disadvantages, centrifugal pumps often require a median sternotomy for implantation. In order to overcome this, some studies have reported a minimally invasive approach through a minithoracotomy and a right or left axillary artery cannulation, showing the feasibility of this technique [22]. Complications of these devices include bleeding, infections and neurological events due to thrombus formation [18].

Impella Ventricular Support System

Impella was created in 1997 and is accessible for clinical use since 2000 [17]. It is a miniaturized ventricular assist device with an axial flow pump that draws blood from the left ventricle via the inlet port and expels it into the ascending aorta via the outlet port, in case of left ventricular support, or less frequently from the right ventricle into the pulmonary artery, in case of right ventricular support. It is generally placed peripherally, primarily through a femoral artery access and less frequently through the axillary artery, but it can also be placed centrally directly into the aorta.

There are different models that can provide antegrade flow from 2 to 5 liters per minute (Impella 2.5, Impella CP and Impella 5.0) for left support and one model for right support. By pumping blood from the left ventricle and into the ascending aorta, Impella increases cardiac output and mean arterial pressure, improving systemic perfusion and increasing coronary flow. Furthermore, it unloads the left ventricle and decreases pulmonary wedge pressure, reducing oxygen consumption and right ventricular afterload [23].

Complications of this device are mainly limb ischemia and bleeding due to the sheath size needed for the vascular access, for instance 14 French for Impella 2.5, which is considerably bigger than the sheath size used for an intra-aortic balloon pump (8 French). Other, less frequent, complications include infections, aortic valve rupture, hemolysis, pump migration, tamponade and left ventricular wall rupture [24].

Contraindications to the placement of an Impella device are the presence of thrombus in the left ventricle, moderate to severe aortic valve regurgitation, mechanical prosthetic valve in aortic position, aortic dissection and ventricular septal defect. This device requires anticoagulation, so any contraindication for anticoagulation should be considered before placing an Impella [17, 23].

There are different studies that assessed the utility of Impella devices in cardiogenic shock. Cheng et al. analyzed 80 Impella devices placed in 64 patients in cardiogenic shock as bridge to decision, durable MCS, or transplantation. Overall, 30- and 60-day survival were 67.2% and 65.6%, respectively and 68.8% of patients were successfully bridged to durable MCS (40.9%), heart transplant (36.4%) or recovery (22.7%) [24]. A meta-analysis of 3933 patients in cardiogenic shock due to acute coronary syndrome revealed that 30-day mortality remains as high as 47.8%, with the use of Impella, which shows that there is a need to improve results with this technology [25].

As mentioned above, in refractory cardiogenic shock, peripherally placed veno-arterial ECMO is a life-saving measure, but it increases afterload and does not unload the left ventricle. One possible strategy to overcome this setback is to use an Impella device combined with ECMO to unload the left ventricle. This is known as ECPELLA (ECMO and Impella) and was studied in analysis that compared 36 patients on ECMO with 30 patients on ECPELLA in cardiogenic shock. Mortality at 30 days was lower in the ECPELLA group (57% versus 78%), however, larger, prospective, randomized studies are needed to adequately evaluate this strategy [26].

Conclusion

Advanced heart failure is a broad-spectrum syndrome that can have different etiologies and different clinical courses. Heart transplantation remains as the gold standard treatment whenever possible, but pharmacological treatment is sometimes insufficient to provide hemodynamic support during the waiting list period. Short-term MCS are a viable option to compensate these patients, but proper selection and classification of patients as well as detailed knowledge of these technologies are critical for this strategy to be successful.

References

[1] Peradejordi M, Favaloro R, Bertolotti A, Abud J, Gomez C, Absi D, Favaloro L, Diez, M, Martinez L, Moscoloni, S. Orthotopic Heart Transplantation: Results from the Hospital Universitario Fundación Favaloro. *Rev Argent Cardiol.*, 2011 Nov-Dec; 79(6): 508-513.

[2] Pineton de Chambrun M, Bréchot N, Combes A. The place of extracorporeal life support in cardiogenic shock. *Curr Opin Crit Care.*, 2020 Aug; 26(4): 424-431.

[3] Baran DA, Grines CL, Bailey S, Burkhoff D, Hall SA, Henry TD, Hollenberg SM, Kapur NK, O'Neill W, Ornato JP, Stelling K, Thiele H, van Diepen S, Naidu SS. SCAI clinical expert consensus statement on the classification of cardiogenic shock: This document was endorsed by the American College of Cardiology (ACC), the American Heart Association (AHA), the Society of Critical Care Medicine (SCCM), and the Society of Thoracic Surgeons (STS) in April 2019. *Catheter Cardiovasc Interv.*, 2019 Jul 1; 94(1): 29-37.

[4] Stevenson LW, Pagani FD, Young JB, Jessup M, Miller L, Kormos RL, Naftel DC, Ulisney K, Desvigne-Nickens P, Kirklin JK. INTERMACS profiles of advanced heart failure: the current picture. *J Heart Lung Transplant.*, 2009 Jun; 28(6): 535-41.

[5] Molina EJ, Shah P, Kiernan MS, Cornwell WK 3rd, Copeland H, Takeda K, Fernandez FG, Badhwar V, Habib RH, Jacobs JP, Koehl D, Kirklin JK, Pagani FD, Cowger JA. The Society of Thoracic Surgeons Intermacs 2020 Annual Report. *Ann Thorac Surg.*, 2021 Mar; 111(3): 778-792.

[6] Schrage B, Dabboura S, Yan I, Hilal R, Neumann JT, Sörensen NA, Goßling A, Becher PM, Grahn H, Wagner T, Seiffert M, Kluge S, Reichenspurner H, Blankenberg S, Westermann D. Application of the SCAI classification in a cohort of patients with cardiogenic shock. *Catheter Cardiovasc Interv.*, 2020 Sep 1; 96(3): E213-E219.

[7] Baran DA, Long A, Badiye AP, Stelling K. Prospective validation of the SCAI shock classification: Single center analysis. *Catheter Cardiovasc Interv.*, 2020 Dec; 96(7): 1339-1347.

[8] Bartlett RH. Extracorporeal life support: history and new directions. *ASAIO J.*, 2005 Sep-Oct; 51(5): 487-9.

[9] Betit P. Technical Advances in the Field of ECMO. *Respir Care.*, 2018 Sep; 63(9): 1162-1173.

[10] Pavlushkov E, Berman M, Valchanov K. Cannulation techniques for extracorporeal life support. *Ann Transl Med.*, 2017 Feb; 5(4): 70.

[11] Rao P, Khalpey Z, Smith R, Burkhoff D, Kociol RD. Venoarterial Extracorporeal Membrane Oxygenation for Cardiogenic Shock and Cardiac Arrest. *Circ Heart Fail.*, 2018 Sep; 11(9): e004905.

[12] McDonagh TA, Metra M, Adamo M, Gardner RS, Baumbach A, Böhm M, Burri H, Butler J, Čelutkienė J, Chioncel O, Cleland JGF, Coats AJS, Crespo-Leiro MG, Farmakis D, Gilard M, Heymans S, Hoes AW, Jaarsma T, Jankowska EA, Lainscak M, Lam CSP, Lyon AR, McMurray JJV, Mebazaa A, Mindham R, Muneretto C, Francesco Piepoli M, Price S, Rosano GMC, Ruschitzka F, Kathrine Skibelund A; ESC Scientific Document Group. 2021 ESC Guidelines for the diagnosis and treatment of acute and chronic heart failure. *Eur Heart J.*, 2021 Sep 21; 42(36): 3599-3726.

[13] Cheng R, Hachamovitch R, Kittleson M, Patel J, Arabia F, Moriguchi J, Esmailian F, Azarbal B. Complications of extracorporeal membrane oxygenation for treatment of cardiogenic shock and cardiac arrest: a meta-analysis of 1,866 adult patients. *Ann Thorac Surg.*, 2014 Feb; 97(2): 610-6.

[14] Montisci A, Donatelli F, Cirri S, Coscioni E, Maiello C, Napoli C. Veno-arterial Extracorporeal Membrane Oxygenation as Bridge to Heart Transplantation: The Way Forward. *Transplant Direct.*, 2021 Jul 8; 7(8): e720.

[15] Giordanino EF. Challenges in optimal bridge to transplantation strategy using short-term mechanical circulatory support devices. *Clin Transplant.*, 2020 Oct; 34(10): e14033.

[16] Giordanino EF, Absi DO, Favaloro LE, Renedo MF, Ratto RD, Rubira DM, Ameri A, Giunta G, Favaloro RR, Bertolotti AM. Short-term mechanical circulatory support devices as bridge to heart transplantation: A prospective single-center experience in Argentina. *Clin Transplant.*, 2020 Jul; 34(7): e13888.

[17] Nagpal AD, Singal RK, Arora RC, Lamarche Y. Temporary Mechanical Circulatory Support in Cardiac Critical Care: A State of the Art Review and Algorithm for Device Selection. *Can J Cardiol.*, 2017 Jan; 33(1): 110-118.

[18] Borisenko O, Wylie G, Payne J, Bjessmo S, Smith J, Yonan N, Firmin R. Thoratec CentriMag for temporary treatment of refractory cardiogenic shock or severe cardiopulmonary insufficiency: a systematic literature review and meta-analysis of observational studies. *ASAIO J.*, 2014 Sep-Oct; 60(5): 487-97.

[19] Mehta V, Venkateswaran RV. Outcome of CentriMag™ extracorporeal mechanical circulatory support use in critical cardiogenic shock (INTERMACS 1) patients. *Indian J Thorac Cardiovasc Surg.*, 2020 Sep 30; 36(Suppl 2): 1-10.

[20] Sef D, Mohite P, De Robertis F, Verzelloni Sef A, Mahesh B, Stock U, Simon A. Bridge to heart transplantation using the Levitronix CentriMag short-term ventricular assist device. *Artif Organs.*, 2020 Sep; 44(9): 1006-1008.

[21] Griffith KE, Jenkins E, Stulak J, Paugh T, Pagani FD. Long-term use of the CentriMag® Ventricular Assist System as a right ventricular assist device: a case report. *Perfusion.*, 2012 Jan; 27(1): 65-70.

[22] Takeda K, Garan AR, Topkara VK, Kirtane AJ, Karmpaliotis D, Kurlansky P, Yuzefpolskaya M, Colombo PC, Naka Y, Takayama H. Novel minimally invasive surgical approach using an external ventricular assist device and extracorporeal membrane oxygenation in refractory cardiogenic shock. *Eur J Cardiothorac Surg.*, 2017 Mar 1; 51(3): 591-596.

[23] Glazier JJ, Kaki A. The Impella Device: Historical Background, Clinical Applications and Future Directions. *Int J Angiol.*, 2019 Jun; 28(2): 118-123.

[24] Cheng R, Tank R, Ramzy D, Azarbal B, Chung J, Esmailian F, Kobashigawa JA, Moriguchi JD, Arabia FA. Clinical Outcomes of Impella Microaxial Devices Used to Salvage Cardiogenic Shock as a Bridge to Durable Circulatory Support or Cardiac Transplantation. *ASAIO J.*, 2019 Sep/Oct; 65(7): 642-648.

[25] Iannaccone M, Albani S, Giannini F, Colangelo S, Boccuzzi GG, Garbo R, Brilakis ES, D'ascenzo F, de Ferrari GM, Colombo A. Short term outcomes of Impella in cardiogenic shock: A review and meta-analysis of observational studies. *Int J Cardiol.*, 2021 Feb 1; 324: 44-51.

[26] Patel SM, Lipinski J, Al-Kindi SG, Patel T, Saric P, Li J, Nadeem F, Ladas T, Alaiti A, Phillips A, Medalion B, Deo S, Elgudin Y, Costa MA, Osman MN, Attizzani GF, Oliveira GH, Sareyyupoglu B, Bezerra HG. Simultaneous Venoarterial Extracorporeal Membrane Oxygenation and Percutaneous Left Ventricular Decompression Therapy with Impella Is Associated with Improved Outcomes in Refractory Cardiogenic Shock. *ASAIO J.*, 2019 Jan; 65(1):21-28.

Chapter 6

Indications and Contraindications for Heart Transplantation

Elian Facundo Giordanino*

Heart Failure and Heart Transplantation, Favaloro Foundation University Hospital, Buenos Aires, Argentina

Abstract

Heart transplantation remains the best treatment for patients with advanced heart failure when other pharmacological and non-pharmacological interventions have failed. Currently, patients have a good post-transplant life expectancy, with a 1-year survival after heart transplantation of approximately 90%. However, not all patients are suitable candidates for this procedure, and knowing the indications as well as the contraindications for heart transplantation is important for appropriate patient selection.

Keywords: heart transplantation, heart failure, contraindications

Introduction

Heart failure is an increasingly prevalent syndrome worldwide with a high impact on quality of life and survival. Although there have been great advances in the treatment of this condition that effectively increase survival, mortality remains unacceptable high, exceeding 40% at 5 years. To put it in

* Corresponding Author's E-mail: efgiordanino@ffavaloro.org.

In: Heart Transplantation
Editor: Elian Facundo Giordanino
ISBN: 978-1-68507-759-4

perspective, this prognosis is worse than a large number of cancers (See Chapter 1) [1, 2]. The picture is even more worrying if we take into account that advanced heart failure patients are a particular subgroup with higher hospitalizations, worse quality of life, and higher mortality, despite optimal medical treatment. Furthermore, in the case of patients with cardiogenic shock, short-term survival can be as low as 50% [3]. However, since its first implementation in 1967, heart transplantation has been the gold standard treatment for this group of patients with advanced heart failure. Currently, the median survival after heart transplantation is approximately 12 years for adult heart transplants and 18 years for pediatric transplants. The decline in survival is greatest during the first year after heart transplantation due to early complications and perioperative mortality. If patients survive the first year, then the conditional median survival is approximately 14 years for adults and 22 years for pediatric patients (Figure 1) [4, 5]. Therefore, if we consider the ominously high 1-year mortality of advanced heart failure patients and compare it with a post-transplant survival of more than 10 years, we realize that there is no other therapy in heart failure with such a disease-modifying impact.

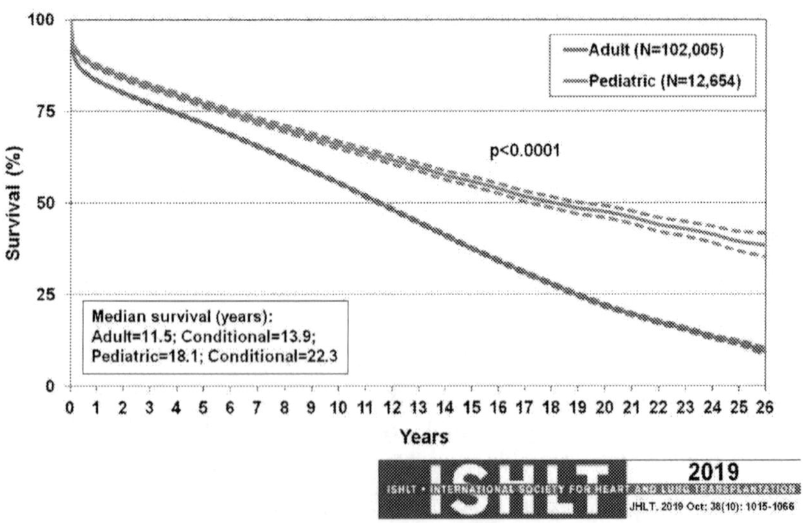

Figure 1. Adult and Pediatric Heart Transplants Survival (January 1992 - June 2017). (Data from ISHLT. 2019. "Overall Heart Transplantation Statistics". Accessed 15 Jan 2022. https://ishltregistries.org/registries/slides.asp).

Unfortunately, heart transplantation is a limited therapeutic option due to the worldwide shortage of donors. Furthermore, not all patients are suitable candidates for this complex procedure. Thus, it is very important to improve patient selection to make the most of this scarce resource, as using an organ for a patient that will not benefit from it is taking the opportunity away from another who might.

The mainstays of adequate patient selection include not only a thorough knowledge of the indications for heart transplantation, but also the consideration of its contraindications. A patient that is "too well" (i.e., asymptomatic, with no hospitalizations) would not benefit from this procedure. However, a patient that is "too sick", with multiple organ failure despite maximum doses of inotropes would not do either and would probably require a bridge to candidacy with a mechanical support device.

Throughout this chapter, the main indications and contraindications for heart transplantations will be discussed.

Indications for Heart Transplantation

At first, heart transplantation was considered a last-resort therapy for patients with advanced heart failure. These patients had to be under optimal pharmacological and device treatment, unable to overcome their heart failure symptoms, and generally hospitalized with inotropic or mechanical circulatory support requirement [6]. Needless to say, these are the patients with the worst postoperative outcomes, and although it continues to be an indication for heart transplantation, there are currently other indications based on earlier stages of the disease in order to achieve better results. In fact, treatment of heart failure has generally moved from a stepwise approach to a more simultaneous one, including the consideration for transplantation [7, 8]. Therefore, outpatients who continue to have symptoms under optimal treatment may be suitable candidates for transplantation provided they meet certain requirements, even if they do not require vasoactive drugs or are hospitalized at the time.

There are multiple indications for heart transplantation and different guidelines have slightly different recommendations, but the general principle remains the same: symptomatic patients with advanced heart failure on optimal pharmacological and non-pharmacological therapy who are considered to have a poor short/medium term prognosis based on clinical course, risk scores or complementary studies [8-10]. The main indications for heart transplantation according to different guidelines are summarized in Figure 2 and are described below.

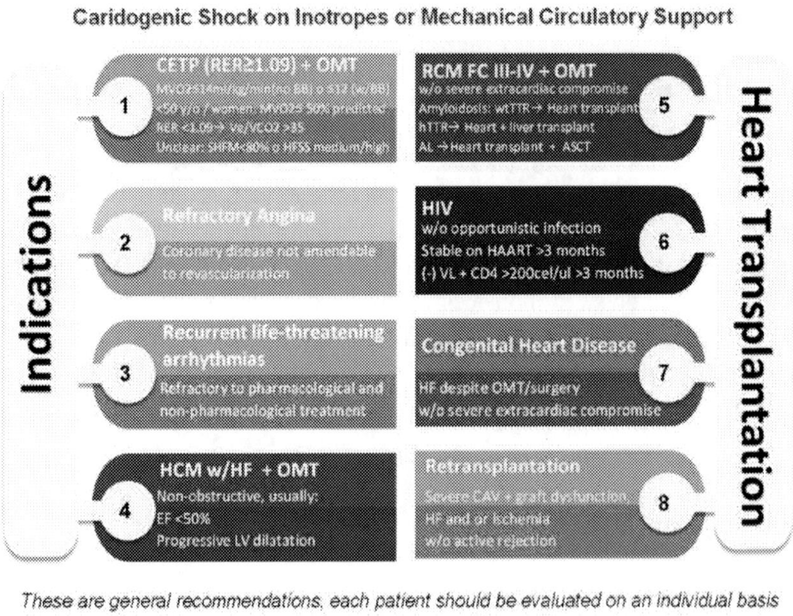

Figure 2. Indications for heart transplantation. AL, light-chain; ASCT, autologous stem cells transplantation; BB, beta blockers; CAV, cardiac allograft vasculopathy; CETP, cardiopulmonary exercise testing; EF, ejection fraction; FC, functional class; HAART, highly active antiretroviral therapy; HCM, hypertrophic cardiomyopathy; HF, heart failure; HFSS, Heart Failure Survival Score; HIV, human immunodeficiency virus; hTTR, hereditary transthyretin; LV, left ventricle; MVO2, maximum oxygen consumption; OMT, optimal medical therapy; RCM, restrictive cardiomyopathy; RER, respiratory exchange ratio; SHFM, Seattle Heart Failure Model; Ve/VCO2, ventilation equivalent of carbon dioxide; VL, viral load; w/, with; w/o, without; wtTTR, wild type transthyretin; y/o, years old. (Data form Mehra MR et al. The 2016 International Society for Heart Lung Transplantation listing criteria for heart transplantation: A 10-year update. *J Heart Lung Transplant*. 2016 Jan;35(1):1-23 and McDonagh TA et al. 2021 ESC Guidelines for the diagnosis and treatment of acute and chronic heart failure. *Eur Heart J.* 2021 Sep 21;42(36):3599-3726.).

Cardiogenic Shock on Inotropes or Mechanical Circulatory Support

Patients in cardiogenic shock who require inotropes and/or mechanical circulatory support due to a condition that is not amendable of recovery, as it would be the situation in some cases of myocarditis or acute myocardial infarction suitable for revascularization, should be considered for heart transplantation as a definitive treatment. However, these patients are often critically ill and cannot be directly transplanted under these conditions. Therefore, hemodynamic stabilization and ideally resolution of multiple organ failure should be achieved before transplantation. In order to do so, in addition to pharmacological treatment with vasoactive drugs, mechanical circulatory support devices may be necessary as a bridge to candidacy or a bridge to transplantation (See Chapter 5) [11, 12].

Recurrent Life-Threatening Arrhythmias

Recurrent life-threatening ventricular arrhythmias are a critical condition that requires prompt therapies. A special situation is the electrical storm, also known as arrhythmic storm. It is defined as three or more episodes of ventricular tachyarrhythmias within 24 hours or, in patients with an implantable cardioverter-defibrillator, as three or more appropriate therapies for ventricular arrhythmias, such as antitachycardia pacing or shocks, within 24 hours [13]. Treatment will depend on the patient's hemodynamic status; in case of hemodynamic instability, it should be treated according to the advanced cardiac life support protocol with electrical cardioversion/ defibrillation. If recurrent life-threatening ventricular arrhythmias persist despite an implantable cardiac defibrillator, antiarrhythmic therapy, or catheter-based ablation, then heart transplantation should be considered. Furthermore, in some cases, mechanical circulatory support may be necessary to stabilize these patients. Given the critical condition of these patients, some allocation policies prioritize this particular situation, as is the case of the United Network for Organ Sharing (UNOS) heart allocation criteria. Patients with ventricular tachyarrhythmias are given a Status 2 condition, and if they require mechanical circulatory support, they are given the highest priority, Status 1 [14].

Refractory Angina

There have been great advances in the field of coronary disease. However, some patients that are unsuitable for further revascularization and persist with refractory angina despite medical therapy should be considered for heart transplantation [15]. It is true that currently there are multiple pharmacological and non-pharmacological options for patients not amendable to revascularization that persist with angina, ranging from additional antiplatelet agents, neurostimulation, enhanced extracorporeal counterpulsation to even gene therapy, which make this indication less and less frequent [16]. Despite this, there are still patients that need heart transplantation due to this condition. In fact, patients with ischemic heart disease with intractable angina are prioritized to Status 4 in the UNOS heart allocation policies [14].

Cardiopulmonary Exercise Testing

Cardiopulmonary exercise testing is a non-invasive method that comprehensively assesses the exercise responses involving mainly the pulmonary, cardiovascular, and skeletal muscle systems. It offers a unique opportunity to physiologically evaluate the circulatory compromise in heart failure patients (See Chapter 2).

This test provides a great amount of information regarding the systems mentioned above, and may even help distinguishing cardiac from respiratory origin of symptoms such as dyspnea. However, one of the most important parameters regarding the evaluation of the heart transplant candidate is the peak volume of oxygen consumption (VO_2max). VO_2max is one of the best predictors for listing a patient for heart transplantation, as it can objectively differentiate patients with limited survival from those at low risk. However, patients should not be listed based solely on VO_2max and this information should be evaluated in the clinical setting of each patient. There are different cut-off values, but the most commonly accepted indication for heart transplantation is a $VO_2max \leq 12$ ml/kg/min (or ≤ 14ml/kg/min in patients not receiving beta blocker therapy due to intolerance) under optimal medical and device treatment [10]. It should be noted that this indication for heart transplantation is for patients who are on the maximum tolerated dose of heart failure medication as well as devices if appropriate. Therefore, if a patient has a $VO_2max \leq 12$ml/kg/min but has not yet been treated with heart failure drugs, that patient should first be treated accordingly and then reassessed. Another important point is to consider VO_2max only if the cardiopulmonary exercise testing has been maximal, that is, if the respiratory exchange ratio (RER) is >1.09 and the anaerobic threshold has been achieved. Otherwise, VO_2max should not be used for clinical decision making. In these cases of sub-maximal cardiopulmonary exercise test, a ventilation equivalent of carbon dioxide (V_E/V_{CO2}) slope of >35 can be used as a criterion for heart transplantation, as it is independent of the RER and is associated with worse outcomes in heart failure patients [10, 17].

There are some special situations that deserve further consideration. In patients younger than 50 years old and in women, a percent of predicted $VO_2max \leq 50\%$ may also be used in conjunction with the absolute value of VO_2max for clinical decision making. In addition, in obese patients with a body mass index >30 kg/m^2, VO_2max can be adjusted to lean body mass, with a cut-off value of <19 ml/kg/min indicating a worse prognosis [10, 18, 19].

Although VO_2max is a very useful tool, it should always be used in conjunction with other clinical data. In some cases, risk scores can also be helpful in making the final decision to include a patient for heart transplantation. The two most commonly used scores are the Seattle Heart Failure Model and the Heart Failure Survival Score. One-year survival of less than 80% calculated by the Seattle Heart Failure Model or a high/medium risk range of the Heart Failure Survival Score are appropriate cut-off points to consider transplantation in conjunction with VO_2max values [10].

Hypertrophic Cardiomyopathy

A small proportion of patients with hypertrophic cardiomyopathy may need heart transplantation when they reach a stage of advanced heart failure. In particular patients with non-obstructive hypertrophic cardiomyopathy that are symptomatic for heart failure despite optimal medical and surgical/device treatment should be listed for transplantation (See Chapter 18).

It is important to be aware that these patients may rapidly progress to end-stage heart failure when they develop systolic dysfunction (left ventricular ejection fraction <50%) with ventricular remodeling similar to dilated cardiomyopathy, including ventricle dilation and wall thinning. Since these patients usually have high ejection fraction, a decrease below 50% is an important predictor of poor prognosis and should prompt careful monitoring. Furthermore, patients with normal ejection fraction but with severe symptoms due to diastolic dysfunction despite optimal medical therapy may also be considered for transplantation [10].

Following heart transplantation, survival of these patients is similar to or even better than for other cardiomyopathies, probably in part due to younger age and fewer comorbidities at the time of listing [5, 20].

Restrictive Cardiomyopathy

Restrictive cardiomyopathies are a special group of diseases characterized by diastolic dysfunction secondary to increased ventricular stiffness. This leads to elevated filling pressures with atrial enlargement, usually without ventricular dilatation. Patients who are unresponsive to medical treatment, including etiology-specific treatment, and continue to have symptoms of severe heart failure, New York Heart Association Functional Classification (NYHA) III–IV, should be considered for heart transplantation [10]. However, throughout evaluation of the etiology and underlying mechanism of restrictive cardiomyopathy should be performed prior to transplantation in order to assess whether specific treatments are available (i.e., sarcoidosis, amyloidosis) and to adequately evaluate the prognosis or potential contraindications related to certain etiologies (see Chapter 18)

Among the different etiologies that may lead to a restrictive cardiomyopathy phenotype, amyloidosis deserves a special consideration regarding heart transplantation. This group of diseases is characterized by the accumulation of misfolded proteins in the extracellular matrix of different tissues, including the heart. There are different types of amyloidosis with different prognoses and treatments that should be carefully evaluated before transplantation [8]. In addition, severe extracardiac involvement is a contraindication for heart transplantation in these patients and should always be ruled out beforehand. Furthermore, these patients should be treated by a multidisciplinary team in experienced centers.

In the case of light-chain amyloidosis (AL), heart transplantation should be followed as soon as possible by autologous stem cells transplantation in order to prevent recurrence [21]. Hereditary or familial transthyretin amyloidosis (hATTR) is caused by a misfolded protein produced in the liver; thus, combined heart and liver transplantation should be performed in these cases [22]. In contrast, wild type transthyretin amyloidosis (wtATTR) with cardiac involvement can be treated by performing isolated heart transplantation [10].

Heart Transplantation in Congenital Heart Disease

Congenital heart disease is increasing in prevalence since better medical and surgical treatment options have allowed for better survival in the last years. In fact, adult congenital heart disease has emerged as a distinct subspecialty in cardiology given the fast-growing populations of adults with this entity. Therefore, chronic heart diseases, particularly end-stage heart failure, are also on the rise. In this context, patients with congenital heart disease that are symptomatic for heart failure despite medical and surgical treatment should be considered for heart or heart-lung transplantation, provided they do not present severe extracardiac compromise (See Chapter 17). This particular population has a worse prognosis than other indications for heart transplantation, and should be treated in experienced centers with a multidisciplinary approach and availability of mechanical circulatory support [23].

Retransplantation

Retransplantation remains the highest mortality group after heart transplantation and should currently be reserved for patients with severe cardiac allograft vasculopathy leading to graft dysfunction and/or symptoms of ischemia or heart failure [10, 24]. Active graft rejection should be ruled out prior to retransplantation, and the benefits and risks of the procedure discussed with the patient. Other indications for heart retransplantation are rare and must be considered on an individual basis.

Transplantation in Patients with Human Immunodeficiency Virus

Previously, infection with human immunodeficiency virus (HIV) was considered a contraindication to heart transplantation. Currently, these patients have a better prognosis due to advances in highly active antiretroviral therapy. Cardiovascular disease has emerged as a growing complication in this population and these patients may have indication for heart transplantation if they develop end-stage heart failure. In order to consider these patients for transplantation, a series of requirements must be met [10, 25]:

- Absence of opportunistic infection.
- Clinical stable on highly active antiretroviral therapy for more than 3 months.
- Undetectable HIV RNA and CD4 counts of more than 200 cells/microliter for more than 3 months.

Additionally, history of neoplasms should be carefully evaluated on a case-by-case basis, since they may constitute a contraindication for transplantation.

A multidisciplinary approach in an experienced center is needed in order to treat this special population and the management of highly active antiretroviral therapy with immunosuppressive regimens can be challenging.

Other Special Situations

Patients with hepatitis B/C virus and end-stage heart failure may be considered for heart transplantation in experienced centers if there is no severe liver disease (i.e., cirrhosis) [26]. Chagas disease is no longer a contraindication for transplantation; indeed, Chagas cardiomyopathy is increasingly becoming an indication for heart transplantation (See Chapter 16).

Finally, these are general recommendations but there are special indications of heart transplantations that are not usually considered in the guidelines and should be evaluated on an individual basis.

Contraindications for Heart Transplantation

When considering a patient for heart transplantation, evaluating the potential contraindications is as important as evaluating its indications. There are different situations that should be taken into account according to different guidelines and there is no universal agreement on which situations should be considered as absolute or relative contraindications for heart transplantation [8-10]. Additionally, some contraindications can be overcome with proper treatment, as is the case of severe pulmonary hypertension with the use of mechanical circulatory support devices (bridge to candidacy, see Chapter 5).

For academic purposes, contraindications will be grouped into four categories: hemodynamic, systemic, psychosocial and individual-related.

Figure 3 summarizes the main contraindications for heart transplantation according to different guidelines.

Individual-Related

As a general rule, patients with a life expectancy of less than 2 years due to extracardiac diseases are considered to have an absolute contraindication for heart transplantation. In addition, patients should be considered for heart transplantation up to the age of 70 and, ideally, up to 65 years old. This constitutes a relative contraindication and some exceptions can be considered on an individual basis as biological age is more important than chronological age [8, 10].

Obesity is a relative contraindication for heart transplantation as it is associated with worse outcomes. Therefore, weight loss should be recommended to achieve a body mass index of 35 kg/m^2 or less [27].

Finally, frailty assessment has gained relevance in recent years and there are different evaluation tools that are used when considering candidacy for transplantation [28]. ISHLT guidelines define frail patients as those with 3 of the following 5 symptoms [10]:

- Unintentional weight loss >4.5Kg in one year
- Muscle loss
- Fatigue
- Slow walking speed
- Low levels of physical activity

However, there is still no general consensus regarding the best tool to assess frailty and it should be considered a relative contraindication along with other conditions.

Systemic

There are different systemic or extracardiac conditions that may be considered as contraindications for heart transplantation. Uncontrolled systemic infections and severe symptomatic cerebrovascular disease are associated with worse prognosis.

In addition, severe peripheral vascular disease is a relative contraindication for transplantation as it limits rehabilitation after the procedure, thus, revascularization should be attempted prior to transplantation whenever possible.

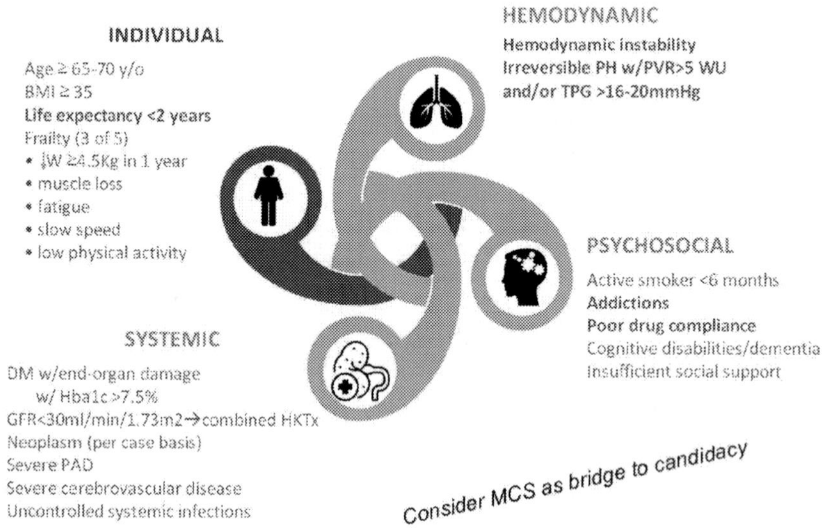

Figure 3. Contraindications for heart transplantation. BMI, body mass index; DM, diabetes mellitus; GFR, glomerular filtration rate; HKTx, heart-kydney transplant; MCS, mechanical circulatory support devices; PAD, peripheral artery disease; PH, pulmonary hypertension; PVR, pulmonary vascular resistance; TPG, transpulmonary gradient; W, weight; w/, with; WU, Wood units; y/o years old. (Data form Mehra MR et al. The 2016 International Society for Heart Lung Transplantation listing criteria for heart transplantation: A 10-year update. J Heart Lung Transplant. 2016 Jan;35(1):1-23 and McDonagh TA et al. 2021 ESC Guidelines for the diagnosis and treatment of acute and chronic heart failure. *Eur Heart J.* 2021 Sep 21;42(36):3599-3726.)

Neoplasms are also considered a contraindication, but they should be evaluated on a case-by-case basis with a multidisciplinary team, including oncology specialists, according to the type of malignancy and the time of remission. In general, active, non-circumscribed neoplasms should be considered as contraindications [8, 10].

Diabetes mellitus with poor glycemic control (HbA1c > 7.5%) or end-organ damage despite optimal medical therapy, is a relative contraindication for transplantation. Additionally, irreversible chronic renal failure with a glomerular filtration rate of less than 30 ml/min/1.73m^2 is a relative contraindication for isolated heart transplantation. In this case, combined heart-kidney transplantation should be considered [10].

Hemodynamic

Hemodynamic instability with multiple-organ failure should be considered as a contraindication for heart transplantation. Patients must be fist stabilized with vasoactive drugs and/or mechanical circulatory support devices as bridge to transplantation [8, 11, 12].

Severe pulmonary hypertension refractory to medical therapy can be considered a contraindication for heart transplantation. Therefore, right heart catheterization with a Swan-Ganz catheter is essential in the evaluation and follow-up of patients considered for transplantation (See Chapter 3). If pulmonary artery systolic pressure is ≥50mmHg with more than 3 Wood units of pulmonary vascular resistance or a transpulmonary gradient ≥15, a challenge with inotropes and/or pulmonary vasodilators (i.e., vasoreactivity test) should be performed. Patients with pulmonary vascular resistance > 5 Wood units and/or transpulmonary gradient >16-20 mmHg despite medical (pulmonary vasodilators) and device (intra-aortic balloon pump and/or left ventricular assist devices) therapy are considered as having irreversible pulmonary hypertension, which is a relative contraindication for heart transplantation. These patients may be considered for destination therapy with a durable left ventricular assist device, especially if pulmonary hypertension persists after 3 to 6 months of effective left ventricle unloading. On the other hand, vasoreactivity test is considered positive if mean pulmonary artery pressure decreases more than 10mmHg and to an absolute value of 40mmHg or less. If the pulmonary vascular resistance is reduced to 2.5 Wood units or less without decreasing systolic arterial pressure below 85mmHg, then the patient can be listed for heart transplantation. It should be noted that if the reduction of pulmonary vascular resistance below 2.5 is achieved by reducing systolic arterial pressure below 85mmHg, the unfavorable prognosis after heart transplantation remains [10, 29]. Finally, combined heart-lung transplantation can be considered in selected cases.

Psychosocial

Patients who demonstrate poor adherence to drug therapy on multiple occasions and those with active substance abuse, including alcohol, have an absolute contraindication for heart transplantation (See Chapter 7) [8, 10]. In addition, active smoking in the previous 6 months is a relative contraindication for heart transplantation as it is associated with worse outcomes [10, 30].

Patients with insufficient social support to achieve compliant care after heart transplantation should be carefully evaluated and social workers are essential to try to achieve better conditions. If this is not possible, then this situation should be considered a relative contraindication. Concomitantly, severe cognitive disabilities or dementia can make transplantation potentially harmful [8, 10].

Conclusion

Heart transplantation is a life-saving treatment for the critically ill population of patients with advanced heart failure. No other treatment has such an important impact on this condition, capable of changing an otherwise ominous clinical course, as is, for example, the case in patients in cardiogenic shock with a short-term mortality of 50%, to a good quality of life and life expectancy, with a median survival of more than 12 years. In order to make the most of this scarce resource, it is of paramount importance to improve patient selection. For this reason, comprehensive knowledge of the indications and contraindications for heart transplantation is of the utmost importance.

References

[1] Jones NR, Roalfe AK, Adoki I, Hobbs FDR, Taylor CJ. Survival of patients with chronic heart failure in the community: a systematic review and meta-analysis. *Eur J Heart Fail.* 2019 Nov;21(11):1306-1325.

[2] Mamas MA, Sperrin M, Watson MC, Coutts A, Wilde K, Burton C, Kadam UT, Kwok CS, Clark AB, Murchie P, Buchan I, Hannaford PC, Myint PK. Do patients have worse outcomes in heart failure than in cancer? A primary care-based cohort study with 10-year follow-up in Scotland. *Eur J Heart Fail.* 2017 Sep;19(9):1095-1104.

[3] Harjola VP, Lassus J, Sionis A, Køber L, Tarvasmäki T, Spinar J, Parissis J, Banaszewski M, Silva-Cardoso J, Carubelli V, Di Somma S, Tolppanen H, Zeymer

U, Thiele H, Nieminen MS, Mebazaa A; CardShock Study Investigators; GREAT network. Clinical picture and risk prediction of short-term mortality in cardiogenic shock. *Eur J Heart Fail.* 2015 May;17(5):501-9.

[4] Moayedi Y, Fan CPS, Cherikh WS, Stehlik J, Teuteberg JJ, Ross HJ, Khush KK. Survival Outcomes After Heart Transplantation: Does Recipient Sex Matter? *Circ Heart Fail.* 2019 Oct;12(10):e006218.

[5] Chambers DC, Perch M, Zuckermann A, Cherikh WS, Harhay MO, Hayes D Jr, Hsich E, Khush KK, Potena L, Sadavarte A, Lindblad K, Singh TP, Stehlik J; International Society for Heart and Lung Transplantation. The International Thoracic Organ Transplant Registry of the International Society for Heart and Lung Transplantation: Thirty-eighth adult lung transplantation report - 2021; Focus on recipient characteristics. *J Heart Lung Transplant.* 2021 Oct;40(10):1060-1072.

[6] Jessup M, Brozena S. Heart failure. *N Engl J Med.* 2003 May 15;348(20):2007-18.

[7] Yancy CW, Jessup M, Bozkurt B, Butler J, Casey DE Jr, Colvin MM, Drazner MH, Filippatos GS, Fonarow GC, Givertz MM, Hollenberg SM, Lindenfeld J, Masoudi FA, McBride PE, Peterson PN, Stevenson LW, Westlake C. 2017 ACC/AHA/HFSA Focused Update of the 2013 ACCF/AHA Guideline for the Management of Heart Failure: A Report of the American College of Cardiology/American Heart Association Task Force on Clinical Practice Guidelines and the Heart Failure Society of America. *Circulation.* 2017 Aug 8;136(6):e137-e161.

[8] McDonagh TA, Metra M, Adamo M, Gardner RS, Baumbach A, Böhm M, Burri H, Butler J, Čelutkienė J, Chioncel O, Cleland JGF, Coats AJS, Crespo-Leiro MG, Farmakis D, Gilard M, Heymans S, Hoes AW, Jaarsma T, Jankowska EA, Lainscak M, Lam CSP, Lyon AR, McMurray JJV, Mebazaa A, Mindham R, Muneretto C, Francesco Piepoli M, Price S, Rosano GMC, Ruschitzka F, Kathrine Skibelund A; ESC Scientific Document Group. 2021 ESC Guidelines for the diagnosis and treatment of acute and chronic heart failure. *Eur Heart J.* 2021 Sep 21;42(36):3599-3726.

[9] Yancy CW, Jessup M, Bozkurt B, Butler J, Casey DE Jr, Drazner MH, Fonarow GC, Geraci SA, Horwich T, Januzzi JL, Johnson MR, Kasper EK, Levy WC, Masoudi FA, McBride PE, McMurray JJ, Mitchell JE, Peterson PN, Riegel B, Sam F, Stevenson LW, Tang WH, Tsai EJ, Wilkoff BL; American College of Cardiology Foundation; American Heart Association Task Force on Practice Guidelines. 2013 ACCF/AHA guideline for the management of heart failure: a report of the American College of Cardiology Foundation/American Heart Association Task Force on Practice Guidelines. *J Am Coll Cardiol.* 2013 Oct 15;62(16):e147-239.

[10] Mehra MR, Canter CE, Hannan MM, Semigran MJ, Uber PA, Baran DA, Danziger-Isakov L, Kirklin JK, Kirk R, Kushwaha SS, Lund LH, Potena L, Ross HJ, Taylor DO, Verschuuren EAM, Zuckermann A; International Society for Heart Lung Transplantation (ISHLT) Infectious Diseases, Pediatric and Heart Failure and Transplantation Councils. The 2016 International Society for Heart Lung Transplantation listing criteria for heart transplantation: A 10-year update. *J Heart Lung Transplant.* 2016 Jan;35(1):1-23.

[11] Giordanino EF. Challenges in optimal bridge to transplantation strategy using short-term mechanical circulatory support devices. *Clin Transplant.* 2020 Oct;34(10):e14033.

[12] Giordanino EF, Absi DO, Favaloro LE, Renedo MF, Ratto RD, Rubira DM, Ameri A, Giunta G, Favaloro RR, Bertolotti AM. Short-term mechanical circulatory support devices as bridge to heart transplantation: A prospective single-center experience in Argentina. *Clin Transplant.* 2020 Jul;34(7):e13888.

[13] Al-Khatib SM, Stevenson WG, Ackerman MJ, Bryant WJ, Callans DJ, Curtis AB, Deal BJ, Dickfeld T, Field ME, Fonarow GC, Gillis AM, Granger CB, Hammill SC, Hlatky MA, Joglar JA, Kay GN, Matlock DD, Myerburg RJ, Page RL. 2017 AHA/ACC/HRS Guideline for Management of Patients With Ventricular Arrhythmias and the Prevention of Sudden Cardiac Death: A Report of the American College of Cardiology/American Heart Association Task Force on Clinical Practice Guidelines and the Heart Rhythm Society. *J Am Coll Cardiol.* 2018 Oct 2;72(14):e91-e220.

[14] Liu J, Yang BQ, Itoh A, Masood MF, Hartupee JC, Schilling JD. Impact of New UNOS Allocation Criteria on Heart Transplant Practices and Outcomes. *Transplant Direct.* 2020 Dec 15;7(1):e642.

[15] Alraies MC, Eckman P. Adult heart transplant: indications and outcomes. *J Thorac Dis.* 2014 Aug;6(8):1120-8.

[16] Kim MC, Kini A, Sharma SK. Refractory angina pectoris: mechanism and therapeutic options. *J Am Coll Cardiol.* 2002 Mar 20;39(6):923-34.

[17] Arena R, Myers J, Aslam SS, Varughese EB, Peberdy MA. Peak VO2 and VE/VCO2 slope in patients with heart failure: a prognostic comparison. *Am Heart J.* 2004 Feb;147(2):354-60.

[18] Stelken AM, Younis LT, Jennison SH, Miller DD, Miller LW, Shaw LJ, Kargl D, Chaitman BR. Prognostic value of cardiopulmonary exercise testing using percent achieved of predicted peak oxygen uptake for patients with ischemic and dilated cardiomyopathy. *J Am Coll Cardiol*. 1996 Feb;27(2):345-52.

[19] Osman AF, Mehra MR, Lavie CJ, Nunez E, Milani RV. The incremental prognostic importance of body fat adjusted peak oxygen consumption in chronic heart failure. *J Am Coll Cardiol.* 2000 Dec;36(7):2126-31.

[20] Maron MS, Kalsmith BM, Udelson JE, Li W, DeNofrio D. Survival after cardiac transplantation in patients with hypertrophic cardiomyopathy. *Circ Heart Fail*. 2010 Sep;3(5):574-9.

[21] Dey BR, Chung SS, Spitzer TR, Zheng H, Macgillivray TE, Seldin DC, McAfee S, Ballen K, Attar E, Wang T, Shin J, Newton-Cheh C, Moore S, Sanchorawala V, Skinner M, Madsen JC, Semigran MJ. Cardiac transplantation followed by dose-intensive melphalan and autologous stem-cell transplantation for light chain amyloidosis and heart failure. *Transplantation.* 2010 Oct 27;90(8):905-11.

[22] Raichlin E, Daly RC, Rosen CB, McGregor CG, Charlton MR, Frantz RP, Clavell AL, Rodeheffer RJ, Pereira NL, Kremers WK, Kushwaha SS, Edwards BS. Combined heart and liver transplantation: a single-center experience. *Transplantation.* 2009 Jul 27;88(2):219-25.

[23] Davies RR, Russo MJ, Mital S, Martens TM, Sorabella RS, Hong KN, Gelijns AC, Moskowitz AJ, Quaegebeur JM, Mosca RS, Chen JM. Predicting survival among high-risk pediatric cardiac transplant recipients: an analysis of the United Network for Organ Sharing database. *J Thorac Cardiovasc Surg*. 2008 Jan;135(1):147-55, 155.e1-2.

[24] Johnson MR, Aaronson KD, Canter CE, Kirklin JK, Mancini DM, Mehra MR, Radovancevic B, Taylor DO, Webber SA. Heart retransplantation. *Am J Transplant*. 2007 Sep;7(9):2075-81.

[25] Koval CE, Farr M, Krisl J, Haidar G, Pereira MR, Shrestha N, Malinis MF, Mueller NJ, Hannan MM, Grossi P, Huprikar S. Heart or lung transplant outcomes in HIV-infected recipients. *J Heart Lung Transplant.* 2019 Dec;38(12):1296-1305.

[26] Kim EY, Ko HH, Yoshida EM. A concise review of hepatitis C in heart and lung transplantation. *Can J Gastroenterol*. 2011 Aug;25(8):445-8.

[27] Russo MJ, Hong KN, Davies RR, Chen JM, Mancini DM, Oz MC, Rose EA, Gelijns A, Naka Y. The effect of body mass index on survival following heart transplantation: do outcomes support consensus guidelines? *Ann Surg*. 2010 Jan;251(1):144-52.

[28] Seese L, Hirji S, Sultan I, Gleason T, Kilic A. Frailty Screening Tool for Patients Undergoing Orthotopic Heart Transplant. *Ann Thorac Surg*. 2021 Feb;111(2):586-593.

[29] Ghio S, Crimi G, Temporelli PL, Traversi E, La Rovere MT, Cannito A, Vizza D, Scelsi L, Raineri C, Guazzi M, Oltrona Visconti L. Haemodynamic effects of an acute vasodilator challenge in heart failure patients with reduced ejection fraction and different forms of post-capillary pulmonary hypertension. *Eur J Heart Fail.* 2018 Apr;20(4):725-734.

[30] Radovancevic B, Poindexter S, Birovljev S, Velebit V, McAllister HA, Duncan JM, Vega D, Lonquist J, Burnett CM, Frazier OH. Risk factors for development of accelerated coronary artery disease in cardiac transplant recipients. *Eur J Cardiothorac Surg*. 1990;4(6):309-12; discussion 313.

Chapter 7

Psychosocial Evaluation in Heart Transplantation

Silvia Elsa Moscoloni and Liliana Martinez*
Heart Failure and Heart Transplantation,
Favaloro Foundation University Hospital, Buenos Aires, Argentina

Abstract

The heart transplant candidate must be evaluated in a comprehensive manner to minimize the possible complications related to this complex treatment. In this sense, the psychological and social evaluations are essential, and can even determine that a patient is not suitable to face a heart transplant. This chapter will address the main aspects of psychological evaluation, social evaluation and the joint approach of both.

Keywords: psychosocial intervention, psychosocial support systems, mental health services

Introduction

Addressing psychosocial problems within a medical structure is complex. We must first use the terms properly. Psychosocial is too broad and ambiguous. When we use it, do we talk about the psychological or the social? Although these concepts are related since a subject cannot be understood without its

* Corresponding Author's E-mail: aps@ffavaloro.org.

In: Heart Transplantation
Editor: Elian Facundo Giordanino
ISBN: 978-1-68507-759-4

environment, the theoretical approach and the look of each one of them is different.

The term tends to be generalized, which oversimplifies it and could even devalue its meaning. We must think of the psychological as the individual, the different in each one of us. We would assume that what was lived, what was inherited and what was learned constitute the personality structure of a subject and his or her behavior. If we refer to the social, we talk about the impact of the environment in a geographical, cultural and political conjunction.

Both the psychological and the social are related, but the response to different situations will be different according to the aforementioned variables. Thus, the form of behavior, the personality structure, the interpersonal relationships as well as the social environment, education, culture, economic support or the social network are not aspects that can be isolated in a health problem.

We get sick when something in our being breaks its biological balance. Our immune system, for instance, does not respond to this breakdown and thus the pathology appears. The emotional, the social, the human bonds can be related to the origin or the consequences of this rupture. We can affirm that a disturbing event in the life of a subject temporarily stops the course of their usual life. Excessive work or family stress that culminates in distress, grief, traumatic situations, relationship difficulties, economic shortages, and/or housing and structural poverty can all awaken a latent pathology or can negatively affect the course of a disease. For this reason, in the case of chronic diseases or even in those with a sudden onset, considering the psychological and social aspects is to understand the patient's problems as a whole. This understanding would lead us to a holistic approach to the subject and a more appropriate response to treatment.

We understand by psychosocial aspects the variables of a psychic, environmental, cultural, family, economic, relational, labor or educational nature that impact on a subject within a specific historical, geographical and political framework, always taking into account the difference of the psychological and the social. The need for a psychosocial approach is delimited by the multiple and varied requirements and changes in the lifestyle of both the patient and their family group within a transplant program.

It is unthinkable to ignore the causes and effects that psychological aspects and social conditioning produce in the development of a disease. In every process of becoming ill, the characteristics of the personality, the form of behavior, the personal history, the affective bonds and the social support play an essential role in the results of the proposed treatments.

Within the interdisciplinary approach, patients who are candidates for intrathoracic transplantation are evaluated by different medical professionals in order to optimize treatment as much as possible according to the results of the studies carried out during the evaluation for transplantation. In this context, psychological and social evaluations are added in order to provide a broader vision of the current conditions of the patient to face the complexity of the transplant treatment.

Our experience has shown us that a psychological evaluation isolated from the patient's social and cultural evaluation dichotomizes its performance and offers us a distorted perspective of the patient's situation. Furthermore, considering social factors in isolation, without including psychic dynamics, leads us to plan unviable actions to solve the patient's problem [1].

Psychology in its different approaches and epistemological currents integrates in its insight and approach the variables of a socio-economic and cultural nature that determine and condition the reality of the subject in the objective dimension of their behavior as well as in their subjective structure.

Social work tries to approach the patient from a subject's perspective, with a social history, and within micro and macro realities that influence and condition them.

It is important to recognize that the diagnostic value of the psychological and social evaluation provides data regarding the possible prognoses and clinical evolution of the patient. Transplantation as a therapy is a treatment that involves a complex reality of a disruptive nature for psychic dynamics, causing in some cases traumatic effects that the patient will process according to their psychic plasticity and their possibilities of functioning in a resilient way.

It is also important to understand the concept of trauma. Laplanche and Pontalis in their dictionary of psychoanalysis defines it as that event in life that is characterized by its intensity, by the inability of the subject to respond adequately to it, as well as by the lasting pathogenic effects that it causes in their psychic organization [2].

Medicine, to better understand the disease, depersonalizes it, separates it from man, from his social environment. It is not seen as the effect of a personal historical process in a single time and space with external conditions, but as an anonymous failure of a function or an organ. The disease is conceived as an intrusive factor. The insight of other non-medical professionals is at the service of recovering this human dimension of the subject's condition, hence the need to approach other specialties.

In Argentina, for example, and in accordance with the legal requirements imposed by transplant regulations, it is necessary to have a mental health professional, Psychologist or Psychiatrist, and a Social Worker as members of the team in order for such team to be considered suitable for a transplant program [3]. Furthermore, the Argentine Society of Transplantation has both a Social Work Advisory Commission and a Mental Health Advisory Commission, which allows interdisciplinary work within the field of transplantology. The same is true for other countries, for instance in the United States it is required by the Centers for Medicare and Medicaid Services [4].

Psychosocial Evaluation

The psychosocial evaluation arises from the need of professionals in the social and psychological area to resolve difficulties that patients presented to effectively carry out the necessary treatments to sustain the transplant situation.

The psychological impossibilities to improve the social situation and the social difficulties to carry out psychological treatment were common situations in professional practice, which made problem solving and professional intervention difficult. Practice indicated that there was a relationship between the two approaches, but it was necessary to substantiate it with statistical data.

In 2005, an analysis of 331 patients evaluated for intrathoracic transplantation was carried out at our center and the relationship between social and psychological diagnoses was assessed. This study showed that:

- Social factors influence psychic symptoms.
- The psychological variable seems more independent than the social ones, to the extent that serious mental illness is not necessarily accompanied by social problems.
- Severe social difficulties would be more linked to the psychic dynamics of individuals.
- Existence of dynamic interdependence between psychosocial variables.

This interdependence founded the need to work together to obtain better adaptive responses to the requirements of transplantation, developing the psychosocial approach in this group of patients in our Institution, without neglecting the specificity and methodology of each discipline.

From these observations a transdisciplinary approach was generated.

The work was organized in:

- Individual interviews of each discipline, with implementation of their own methodology and intervention techniques.
- Joint family interviews.
- Discussion of cases. Exchange of observations and joint planning of the follow-up form.
- Joint treatment and group approach.

Although diagnoses are by discipline, the construction of one implies the knowledge and evaluation of the other. The reports are, therefore, psychosocial and include:

- Result of individual psychological evaluation
- Result of the individual social evaluation
- Result of the joint family evaluation.
- Joint conclusion: follow-up form.

Psychological Evaluation

The psychological approach focuses on the different moments that the patient goes through.

Evaluation

The pre-transplant psychological evaluation is a diagnostic instrument that aims to provide the medical team with knowledge about the patient's personality, behavior, and difficulties in coping with problems. This helps predict behaviors after transplantation. Diagnostic interview is conducted on an outpatient basis prior to patient's hospitalization for clinical evaluation. In this semi-directed interview, an anamnesis of the patient's life history is made. The following information is gathered:

- Demographic data: age, education, occupation, marital status, social coverage, address and contact information.
- Household members' data. Number of people they live with and their relationship.
- Family data. Parents, brothers, husbands/wives, children.
- Psychological history. Consumption of psychotropic drugs. History of previous or current treatments. Type and rhythm of sleep.
- Addictions. Current or previous. Time since suspension.
- History of diseases and their treatments.
- History of previous surgeries.
- Family mental history.
- Triggers for the current illness.
- Level of knowledge of the possibility of transplantation.
- Level of knowledge of the significance of transplantation.
- Adherence to medical treatment.
- Degree of information about the requirements for transplantation.
- Description of their state of mind. Anguish, fears including fear of emotional separation.

In return, containment and general guidance on medical treatment is provided and a follow-up schedule is established for the time on the waiting list for transplantation. A report is made jointly with the Social Worker and the diagnoses are grouped into categories according to the aptitude of the patient to face the situation of transplantation. Categories are described in Table 1.

Pre-Transplant Follow-Up

It is carried out on an outpatient basis or during hospitalization in case the clinical situation of the patient justifies waiting for the organ while hospitalized. It is focused on psychoprophylaxis techniques, on the situation that the patient is going through and on the emotional conditions that derive from it. It also generates an environment of empathic relationship that favors the emotional expression of the patient.

Post-Transplant Follow-Up

Post-transplant follow-up is carried out during hospitalization and consists of accompanying the patient and the medical team in the adaptation of the patient to their transplant condition. Some of the most important points during this stage are:

- Reduce reactive symptoms to the situation (Anxiety, anguish, fears)
- Regularize the rhythm of sleep.
- Promote rehabilitation.
- Work on changes in their routines, medications, medical check-ups, endomyocardial biopsies, the possibility of rejection and family reintegration.
- Schedule post-discharge follow-up, if required.

Table 1. Categories of psychological evaluation

Psychological categories	
C1, Without Contraindication.	This category includes patients with good mental dynamics, without a psychiatric history, without addictions, with awareness of illness and good family support.
C2, Needs Follow-up.	Patients with symptoms of mental disturbance, relatively low awareness of the disease, history of difficulties in adherence or relatively low family support.
C2, High Psychological Risk.	Patients with the aforementioned difficulties plus a history of addictions, psychiatric symptoms under treatment or with difficulties in family and social support.
C3, Admission is not recommended.	Patients with active addictions, without awareness of the disease, difficulties in adherence, poor family support or psychosis.
C0.	Patients that cannot be evaluated due to its current clinical condition

Social Evaluation

The transplant teams are made up of different professionals whose object of study covers not only the physical dimension but also the psychic and social dimensions. Social evaluation is carried out within this interdisciplinary approach.

According to the World Health Organization, health is defined as a "state of complete physical, mental and social well-being and not merely the absence of disease" [5].

Quality of life, related to health, takes into account objective and subjective components for its definition. The objective components are those that can be quantified based on external criteria (physical, mental and social) and the subjective components are those that depend on the personal assessment that each subject makes of their physical, mental and social experience. Quality of life is temporary and transitory in nature and depends on the patient's previous state before a given treatment. The Social Worker aims to improve the quality of life of the patient and their role is inserted in an interdisciplinary work with the transplant team. This work implies a questioning of the criteria of causality, basically those of linear causality, and attempts against the possibility of fragmentation of the phenomena to be addressed. It also implies the recognition that disciplinary fields are not a 'reflection' of different real objects, but a historically determined construction of theoretical objects and methods [6].

Numerous studies show that those patients with social problems have greater difficulties in the post-transplant recovery, as well as greater mortality on the waiting list [7, 8].

The objective of this intervention is to know the social situation of the patient, analyze the social resources necessary to comply with the pharmacological and non-pharmacological treatment required by the transplant program and facilitate the mechanisms for accessing those treatments. It also acts as a link between a specific need and its corresponding resource and facilitates the necessary tools for an adequate evolution in an unfavorable social context.

The social requirements necessary for the adequate fulfillment of this program do not only include the satisfaction of basic needs, but also the analysis of other variables such as family and social support as well as the development of survival strategies which affect the patient, their family group and their quality of life. Knowing the social reality of the patient allows generating actions aimed at modifying those aspects that negatively affect their quality of life and can condition their evolution.

Social Evaluation Process

The social evaluation of candidates to intrathoracic transplantation is carried out prior to the initiation of the pre-transplant evaluation. It is done through individual, family and home interviews. The latter can be carried out by professionals of the transplant team or be requested from the local social service.

The aspects to be surveyed are:

- *Personal data*: Address, level of education, nationality, current occupation, work history, income.
- *Social security*: Access to social security programs or benefits.
- *Daily life*: daily activities.
- *Current disease and treatment*: Diagnosis, treatment, referral center, adherence, social difficulties.
- *Day of transplant procedure*: Transfer for surgery, accommodation near the center.
- *Family and social data*: household members, significant non-household members, type of family, identification of the main caregiver, social networks and special situations in family life.
- *Employment status*: Patient or family member in charge. Current status (medical license, retired).
- *Economic situation*: Income to meet basic needs. The income must be stable and sufficient to cover expenses related to the transplantation process (transfers, accommodation, food, pharmacological treatment)
- *Health insurance*: types, policies
- *Housing conditions*: location, accessibility, type of house, house utilities, number of rooms, animals.
- *Basic needs*: living place, food.

Once the social evaluation is finished a report is issued with its conclusion and the diagnostic category of the patient and their family. This is useful for using a common language among all members of the medical team. The report also incorporates the social review, which synthesizes the aspects that made the patient fit into a certain category. The diagnostic categories are described in Table 2.

Table 2. Categories of social evaluation

Social Categories
Suitable
Supportive family or social group
Patient or family member in charge with stable employment or with a reasonable social benefit
Enough income to meet basic needs
Proper house conditions and utilities
Relatively Suitable
Social problems with a possible solution. Arrangement of social assistance in the short or medium term (6 months)
Patients who lack one or more social requirements but with the possibility of accessing social assistance that allows them to overcome the situation
Social Risk
Patients could solve their problems, but the instability of the social context makes it difficult to find the solution in the medium term. They may become *Not Suitable* or *Relatively Suitable.*
They have no health-insurance access to some drugs and do not always have the money to buy them.
They are not able to eat the 4 daily meals at this time.
They have job instability or short-term employment contracts
They have severe housing and structural problems
They have financial difficulties for their transfer or residence near the transplant center
Not Suitable
Patients who lack two or more social requirements with important limitations to solve them, being the solution in the long-term
Temporary: They could have a solution in the long-term, as long as they commit to the task and are provided with the social resources
Final: The social assistance would not improve their situation, since their problem is structural (it depends on their history, context, lack of personal and family resources to face the situation)

It should be noted that these categories are dynamic, and the Social Worker helps patients in all the categories, including those in the "not suitable" category, according to their needs. The time required to solve the different problems is an estimate and depends on the response of the patient and their support group.

Pre-Transplant Follow-Up

Interventions at this stage aim to generate tools to improve the social situation of patients, focusing on those areas that have been detected as being at risk. These actions are multisectoral and include local and national resources.

These interventions are centered on:

- Accompaniment
- Support
- Information
- Orientation
- Management

The demand for this service is spontaneous, which guarantees patient access in the event of any difficulty arising.

Post-Transplant Follow-Up

Once transplantation has been performed, the duties of the Social Worker continue, focused on solving administrative problems and on social, labor, educational and family reintegration.

Psychosocial Group Interventions

Group intervention in patients awaiting transplantation contributes to the development of adequate survival strategies. These are understood as social processes that allow generating, selecting and combining paths for the satisfaction of needs and to face the difficulties and requirements of post-transplantation as well as its consequences in the clinical evolution [9].

In our experience, the main task was focused on providing information and guidance to both the patient and their family about heart transplantation and responding to the concomitant emotions related to the surgery and life after heart transplantation.

The objective of psychosocial group interventions is to provide patients on the waiting list with a space of containment, belonging and identification to sustain the wait, regardless of their family and cultural context.

Conclusion

Psychosocial evaluation in heart transplantation is of utmost importance. Although the psychological and social approaches have individual characteristics, the joint evaluation of both disciplines provides a better understanding of the patient's situation. Ultimately, this special strategy helps the patient and the heart transplant team achieve the best possible results for each situation.

References

[1] Favaloro R R, Perrone S V, Moscoloni S E, Gomez C B, Favaloro L E, Sultan M G, San Martino J. Value of pre-heart-transplant psychological evaluation: long-term follow-up. *Transplant. Proc*. 1999 Nov;31(7):3000-1.

[2] Laplanche J, Pontalis J B. *The Language of Psychoanalysis*. London: The Hogarth Press and the Institute of Psycho-Analysis, 1973, 465-468.

[3] INCUCAI. Resolutions 062/17, 063/17 and 065/17. [online]. 2021 [cited 2021-Dec-21]. Available from: https://www.argentina.gob.ar/sites/default/files/norm-panc-reso-incucai_063_17.pdf.

[4] Medicare Program; Hospital Conditions of Participation: Requirements for Approval and ReApproval of Transplant Centers To Perform Organ Transplants. Rules and Regulations. Federal Register 2007 March 30;72(61). [online]. 2021 [cited 2021-Dec-23]. Available from: https://www.cms.gov/Regulations-and-Guidance/Legislation/CFCsAndCoPs/Downloads/trancenterreg2007.pdf.

[5] Constitution of the World Health Organization. In: World Health Organization: Basic documents. 45th ed. Geneva: World Health Organization; 2005.

[6] Stolkiner A. La Interdisciplina: entre la epistemología y las prácticas [Interdiscipline: between epistemology and practices] [online]. 1999 [cited 2021-Dec-21]. Available from: http://www.campopsi.com.ar/lecturas/stolkiner.htm.

[7] Sirri L, Potena L, Masetti M, Tossani E, Magelli C, Grandi S. Psychological predictors of mortality in heart transplanted patients: a prospective, 6-year follow-up study. *Transplantation*. 2010 Apr 15;89(7):879-86.

[8] Dew M A, Roth L H, Thompson M E, Kormos R L, Griffith B P. Medical compliance and its predictors in the first year after heart transplantation. *J. Heart Lung Transplant.* 1996 Jun;15(6):631-45.

[9] Abbey S, Farrow S. Group therapy and organ transplantation. *Int. J. Group Psychother.* 1998 Apr;48(2):163-85.

Part II: Perioperative Management of Heart Transplantation

Chapter 8

Surgical Techniques for Heart Transplantation

Daniel Oscar Absi*
Heart Failure and Heart Transplantation, Favaloro Foundation University Hospital, Buenos Aires, Argentina

Abstract

The first successful human heart implant was performed on December 3, 1967, by Dr. Christiaan Barnard in Cape Town, South Africa. Since then, many have changed in the heart transplant field, but the surgical details of successful heart transplant remained similar over the years. Patients with congenital heart diseases, as well as those bridged to transplant with ventricular assist devices, pose unique surgical and management challenges. This chapter outlines an approach to the most relevant issues related to heart transplant from the surgical perspective.

Keywords: heart transplantation, cardiac surgical procedures, tissue and organ harvesting

Introduction

Lower and Shumway described in 1960 the key technical aspects for the success of orthotopic heart transplantation [1]. Since its clinical inception in the early sixties, heart transplantation has benefited thousands of patients with heart failure worldwide and represents one of the seminal accomplishments for the field of cardiac surgery. Changes in the field of heart transplantation

---

* Corresponding Author's E-mail: dabsi@ffavaloro.org.

In: Heart Transplantation
Editor: Elian Facundo Giordanino
ISBN: 978-1-68507-759-4

have been many in the past forty years, including improved rejection monitoring and immunosuppression therapies, biventricular pacing, as well as major advances in the application of mechanical support devices as a bridge to transplant or candidacy in patients with end stage heart failure. Despite these many changes and others, the surgical details of successful heart transplantation have changed little over this period. In this chapter we review in detail donor selection, organ procurement and preservation, and implantation techniques.

Organ Procurement

Meticulous preoperative management of the donor is critical for successful organ recovery and post-implant function. Poor preservation at the time of procurement can lead to early graft dysfunction, or more critically, graft failure. Dissection between the organs being procured has to be very precise and the lack of understanding of this aspect of the operation can adversely impact implantation.

When performing organ procurement, there is a critical list of confirmations and verifications that must be carried out. First, the donor must be properly identified. Second, the ABO compatibility of the donor and recipient must be documented. Finally, health information must be carefully reviewed to ensure that previously unreported health issues do not arise [2, 3].

All potential donors are evaluated with chest X-ray, electrocardiogram, standard laboratory tests and more specific tests such as toxicological screening and viral serology. Concomitantly, the clinical status of the donor must be assessed, including current interventions and changes since the accepting team last reviewed the clinical data. Pharmacological as well as fluid management should be decided together with the local providers to maintain stability and avoid potential complications. For example, brain death may be associated with endocrinological derangements in the hypothalamic pituitary axis such as diabetes insipidus and require treatment with intravenous fluid and vasopressin infusion. In fact, hormonal analogues are being increasingly used to treat autologous secretion deficit and have been shown to decrease vasopressor requirement and improve hemodynamic stability in potential organ donors [4-6].

Nowadays, many recipients have had previous surgeries and more time is required for the implanting surgeon to provide adequate exposure for the implant. Adequate communication between all procurement teams can minimize donor organ ischemic time and lower the risk of a donor becoming unstable. Echocardiogram and coronary angiogram should also be reviewed carefully. Coronary angiogram is not routinely performed, unless the donor is over 40 years old, has strong risk-factors for coronary artery disease, or abnormalities on the echocardiogram.

It should be taken into account that harvest of lungs for transplantation usually occurs at the same time that heart retrieval. Therefore, there are certain technical modifications to ensure that all recipients receive adequate tissue to allow for successful transplantation in these cases [2].

Thoracic Organs Harvesting

The donor is positioned supine with tucked arms and is prepped with chlorhexidine or iodine and sterile drapes are placed. Subsequently, median sternotomy is performed in continuity with the abdominal midline incision for abdominal organs harvesting. The pleural reflections are fully along bilaterally and the pericardium is opened vertically from the diaphragm to the aorta. Additionally, both lungs are checked searching for unsuspected lesions. The heart is also inspected for chamber distension, coronary calcification, myocardial contusions and ventricular function [4].

Although there are different surgical techniques for thoracic organ harvesting, there are some universal principles. Systemic and pulmonary venous return should be occluded or vented; cardioplegia solution should be used properly to ensure effective cardiac arrest; and every effort should be made to avoid injuring any structure used in the implant [7]. Only minimal dissection is recommended until cardiopulmonary perfusion and preservation occurs in order to avoid hemodynamic instability secondary to the manipulation of the heart and related vascular structures. Subsequently, the aorta is carefully mobilized from the main pulmonary artery and the anterior aspect of the aorta, the arch, and the great vessels are exposed. The innominate vein is mobilized from the arch, allowing exposure of the great vessels [3].

In case of harvesting lungs and heart, the anatomy should be well defined beforehand. As the heart is moved to the left and the right pulmonary veins are exposed, Waterston's groove (the interface of the left and right atria) is fully opened to properly define the interface of the left atria and right pulmonary veins.

Once all the different organs harvestings have been performed, the preparations for cannulation and organ procurement start A purse-string suture is placed into the anterior ascending aorta and in the main pulmonary artery. The donor is heparinized and perfusion cannula are placed into the aorta and pulmonary artery. All central lines should be pulled back so that they are above the azygous vein. Subsequently, the inferior vena cava is divided on its anterior wall and the inferior left pulmonary vein is divided in case that lung procurement is not performed, otherwise the left atrial appendage is amputated. The aorta is then cross clamped at its distal ascending portion and cardioplegic solution is infused. It is important to measure the aortic root pressure and be sure that adequate delivery of the preservation solution at a consistent pressure of 60-80 mmHg is being performed [4, 8].

There are three key components to myocardial preservation: First, adequate and aggressive ventricular degravitation. This is a very important step to reduce myocardial oxygen consumption and ensure a more homogeneous distribution of the preservation solution. Second, rapidly achieve electromechanical activity cessation. Finally, control organ hypothermia and maintain it between 8 and 10 degrees Celsius. Additionally, the infusion is complemented with topical cold saline or slush, not ice.

Cardiectomy is performed after the infusion of the preservation solution has been completed. Of note, if the lungs and heart are harvested, delivery of lung preservation solution into the coronaries should be avoided by sectioning the aorta immediately after completion of cardioplegia administration and performing a large incision in the left atrial appendage or opening the interatrial groove in order to aspirate the return from the pulmonary veins. Afterwards, the superior vena cava is widely opened together with the azygous vein and complete section of the inferior vena cava is performed. All head vessels are divided from the aortic arch and the descending aorta is divided at the level of the ligamentum arteriosum, which exposes the pulmonary artery. The latter is opened at the level of the perfusion cannula leaving the orifice of the left and right pulmonary arteries intact in case lung procurement is also done, or dividing both branches in case it is not. Subsequently, the heart is lifted exposing the inferior left atrium and the pulmonary veins are transected at the pericardial reflection. A cuff of left atrium is created by connecting incisions in the transected pulmonary veins. If lungs are also harvested, the heart is moved to the left and the dissection in the Waterston's groove is exposed. The left atrium is then divided at a point equal between the right pulmonary veins and the fused margin of the left and right atria, leaving sewing tissue for both organs. Afterwards, the heart is lifted to the right and the procedure is repeated with an incision to the right and left atrium/pulmonary vein junction and extended to the base of the left atrial appendage. The heart valves are then examined carefully, as well as other anatomic findings, and the organ is placed in preservation solution for transportation (Figure 1) [4, 9].

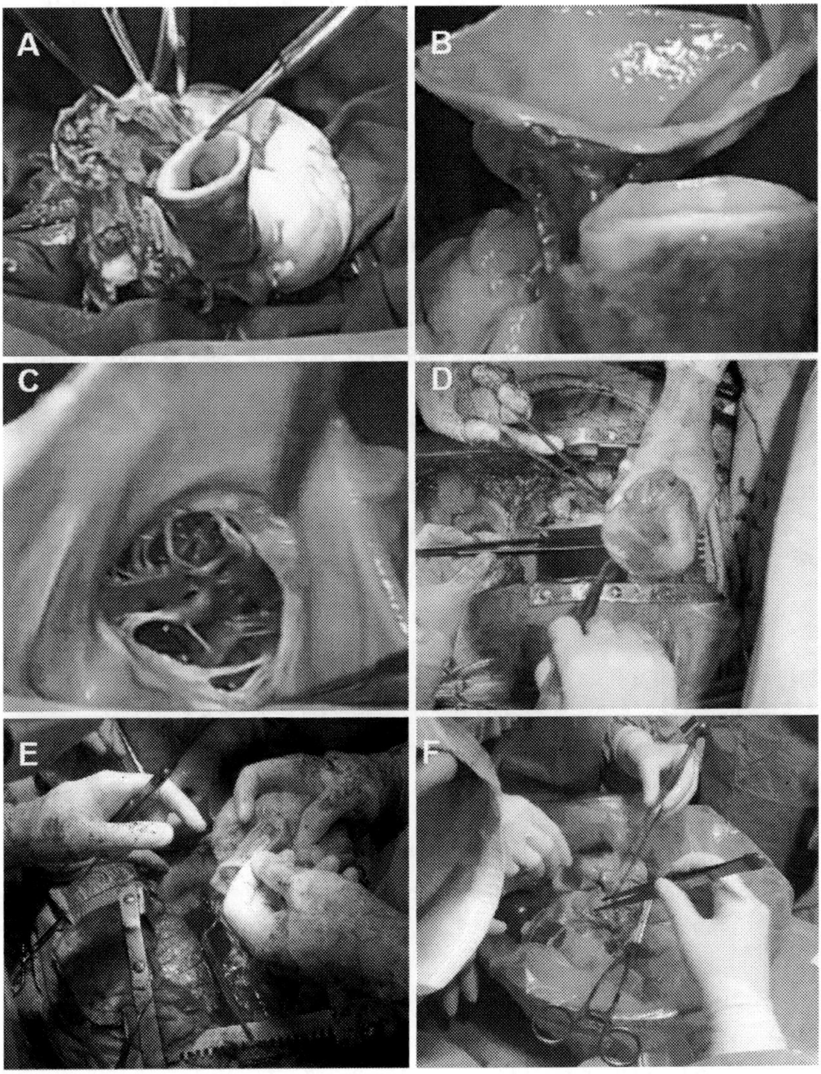

Figure 1. Graft examination. A. and B. Heart and great vessels. C. Valve examination. D. and E. Coronary arteries examination. F. Preparation for transportation.

Ischemic times are of great importance when procuring a heart, for instance, younger donors allow for longer ischemic times [10, 11]. A possible strategy is using ex vivo normothermic machine perfusion, organ care system (OCS), instead of hypothermic static storage, which constitutes a shift of paradigm in organ preservation. With OCS, the coronary arteries of a beating heart are continuously perfused with oxygenated, nutrient-rich blood. Its feasibility was demonstrated in the PROCEED II, a prospective, open-label, multicenter, randomized trial that showed non-inferiority of the OCS compared with cold static storage in terms of graft dysfunction and recipient mortality [12]. Afterwards, the OCS Heart EXPAND Trial was published and evaluated the effectiveness of this system to resuscitate, preserve and assess donor hearts that did not meet current standard donor heart criteria for transplantation, in order to improve donor heart utilization. It demonstrated that graft recovery and assessment, as well as more long-distance donor procurement with a reduced total ischemic time, were possible [13]. After this trial, utilization of extended criteria donors´ hearts improved with good short-term post-transplant outcomes and, importantly, a low rate of primary graft dysfunction. However, the main disadvantages of the OCS are a complex and time-consuming procedure and the cost when compared with standard cold static storage preservation [14].

Orthotopic Heart Transplantation

Timing and organization are of paramount importance, especially to limit ischemic time. The following factors should be considered in order to achieve the best possible coordination of donor and recipient operations [15]:

- Time needed by other procurement teams before cross-clamping the donor heart
- Time of transportation
- Surgical preparation times: monitoring lines and catheters, anesthesia induction, among others
- Time for explantation
- Time for recipient's surgery: patients with previous sternotomies or mechanical circulatory support may require more time

Recipient Operation Setup

Right pulmonary artery catheterization with a Swan-Ganz catheter is important for proper patient management in the perioperative stage and allows adequate identification of those who will benefit from pulmonary vasodilator therapy such as nitric oxide. Furthermore, in those patients with previous sternotomy, the groin should be prepped for rapid cannulation of the femoral vessels in case of heart injury during reentry. After the initial preparations, a full standard median sternotomy is performed approximately 2 hours before the estimated time of organ arrival. Cannulation for cardiopulmonary bypass is performed in the ascending aorta, superior vena cava or right atrium and inferior vena cava through the right atrium. Hypothermia should be moderate, 28 to 30° Celsius, and the aorta cross-clamped proximal to the aortic cannula [7, 15].

There are currently two main techniques for heart transplantation. The first one is the biatrial technique, described by Lower and Shumway, and the second one is the bicaval technique, described by Sievers and Sarsam [1, 16, 17]. The bicaval technique is the most widely used in the modern era, but the biatrial technique is useful in certain circumstances, for example, when dissection of the vena cava is hazardous, such as in re-do operations with dense adhesions. Both techniques are safe and effective in patients with end stage heart failure.

Recipient Preparation for Biatrial Heart Transplantation

An incision in the right atrial appendage is made from the inferior vena cava cannula toward the aorta root, and the left atrium is accessed via the fossa ovalis. Subsequently, the great vessels are sectioned above the valvular plane and the interatrial septum at the level of the coronary sinus. The heart is removed together with the atrial appendage, creating the cuffs of left and right atrium, aorta, and pulmonary artery (Figure 2). At this point, meticulous hemostasis should be performed on the posterior pericardial region and the margins of the left atrial cuff, as these areas will be difficult to see after implantation [3, 15].

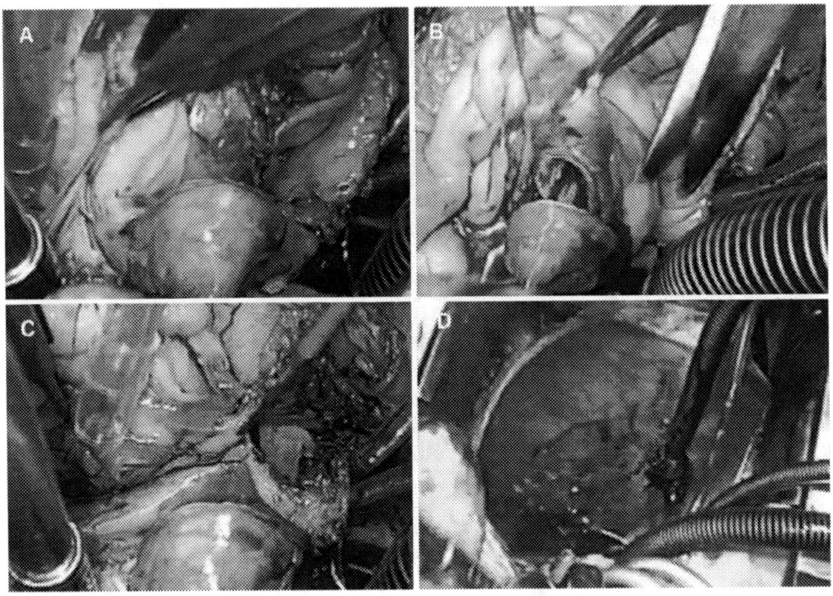

Figure 2. Explant. A. Sectioning of the pulmonary artery. B. Sectioning of the aorta. C. Left atrium D. Heart removed from the thoracic cavity.

Implantation of the Donor Heart in the Biatrial Technique

The four pulmonary veins are connected through incisions, trimming off excess tissue, creating the left atrial cuff. The donor and recipient left atria are anastomosed beginning at the level of the left atrial appendage. Next, the donor's right atrium is sectioned from the inferior vena cava and towards the atrial appendage trying to match the size of the cuff of the recipient's right atrium, and donor and recipient right atria anastomosis is performed beginning at the midpoint of the interatrial septum. The donor's superior vena cava is then oversewn.

Subsequently, the aorta and the pulmonary artery of donor and recipient are anastomosed. It is important to try to leave the aorta sufficiently long, to allow mobilization and inspection of the surrounding structures, and the pulmonary artery short, to avoid kinking with right ventricular contraction. This also allows for the anastomosis of aortas of different sizes between donor and the recipient. In addition, a bolus of corticosteroids should be infused at this time, before releasing the aortic clamp, to induce immunosuppression. Finally, deairing of the cavities must be performed with an air vent in the ascending aorta. While the heart is reperfusing, pulmonary arteries of donor and recipient are anastomosed beginning in the midportion of the posterior wall [3, 15].

Recipient Preparation for Bicaval Heart Transplantation

After cardiopulmonary bypass, the great vessels are separated as previously mentioned. The main difference with this technique is that the entire right atrium is removed by dividing the superior vena cava at the level of the cavo-atrial junction and the inferior vena cava above its junction with the right atrium. The left atrium is excised, leaving a cuff of posterior left atrial tissue containing the four pulmonary veins [15].

Implantation of the Donor Heart in the Bicaval Technique

Donor's superior vena cava is divided at the level of the azygous vein. The sequence for the anastomosis in this technique is: left atrial, then superior and inferior vena cava, and finally the great vessels. In order to do so, the remaining recipient's left atrial cuff is anastomosed to the donor left atrium beginning at the level of the left superior pulmonary vein. The heart is then lowered into the pericardial space. An everting suture can be used to anastomose the donor and recipient left atria to prevent thrombus formation, and a left ventricular vent can be used to deareate. Subsequently, the inferior vena cava is anastomosed, taking care not to injure the ostium of the coronary sinus; superior vena cava is also anastomosed, paying attention not to create a tight union at the level of the anastomosis. Finally, pulmonary artery and aortic anastomosis are performed (Figure 3) [15].

Final Steps

Once the heart is adequately decompressed on cardiopulmonary bypass, careful hemostasis should be performed and deaeration techniques implemented. The latter include aspiration of the left atrium with a needle, mobilization of the heart on mechanical ventilation, and decreasing pump flow to allow ejection of the heart.

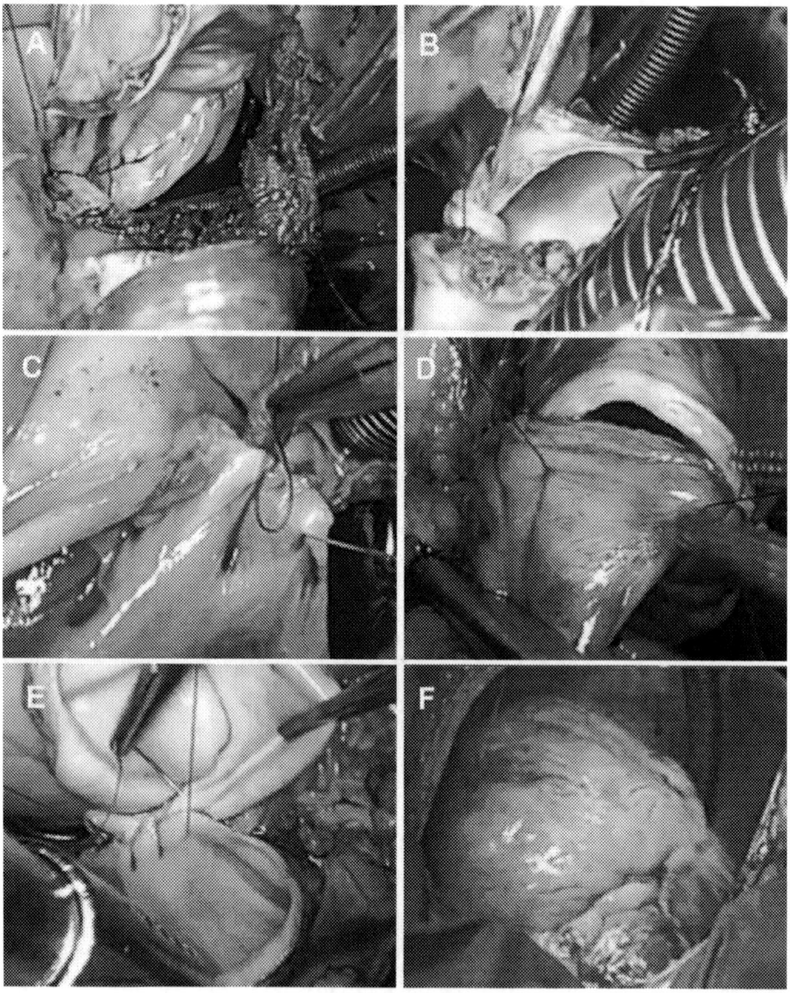

Figure 3. Implantation of the heart in the bicaval technique. A. Left atrial anastomosis B. and C. Superior and inferior vena cava anastomosis D. and E. Great vessels anastomosis. F. Implanted heart.

Inotropic support is initiated and normothermia and reperfusion are achieved, allowing weaning from cardiopulmonary bypass. Temporary pacemaker wires are also placed in the right atrium and right ventricle to ensure proper perioperative management [3]. Intraoperative transesophageal echocardiography is important to confirm cardiac function and valve competence. Because the recipient's pericardium is often dilated due to underlying disease, it is generally recommended to drain the pericardium with both a posterior and an anterior drainage tube to decrease the risk of developing postoperative pericardial effusions due to size mismatch between the donor heart and the relatively large pericardial space. In some cases, the pericardium can be loosely closed over the right ventricle with two or three interrupted sutures [15].

The bicaval technique preserves normal atrial morphology, sinus node function, and valve function. As a result, it has been consistently associated with a lower incidence of atrial arrhythmias and the need for pacemaker implantation. However, possible disadvantages include longer ischemia time and the possibility of narrowing the caval anastomosis [7, 18, 19].

Heart Transplantation in Patients with Left Ventricular Assist Devices

More and more patients are being bridged to heart transplantation with left ventricular assist devices, which constitutes a more complex scenario at the time of transplantation [20-22]. One of the main problems is bleeding, since these patients are anticoagulated and have had previous sternotomies. Intravenous vitamin K and fresh frozen plasma should be given to partially reverse the anticoagulation before the surgical procedure. However, despite these measures and careful hemostasis, it is sometimes necessary to leave to chest open and packed and delay closure 24 to 48 hours. Some strategies when implanting these devices might facilitate their explants at the time of transplantation. Outflow graft anastomosis should be performed on the lateral wall of the aorta to leave room for aortic cannulation and anastomosis when performing transplantation. Additionally, it should be directed to the right atrium in order to avoid its damage when performing the sternotomy. In some centers, barriers such as expanded polytetrafluoroethylene mesh or Cormatrix are increasingly being used to prevent injury during resternotomy. Peripheral cannulation for cardiopulmonary bypass before sternotomy is another safety measure. When initiating cardiopulmonary bypass, pump speed should be decreases in order to avoid cavitation in the left ventricle. The pump is turned off after it has been completely mobilized while on cardiopulmonary bypass and the outflow graft is clamped and sectioned near its insertion in the aorta. After removing the inflow cannula from the apex, a left ventricular vent can be placed through the remaining hole. The power cord is trimmed and the device is removed from the surgical field [23, 24].

Heterotopic Heart Transplantation

In 1974, Dr. Christiaan Barnard first used heterotopic heart transplantation in humans, using a donor heart in parallel with the native heart. Heterotopic heart transplantation is currently rarely used, but in a left assist configuration could expand the donor pool and also enable transplantation in highly selected groups of patients who are currently ineligible for a heart transplant or have left ventricular assist device therapy contraindications. Some of its current indications include recipient's irreversible high pulmonary vascular resistance and severe cases of donor-recipient size mismatch. Additionally, preservation of the native heart constitutes a safety measure in case of graft dysfunction [7, 25-28].

Technical Considerations and Organ Harvesting

There are some modifications to the heart harvesting technique when considering a heterotopic heart transplantation. A longer segment of the ascending aorta must be taken in order to perform the anastomosis in the recipient's heart. Similarly, a longer section of the superior vena cava up to the level of the innominate vein is also needed, as it will then be used as a pathway for endomyocardial biopsies. After cardioplegia infusion through the aortic line, the inferior vena cava and the junction of the left pulmonary vein with the left atrium are transected. In case there is also lung procurement, the incision is performed in the left atrial appendage. After heart decompression, the aorta is cross-clamped and the rest of the cardioplegic solution is infused. It is important to avoid a small donor left atrium size that could be an obstruction in the flow path to the left ventricle [25].

Heterotopic Heart Implantation

After median sternotomy, the recipient's pericardium is incised longitudinally, as usual, and three transverse incisions are added: one near the diaphragm, another at the level of the right pulmonary artery, on the right side, and the last one halfway in between. This prevents constriction of the graft by the pericardium, allowing it to be placed comfortably on the right chest. Afterwards, cannulation of the superior and inferior vena cava, as well as the aorta is performed for cardiopulmonary bypass together with moderate hypothermia. A cross-clamp is placed on the aorta and implantation begins. The donor's left atriotomy is anastomosed to a large incision of the recipient's left atrium, at the level of the Waterson's groove. Pericardial constrictions should be avoided at this point. Subsequently, the distal end of the donor aorta is anastomosed to the lateral portion of the recipient aorta and the aortic cross-clamp is removed [25, 29].

In the left ventricular assist configuration, the distal end of the donor's main pulmonary artery is anastomosed to the recipient's right atrium. This only serves to decompress the donor right side of coronary venous return. In the biventricular assist configuration, the distal end of the donor pulmonary artery is anastomosed to the recipient pulmonary artery using a graft to avoid tension in the anastomosis, and the donor's right atrium is anastomosed to recipient's right atrium.

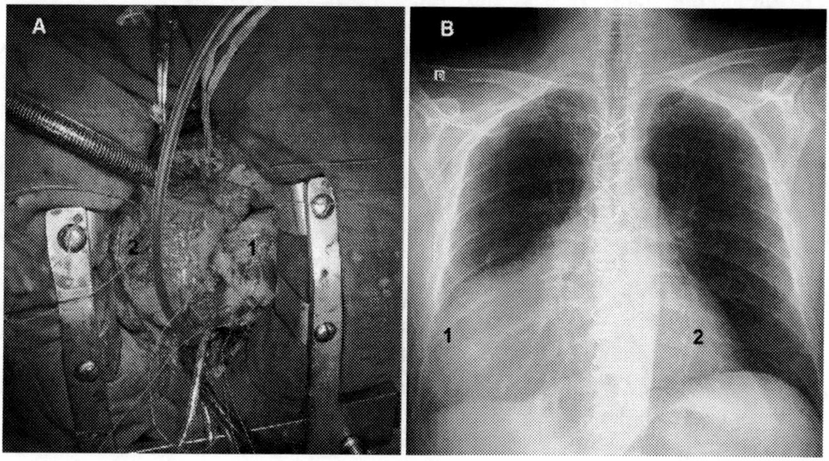

Figure 4. Heterotopic heart transplantation. A. Implant completion (view from patient's head). B. Chest radiography. 1. Heterotopic graft 2. Native heart.

Finally, in the left ventricular assist configuration, an end-to-side anastomosis between the donor's superior vena cava and the recipient's superior vena cava is performed, mainly to establish a conduit for future endomyocardial biopsies, with four metallic clips placed around it as markers to be used under fluoroscopy [30]. Deairing in Trendelemburg's position, rewarming and inotropic support are performed similarly to orthotopic heart transplantation, and the patient is weaned from cardiopulmonary bypass. It is important to assess all the anastomoses, avoid pericardial constrictions, evaluate left ventricular function of the donor's heart and right ventricular function of the recipient's heart and the effect of the graft on the right lung (Figure 4).

Conclusion

There have been great advances in recent years in the field of heart transplantation, however, the fundamental principles of this technique remain similar. Different scenarios require different strategies to overcome any potential complications, and proper knowledge of these situations can prevent serious complications. Adequate harvesting of the donor's heart, thorough preparation of the recipient, and careful execution of the procedure are key to ensuring satisfactory outcomes from this amazing technique.

References

[1] Lower R R. Shumway N E. Studies on orthotopic homotransplantation of the canine heart. *Surg. Forum*. 1960;11:18-9.

[2] Bolman III R M, Molina J E, Anderson R W. Heart transplantation, In Simmons R L, Finch ME. Ascher NL, Hernriksen A J, Najarian J S. Manual of Vascular. *Organ Donation, and Transplantation*. New York, Springer-Verlag, 1984, 105-143; 209-231.

[3] Bolman R M 3rd. Cardiac transplantation: the operative technique. *Cardiovasc. Clin.* 1990;20(2):133-45.

[4] Camp P C Jr. Heart Transplantation: Donor Operation for Heart and Lung Transplantation. *Oper. Tech. Thorac. Cardiovasc. Surg.* 2010 Jun 1;15(2):125-137.

[5] Salim A, Vassiliu P, Velmahos G C, Sava J, Murray J A, Belzberg H, Asensio J A, Demetriades D. The role of thyroid hormone administration in potential organ donors. *Arch. Surg.* 2001 Dec;136(12):1377-80.

[6] Nicolas-Robin A, Amour J, Ibanez-Esteve C, Coriat P, Riou B, Langeron O. Effect of glucose-insulin-potassium in severe acute heart failure after brain death. *Crit. Care Med.* 2008 Oct;36(10):2740-5.

[7] Esmailian F, Perry P, Kobashigawa J. Donor Organ Preservation and Surgical Considerations in Heart Transplantation, In Kobashigawa J. *Clinical Guide to Heart Transplantation. Cham.*, Springer, 2017, 73-80.

[8] Baumgartner W A. Operative techniques in heart transplantation, In Baumgartner W A. *Heart and Heart-Lung Transplantation*. Philadelphia, Saunders, 1990, 113-133.

[9] Shumway S J. Operative techniques in thoracic organ procurement, In Shumway S J, Shumway N E. *Thoracic Transplantation.* Cambridge, Blackwell Science, Inc, 1995, 187-192.

[10] Lund L H, Edwards L B, Kucheryavaya A Y, Dipchand A I, Benden C, Christie J D, Dobbels F, Kirk R, Rahmel A O, Yusen R D, Stehlik J; International Society for Heart and Lung Transplantation. The Registry of the International Society for Heart and Lung Transplantation: Thirtieth Official Adult Heart Transplant Report--2013; focus theme: age. *J. Heart Lung Transplant.* 2013 Oct;32(10):951-64.

[11] Russo M J, Chen J M, Sorabella R A, Martens T P, Garrido M, Davies R R, George I, Cheema F H, Mosca R S, Mital S, Ascheim D D, Argenziano M, Stewart A S, Oz MC, Naka Y. The effect of ischemic time on survival after heart transplantation varies by donor age: an analysis of the United Network for Organ Sharing database. *J. Thorac. Cardiovas.c Surg.* 2007 Feb;133(2):554-9.

[12] Ardehali A, Esmailian F, Deng M, Soltesz E, Hsich E, Naka Y, Mancini D, Camacho M, Zucker M, Leprince P, Padera R, Kobashigawa J; PROCEED II trial investigators. Ex-vivo perfusion of donor hearts for human heart transplantation (PROCEED II): a prospective, open-label, multicentre, randomised non-inferiority trial. *Lancet.* 2015 Jun 27;385(9987):2577-84.

[13] Schroder J N, D'Alessandro D, Esmailian F, Boeve T, Tang P, Liao K, Wang I, Anyanwu A, Shah A, Mudy K, Soltesz E, Smith J W. Successful Utilization of Extended Criteria Donor (ECD) Hearts for Transplantation - Results of the OCS™ Heart EXPAND Trial to Evaluate the Effectiveness and Safety of the OCS Heart System to Preserve and Assess ECD Hearts for Transplantation [abstract]. *J. Heart Lung Transplant.* 2019;38(4):S42.

[14] John R. Donor management and selection for heart transplantation. *Semin. Thorac. Cardiovasc. Surg.* 2004 Winter;16(4):364-9.

[15] John R, Liao K. Orthotopic heart transplantation. *Oper. Tech. Thorac. Cardiovasc. Surg. 2010* Jun 1;15(2):138-146.

[16] Sievers H H, Weyand M, Kraatz EG, Bernhard A. An alternative technique for orthotopic cardiac transplantation, with preservation of the normal anatomy of the right atrium. *Thorac. Cardiovasc. Surg.* 1991 Apr;39(2):70-2.

[17] Sarsam M A, Campbell C S, Yonan N A, Deiraniya A K, Rahman A N. An alternative surgical technique in orthotopic cardiac transplantation. *J. Card. Surg.* 1993 May;8(3):344-9.

[18] John R, Kamdar F, Liao K, Colvin-Adams M, Boyle A, Joyce L. Improved survival and decreasing incidence of adverse events with the HeartMate II left ventricular assist device as bridge-to-transplant therapy. *Ann. Thorac. Surg.* 2008 Oct;86(4): 1227-34; discussion 1234-5.

[19] Aziz T, Burgess M, Khafagy R, Wynn Hann A, Campbell C, Rahman A, Deiraniya A, Yonan N. Bicaval and standard techniques in orthotopic heart transplantation:

medium-term experience in cardiac performance and survival. *J. Thorac. Cardiovasc. Surg.* 1999 Jul;118(1):115-22.

[20] Davies R R, Russo M J, Morgan J A, Sorabella R A, Naka Y, Chen J M. Standard versus bicaval techniques for orthotopic heart transplantation: an analysis of the United Network for Organ Sharing database. *J. Thorac. Cardiovasc. Surg.* 2010 Sep;140(3):700-8, 708.e1-2.

[21] John R, Pagani F D, Naka Y, Boyle A, Conte J V, Russell S D, Klodell C T, Milano C A, Rogers J, Farrar D J, Frazier O H. Post-cardiac transplant survival after support with a continuous-flow left ventricular assist device: impact of duration of left ventricular assist device support and other variables. *J. Thorac. Cardiovasc. Surg.* 2010 Jul;140(1):174-81.

[22] Kamdar F, John R, Eckman P, Colvin-Adams M, Shumway S J, Liao K. Postcardiac transplant survival in the current era in patients receiving continuous-flow left ventricular assist devices. *J. Thorac. Cardiovasc. Surg.* 2013 Feb;145(2):575-81.

[23] Southerland K W, Milano C A. Heart Transplantation After Left Ventricular Assist Device. *Oper. Tech. Thorac. Cardiovasc. Surg.* 2014 Mar 1;19(1):47-63.

[24] Ihnken K A, Ramzy D, Esmailian F, Trento A, Arabía FA. Surgical Technique to Facilitate Explantation of Mechanical Circulatory Support Devices: LVADs, BiVADs, and TAHs Before Heart Transplantation. *ASAIO J.* 2016 Mar-Apr; 62(2):211-3.

[25] Copeland J, Copeland H. Heterotopic Heart Transplantation: Technical Considerations. *Oper. Tech. Thorac. Cardiovasc. Surg.* 2016;21(3):269-280.

[26] Kadner A, Chen R H, Adams D H. Heterotopic heart transplantation: experimental development and clinical experience. *Eur. J. Cardiothorac. Surg.* 2000 Apr;17(4): 474-81.

[27] Reichenspurner H, Hildebrandt A, Boehm D, Kaulbach H G, Willems S, Odell J A, Horak A, Reichart B. Heterotopic heart transplantation in 1988--recent selective indications and outcome. *J. Heart Transplant.* 1989 Sep-Oct;8(5):381-6.

[28] Mehra M R, Kobashigawa J, Starling R, Russell S, Uber PA, Parameshwar J, Mohacsi P, Augustine S, Aaronson K, Barr M. Listing criteria for heart transplantation: International Society for Heart and Lung Transplantation guidelines for the care of cardiac transplant candidates--2006. *J. Heart Lung Transplant.* 2006 Sep;25(9):1024-42.

[29] Copeland H, Kalra N, Gustafson M, Coehlo-Anderson R, Friedman M, Copeland JG. A case of heterotopic heart transplant as a "biologic left ventricular assist" in restrictive cardiomyopathy. World J. Pediatr. Congenit. Heart Surg. 2011 Oct 1;2(4):637-40.

[30] Arzouman D A, Arabia F A, Sethi G K, Copeland J G. Endomyocardial biopsy in the heterotopic heart transplant patient. *Ann. Thorac. Surg.* 1998 Mar;65(3):857-8.

Chapter 9

Graft Dysfunction and Postoperative Management of Heart Transplantation

María Florencia Renedo*

Heart Failure and Heart Transplantation, Favaloro Foundation University Hospital, Buenos Aires, Argentina

Abstract

Postoperative care of the heart transplant recipient is complex and requires specialized physicians, nurses and providers at transplant centers in order to achieve successful outcomes. Although management of the postoperative phase has improved in the last years, these patients continue to experience significant morbidity and a mortality, primarily related to early failure of the allograft.

The aim of this chapter is to describe the main complications after heart transplantation with a special focus on graft failure.

Keywords: heart transplantation, postoperative care, primary graft dysfunction

Introduction

Despite advances in pharmacological and non-pharmacological therapies for heart failure (HF), morbidity and mortality remain high, and patients often progress to end-stage HF. During the last decades, heart transplantation (HTx)

---

* Corresponding Author's E-mail: mfrenedo@ffavaloro.org.

In: Heart Transplantation
Editor: Elian Facundo Giordanino
ISBN: 978-1-68507-759-4

has been considered a standard therapy for selected patients with advanced HF. However, although HTx has become the treatment of choice for end-stage heart failure, challenges remain to improve short- and long-term outcomes. In the current era, 1-year survival after HTx is almost 90% and it has a conditional half-life of approximately 13 years. Although there is an increase in the number of patients with advanced HF, the number of organ donors remains a constant and limiting factor. Heart transplant candidates in the current era are also more complex. They are older, are on mechanical circulatory support and with human leukocyte antigens (HLA) antibody sensitization. Due to all of these issues, these patients are at increased risk for several complications that may impair their outcomes, including graft dysfunction and rejection. Advances in the management of these potential complications can improve quality of life and survival for this high-risk population [1-3].

This chapter will provide a practical review of the perioperative care of HTx patients and an update of the main considerations for the management of the most relevant post-transplant complications, including primary graft dysfunction (PGD). Graft rejection and infections are discussed in Chapters 11 and 13.

Postoperative Management

Heart transplantation survival rates have increased and complication rates have decreased due to better immunosuppressive agents, improvement in organ procurement and surgical technique, and overall increase in experience with perioperative management of HTx. However, although the survival of HTx recipients is steadily improving, patients continue to experience significant post-transplantation morbidity and mortality. The collaboration of primary care physicians, intensive cardiovascular care physicians and all the related specialties is very important to optimize the postoperative management of HTx recipients [3, 4].

After completion of HTx, the recipient is transferred to the cardiovascular intensive care unit (CVICU) for continuous monitoring and recovery. The initial postoperative management is similar to other cardiac surgery, but there are some potential complications that are unique to HTx patients that may require specific interventions. Fluid resuscitation may be used to optimize the preload, inotropes to support contractility and vasopressors to maintain mean arterial pressure (MAP). Furthermore, mechanical circulatory support (MCS) may be required to stabilize these patients in case of severe PGD [5].

The patient will arrive to the CVICU with several invasive lines. The International Society for Heart and Lung Transplantation (ISHLT) recommends monitoring with a Swan-Ganz catheter, electrocardiogram, oxygen saturation, invasive MAP as well as a bladder catheter for measurement of urine output [1]. There are different causes of early hemodynamic compromise, such as bleeding, primary and secondary graft dysfunction, arrhythmia, vasoplegia, and pulmonary hypertension (PH). Subsequently, other complications can arise, including respiratory failure, kidney failure, fluid overload, and infections [3, 6].

Additionally, there are certain laboratory parameters that should be checked frequently after HTx. Complete blood count and coagulation tests are useful for guiding transfusion of blood products; alterations in electrolyte panel should also be corrected; and arterial blood gases can be used to adjust ventilator settings and direct fluid resuscitation [6].

Physiology of the Donor Heart

The donor heart is completely denervated at the time of HTx. In the current era, donor heart implantation is performed using the bicaval anastomosis (BC) technique, which is associated with less atrial scarring compared to biatrial (BA) anastomosis, reducing the risk of supraventricular arrhythmias in the late follow-up (See Chapter 8). Due to denervation and lack of vagal tone, HTx recipients usually have a higher resting heart rate and certain cardiac medications are ineffective (i.e., digoxin and atropine) or demonstrate an exaggerated response (i.e., adenosine). The β-receptor density on the donor increases the sensitivity to circulating epinephrine and norepinephrine. Heart transplant recipients have also an abnormal heart rate in response to exercise and, following exercise, heart rate returns to baseline more slowly due to the gradual decline in circulating catecholamines. Patients are also unlikely to experience angina in response to ischemia. Cardiac reinnervation may be possible several years after transplant, but it may be incomplete and heterogeneous [7, 8].

Vasoactive Medications

The goals of hemodynamic management in the post-transplant period are to optimize preload, contractility, and afterload of both the right and left ventricles. Vasoplegic shock is common in the postcardiotomy period; infusions of vasopressors, such as norepinephrine, phenylephrine, and vasopressin, should be titrated to maintain adequate MAP. Methylene blue may also be considered for refractory vasoplegia. Commonly used inotropes include isoproterenol, epinephrine, dopamine, milrinone, and dobutamine.

Table 1. Inotropic and Vasopressor Agents for Heart Transplant Patients Initial Hemodynamic Support

Vasoactive	Mechanism	Primary effects	Adverse effects
Inotrope			
Dobutamine	β agonist weak β2 agonist	↑ Inotropism ↑ Cardiac output Vasodilator	Tachycardia and arrhythmias
Epinephrine	β agonist α agonist (↑doses)	↑ Inotropism ↑ Chronotropism ↑ SVR (↑doses)	Tachycardia and arrhythmias
Isoproterenol	Nonselective β agonist	↑ Chronotropism ↓ PVR (small effect)	Tachycardia and arrhythmias
Vasoactive	Mechanism	Primary effects	Adverse effects
Milrinone	Phosphodiesterase III inhibitor	↓ SVR and PVR ↑ Lusitropism ↑ Inotropism	Hypotension
Vasopressor			
Dopamine	α agonist β agonist (↑doses)	↑ Inotropism ↑ Chronotropism ↑ SVR (small effect)	Arrhythmias
Norepinephrine	α1 agonist	↑ SVR and MAP	Vital organs /extremities ischemia ↑ PVR
Vasopressin	V1 (vasomotor) V2 (renal) agonist	↑ SVR and MAP	Vital organs ischemia

MAP, mean arterial pressure; PVR, pulmonary vascular resistance; SVR, systemic vascular resistance. (Data from Subramani S et al. Early Graft Dysfunction Following Heart Transplant: Prevention and Management. Review. *Seminars in Cardiothoracic and Vascular Anesthesia.* 2020; 24 (10): 24-33).

Inhaled pulmonary vasodilators, if started in the operating room, may be continued during early postoperative period [4]. Myocardial function after HTx is often labile and continuous inotropic support is needed during this period. Similar to other cardiac surgeries, low cardiac output and myocardial dysfunction are frequently encountered after HTx and are associated with multiple causes, including reperfusion injury, inadequate myocardial protection, inflammatory response, PH and duration of ischemic time. However, other causes should be considered in cases where significant vasoactive support is needed, such as cardiac tamponade and acute rejection. Otherwise, myocardial dysfunction is frequently managed with infusions of isoproterenol, dobutamine or milrinone. Isoproterenol is very useful, especially in patients requiring heart rate support, as it has inotropic, chronotropic, and vasodilatory effects. Dobutamine, a pure β-agonist, can also be used. Finally, milrinone provides inotropic support in addition to afterload reduction and is often used in patients with PH. This inotropic support is often continued for at least 3 to 5 days after HTx and is slowly withdrawn as the heart recovers [5] (Table 1).

Mechanical Circulatory Support

De novo temporary MCS such as intra-aortic balloon pump (IABP), ventricular assist device (VAD) or extracorporeal membrane oxygenation (ECMO) may be placed intraoperatively if the patient cannot be weaned from cardiopulmonary bypass or if profound ventricular dysfunction and hemodynamic instability occur despite maximal pharmacological therapy. Therefore, a small percentage of patients will arrive to the CVICU with some type of MCS. Once no longer needed, MCS can be removed after coagulopathy has been corrected [4].

Ventilator Management

Patients should remain intubated and mechanically ventilated in the immediate postoperative period. Goals of ventilator management include avoidance of hypoxia, hypercapnia, and acidosis, which may lead to increased PAP and exacerbate RV dysfunction, and avoidance of high inspiratory pressures and positive end-expiratory pressure (PEEP), as well as auto-PEEP, which may impair venous return. Once the patient is hemodynamically stable, the respiratory support should be weaned and the patient extubated as soon as possible. Mechanical ventilation can contribute to increased intrathoracic pressures and subsequent HP. Moreover, inadequate ventilation can lead to hypercapnia, respiratory acidosis, and increased pulmonary vascular resistance, which can also adversely affect cardiac function. When the patient achieves hemodynamic stability and the respiratory support can be weaned, the patient begins pressure support testing. Trying to achieve early extubation is important as it reduces the risk of developing ventilator-associated complications, such as ventilator-associated pneumonia and deconditioning [4, 5].

Volume Management

Preoperative volume status its variable as patients may be with volume overload due to heart failure or euvolemic if they are previously compensated. Intraoperatively, ultrafiltration performed during cardiopulmonary bypass, bleeding, fluid administration, and transfusion may cause significant volume changes. Therefore, it is important to assess volume status using a Swan-Ganz catheter and/or echocardiography. Volume overload should be avoided, and renal replacement therapy should be instituted promptly if adequate volume removal is not achieved with diuretics [4].

Immunosuppression Management

Immunosuppressive therapy is key for graft survival after HTx. Rejection can occur at any time, from hyperacute rejection immediately upon allograft reperfusion to acute rejection throughout the post-HTx period and, finally, to chronic rejection in the form of cardiac allograft vasculopathy (See Chapter 11). Immunosuppression can be divided into three distinct phases: induction therapy, maintenance therapy, and treatment of rejection [2, 4].

Induction therapy is given in the early stages after HTx and may reduce the incidence of acute and chronic rejection. However, overall survival benefit has not been demonstrated. In fact, the ISHLT does not recommend the routine use of induction agents. Nevertheless, a great proportion of patients currently receive induction therapy, mainly to delay the initiation of nephrotoxic calcineurin inhibitors (CNIs) in patients with renal insufficiency or in those with the highest risk for rejection (i.e., sensitized patients, re-transplantation, or multiparous women) [2,7]. There are different induction drugs. Anti-thymocyte globulin (ATG) is a polyclonal antibody that induces T-cell death through CD3-mediated cytolysis. Basiliximab is a chimeric (mouse/human) monoclonal antibody against the Interleukin-2 receptor, which reduces T-cell proliferation. ATG may cause systemic inflammation and cytopenias. In addition, infections are more frequent with ATG than with basiliximab or with no induction [2]. Finally, all patients receive methylprednisolone 1000 mg in the operating room.

Table 2. Immunosuppression Scheme in Heart Transplantation

Scheme	Treatment	Drug	Doses	Posology	Observations
Induction					
Low risk	*Option # 1*	Methylprednisolone	1 gram	IV	At release of aortic cross-clamp
	Option # 2	Methylprednisolone	1 gram	IV	At release of aortic cross-clamp
		RATG	1-1.5 mg/Kg	IV (6 h)	At release of aortic cross-clamp
	Option # 3	Methylprednisolone	1 gram	IV	At release of aortic cross-clamp
		Basiliximab	20 mg 1° and 4 ° days	IV	At release of aortic cross-clamp
High risk (PRA > 10%)	Scheme should be decided considering the immunological and clinical risks	Methylprednisolone	1 gram	IV	At release of aortic cross-clamp
		RATG *	1-1.5 mg/Kg	IV (6 h)	At release of aortic cross-clamp. Continue 3 to 5 days
		Plasmapheresis	1 session day		At release of aortic cross-clamp. Continue 3 to 5 days
Maintenance					
	Steroids	Methylprednisolone	1° day: 125mg q8 h	IV	Day # 2: 125 mg q12 h Day # 3: 125 mg/day
		Prednisone	1 mg/kg/day for 48 h	Oral	Progressive decrease. Objective: discontinuation at 6-12 months after HTx
	Calcineurin inhibitors	Tacrolimus	0,10-0,20 mg/kg/day (in 2 doses)	Oral	Dose adjustment according to target dosage
		Ciclosporin**	2-3 mg/kg/day (in 2 doses)	Oral	Dose adjustment according to target dosage

Table 2. (Continued)

Scheme	Treatment	Drug	Doses	Posology	Observations
	Antiproliferatives	Mycophenolate mofetil (MMF)	2-3gr/day (in 2 doses)	Oral	If > 70 Kg: 3 gr/day
		Mycophenolate sodium	1,5-2 gr/day (in 2 doses)	Oral	When digestive intolerance to MMF is present
		Azathioprine	50-150 mg/d	Oral	Replace MMF in Chagas disease
	mTOR Inhibitors***	Sirolimus (rapamycin)	1-2 mg/day	Oral	Dose adjustment according to target dosage
		Everolimus	0,75 mg bid	Oral	Dose adjustment according to target dosage

HTx, heart transplantation; IV, intravenous; MMF, mycophenolate mofetil; PRA, panel-reactive antibody; RATG, rabbit anti-thymocyte globulin. (Data from Costanzo MR et al. The International Society of Heart and Lung Transplantation Guidelines for the care of heart transplant recipients. J Heart Lung Transplant. 2010 Aug;29(8):914-56 and Chang DH et al. Heart Transplant Immunosuppression Strategies at Cedars-Sinai Medical Center. *Int J Heart Fail*. 2021 Jan;3(1):15-30).

Maintenance therapy in the early postoperative therapy includes three-drug immunosuppression regimens consisting of steroids, CNIs, and antiproliferative agents. Steroids are tapered to discontinuation in the first 6 to 12 months after HTx. Regarding CNIs, tacrolimus is titrated to initial serum levels of 15–20 ng/ml or cyclosporine 1.5 to 5 mg/kg every 12 h titrated to a level of 300 ng/ml. Finally, antiproliferative agents such as mycophenolate mofetil 1000 to 1500 mg twice daily or azathioprine 2 mg/kg daily are also used [7]. Although mycophenolate mofetil is associated with a lower incidence of rejection and mortality compared with azathioprine, some reports showed that in recipients with Chagas disease, the incidence of Chagas reactivation was increased with mycophenolate mofetil compared to azathioprine. For this reason, azathioprine may be preferred in these patients [9, 10]. The immunosuppression scheme used in our center is shown in Table 2.

Postoperative Complications

Most complications occur during the first months after surgery, therefore, optimizing postoperative management is imperative for the long-term survival of HTx recipients [8, 11].

Hyperacute Rejection

Hyperacute rejection may occur upon the reperfusion of the allograft due to preformed antibodies against the donor. Currently, this complication is very rare thanks to a better understanding of the immune response and to an exhaustive immunological evaluation prior to HTx (See Chapter 11). However, when hyperacute rejection does occur, significant allograft dysfunction is usually present and inotropic or even MCS support may be necessary. Therefore, early diagnosis and treatment are essential in this scenario. High-dose immunosuppressive drugs including corticosteroids, ATG, plasmapheresis and intravenous immunoglobulin should be administered [4].

Bleeding

Bleeding can have an important negative impact after HTx as it results in decreased preload, increased afterload, and compromised contractility. It may occur secondary to coagulopathy due to prolonged cardiopulmonary bypass, preoperative antithrombotic medication, hypothermia, incomplete heparin reversal, or due to surgical reasons. Therefore, chest tube output should be closely monitored. Swan-Ganz catheter shows a pattern of hypovolemia with hypotension, low filling pressures, and low cardiac output. On echocardiography, both ventricles may appear with decreased chamber dimensions secondary to a decreased preload.

Management often involves correction of underlying coagulopathies and acidosis, transfusion of blood products and hemodynamic support. Transfused blood products should be irradiated and leukodepleted. Protamine can be administered for elevated partial thromboplastin time, and infusions of protamine or antifibrinolytics (tranexamic acid or aminocaproic acid) may be continued postoperatively in case of severe bleeding [4, 5].

Tamponade

Cardiac tamponade should be ruled out in patients with low cardiac output in the context of persistent postoperative bleeding. However, the classic presentation of tamponade, with tachycardia and equalization of pressures, may be absent after HTx. Echocardiography is useful in this scenario, but it should be noted that transthoracic echocardiography may not be able to identify posterior or isolated collections, thus, transesophageal echocardiography may be necessary. The typical pattern of collapse of the right cavities that is seen with concentric pericardial effusion may be absent and variations in transvalvular velocities and septal shift during the respiratory cycle may not be evident in mechanically ventilated patient. Furthermore, if the patient is on veno-arterial ECMO, cardiac chambers may be decompressed due to ECMO flow. The diagnosis of tamponade by echocardiography or in cases where clinical suspicion is high in a hemodynamically unstable patient should prompt urgent surgical reexploration [4, 6].

Vasoplegia

Vasoplegia is characterized by severe hypotension secondary to vasodilation, leading to inadequate end-organ perfusion or shock. Cardiac output may be normal or even elevated. There are multiple factors contributing to this syndrome, such as the systemic inflammatory response secondary to surgery or cardiopulmonary bypass support. In addition, factors such as high body mass index, prior cardiac surgery, MCS, long cardiopulmonary bypass time and ischemic time have also been implicated in the development of vasoplegia.

Treatment usually includes the use of vasopressors targeting a minimal MAP of 65 to 70 mmHg. The most frequently used drugs are norepinephrine, phenylephrine, epinephrine, and dopamine. There is no clear evidence that one agent is better than another, but dopamine is associated with the development of arrhythmias and phenylephrine lacks inotropic effect [4]. Therefore, in our center and in several other institutions, norepinephrine is the first-line agent used. Additionally, vasopressin and methylene blue can be considered. Vasopressin binds to the arginine vasopressin receptor, oxytocin receptor, and purinergic receptor. Its use has been associated with a reduction in the need for catecholamine infusions. However, mesenteric ischemia has been reported when high doses are used. Finally, methylene blue has been shown to reduce vasopressor requirements in this setting, but there is limited evidence supporting its indication [4, 5].

Right Ventricular Dysfunction

Patients with preoperative PH are at high risk of developing acute right ventricular failure (RVF) after HTx because the right ventricle of the recently implanted heart must now eject against an increased afterload. For this reason, high and irreversible PH is a contraindication for HTx (see Chapter 6). RVF may be secondary to PH or associated with ischemia, arrhythmias, cold ischemic time, reperfusion injury, mechanical obstruction at the level of the pulmonary artery anastomosis, donor-recipient size mismatch or PGD. In fact, when acute RVF occurs in the first 24 hours without an identifiable cause, it is classified as primary right ventricular graft failure (PGD-RV) [12].

Diagnosis of RVF should be suspected in a hemodynamically unstable patient with a San-Ganz catheter profile that shows elevated CVP, decreased CO, and normal PCWP. Treatment includes sildenafil, nitroglycerin, dobutamine, milrinone, or inhaled nitric oxide to lower pulmonary vascular resistance (PVR) and help unload the RV [1, 6-7]. Adequate ventilation using low pressures while avoiding auto-PEEP as well as correction of acid-base and electrolytes disturbances are also useful for the management of this syndrome. In patients with continued RV failure refractory to pharmacological therapy, prompt consideration for temporary MCS is advised [4, 13].

Acute Renal Failure

Acute kidney injury is associated with increased 1-year mortality. ISHLT registries show that it occurs at a rate of 25% at 1 year and 51% at 5 years [14]. Cardiopulmonary bypass and initiation of CNIs frequently cause acute renal failure in the first 48 hours after HTx. Intensive use of diuretics and even renal replacement therapy may be necessary when there is volume overload until renal function improves. On the other hand, in cases of hypovolemia, it is important to maintain a MAP of at least 65 to 70 mmHg and a CVP of 5 to 12 mmHg through the use of fluids, inotropes and/or vasopressors. Additionally, the use of ATG over 3 to 5 days allows delayed initiation of CNIs. Close monitoring of renal function and levels of immunosuppression in conjunction with a multidisciplinary care team is essential for the overall care of the HTx patient [4].

Arrhythmias

Arrhythmias and conduction abnormalities after HTx may be related to different causes, such as transplant physiology, surgical technique, rejection or cardiac allograft vasculopathy. Improvements in the management of HTx such as utilization of the BC technique and the minimization of ischemic time have positively affected the natural history of arrhythmia occurrence in this population. For instance, atrial fibrillation (AF) or flutter (AFL) has been reported in 10% to 25% of patients after HTx, an incidence significantly lower than that reported with other forms of cardiac surgery [15]. During procurement in HTx, there are hemodynamic, electrical, and biochemical disturbances that may have pro- or antiarrhythmic effects, such as organ retrieval, long ischemia times, graft manipulation, and the use of proarrhythmic inotropic treatment. The BA technique was one of the initial methods for orthotopic HTx, but was noted to cause significant disruption of the atrial anatomy and subsequent postoperative arrhythmias. In the 1990s, the BA technique was replaced by the BC method, where the donor's right heart is sutured using a bicaval anastomosis, leaving the right atrium generally intact [5, 16]. Different types of arrhythmias may appear after HTx.

Atrial Arrhythmias

The most common atrial arrhythmias after HTx are AF, AFL, and supraventricular tachycardias. AF is the most common early arrhythmia, whereas AFL or macroreentrant atrial tachycardia appear more frequently in long-term follow-up. It should be noted that the appearance of AF beyond 2 weeks after HTx may be secondary to graft rejection and should be evaluated accordingly. Early anticoagulation after HTx can be problematic due to the need for frequent endomyocardial biopsies. In these cases, patients can be maintained on subcutaneous low molecular weight heparin during this period [5, 17].

Ventricular Arrhythmias

Ventricular tachycardia and fibrillation are the most worrisome but least common arrhythmias. Non-sustained ventricular tachycardia is more frequent in the early postoperative period and is usually managed with electrolyte optimization and antiarrhythmic medication. In addition, amiodarone can be considered as the first-line antiarrhythmic drug. It should be noted that although patients are initially treated with cardioversion for sustained ventricular arrhythmias, they may require additional studies, including angiogram to assess coronary anatomy and endomyocardial biopsy to rule out rejection [5, 16].

Bradycardia and Conduction System Disease

Bradycardia and sinus node dysfunction are frequently encountered in the early period after HTx. Incomplete and complete right bundle branch block are also common findings.

Sinus node dysfunction may be related to sympathetic denervation, sinus node ischemia/injury, tachycardia-bradycardia syndrome, or prior use of antiarrhythmic drugs. The use of amiodarone before HTx can affect the new allograft and contribute to post-transplant bradycardia that can persist for several weeks. In contrast, sinus node injury has been shown to be reduced with the BC technique.

Symptomatic sinus node dysfunction can be initially managed with temporary pacing or with drugs such as isoproterenol and theophylline to increase the heart rate while awaiting the return of normal sinus node function. Permanent pacemakers are generally indicated only for symptomatic bradycardia that does not resolve after the third week of transplantation [5, 15].

Graft Dysfunction

During organ procurement and transportation, several phenomena can affect the graft, including local inflammation, acidosis and ATP depletion. In addition, reperfusion injury occurs secondary to the release of free radicals and inflammatory cytokines. This results in a delayed recovery of graft contractility that impact both systolic and diastolic function after HTx. Although early graft dysfunction is relatively common, there were different definitions and classifications not universally accepted. It was not until recently, in 2014, when an ISHLT consensus established the standards for the diagnosis, definition, classification and treatment of early graft dysfunction [12]. There are two main entities among early graft dysfunction, secondary graft dysfunction (i.e., due to PH, graft rejection, surgical complication) and PGD, when there is no known cause. PGD must be diagnosed during the first 24 hours after HTX, and is usually more concerning as it can occur unpredictably and there is no etiological therapy available.

Primary Graft Dysfunction

This entity refers to the dysfunction of the donor graft which fails to meet the circulatory requirements of the recipient immediately after HTx. It is divided into PGD-left ventricle (LV), when it affects the left or both ventricles, and PGD-right ventricle (RV), when it affects only the RV. Additionally, PGD-LV is further classified into mild, moderate, or severe depending on the level of cardiac function and the extent of hemodynamic support required [12, 18].

Mild PGD is diagnosed when there is ventricular dysfunction demonstrated by echocardiography (left ventricular ejection fraction <40%) or by hemodynamic parameters on the Swan-Ganz catheter (right atrial pressure [RAP] >15 mmHg and wedge pressure [PCWP] > 20 mmHg in the setting of a cardiac index [CI] < 2.0 L/min/m2) lasting at least 1 h. The dose of inotropes needed should be low, with an inotrope score less than 10 [12, 19]. Moderate PGD is identified by the same echocardiographic and hemodynamic parameters but with the addition of requiring high dose inotropes (inotropes score >10) or IABP to maintain stability. Finally, severe PGD is one that requires short-term MCS, such as veno-arterial ECMO or VADs.

In contrast, PGD-RV is not divided into different categories, but is diagnosed based on the requirement of right side MCS or a Swan-Ganz catheter profile with RAP > 15 mmHg, PCWP < 15 mmHg, CI < 2.0 L/min/m2 in the context of a transpulmonary gradient < 15 mmHg and/or systolic pulmonary artery pressure < 50 mmHg (Table 3) [12, 20]

Epidemiology and Pathogenesis

This syndrome is a potentially fatal complication following HTx that affects both short- and long-term survival. Early mortality due to PGD can be as high as 66% in the first 30 days. This risk varies according to the etiology of the heart disease that led to HTx, being higher in retransplant patients and congenital heart disease (approximately 20%) and lower in ischemic and non-ischemic dilated cardiomyopathy (approximately 10%). Therefore, despite some improvements in the management of PGD in recent years, early mortality remains significantly high [12, 21].

Table 3. Primary Graft Dysfunction Severity Scale

PGD-LV	Mild	LVEF ≤ 40% by echocardiography or RAP > 15 mmHg, PCWP > 20 mmHg, CI < 2.0 L/min/ m^2 requiring low-dose inotropes
	Moderate	LVEF ≤ 40% or RAP > 15 mmHg, PCWP > 20 mmHg, CI < 2.0 L/min/ m^2 hypotension with MAP < 70 mmHg + High dose inotropes - Inotrope score* > 10 or Need of IABP
	Severe	Need of MCS including VA ECMO, LVAD, BiVAD or percutaneous LVAD
PGD-RV		Need for RVAD or Hemodynamics with RAP > 15 mmHg, PCWP < 15 mmHg, CI < 2.0 L/min/$m^2$and + TPG < 15 mmHg ± PA systolic pressure < 50 mmHg

*Inotrope score: dopamine (x1) + dobutamine (x1) + amrinone (x1) + milrinone (x15) + epinephrine (x 100) + norepinephrine (x 100) (with each drug dosed in ug/kg/min). BiVAD, biventricular assist device; CI, cardiac index; IABP, intra-aortic balloon pump; LV, left ventricle; LVAD, left ventricular assist device; LVEF, left ventricular ejection fraction; MAP, mean arterial pressure; PA, pulmonary artery; MCS, mechanical circulatory support; PCWP, pulmonary capillary wedge pressure; PGD, primary graft dysfunction; RAP, right atrial pressure; RV, right ventricle RVAD, right ventricular assist device; TPG, transpulmonary pressure gradient; VA ECMO, veno-arterial extracorporeal membrane oxygenation. (Data from Kobashigawa J et al. Report from a consensus conference on primary graft dysfunction after cardiac transplantation. *J Heart Lung Transplant.* 2014 Apr;33(4):327-40).

Regarding the pathogenesis of PGD, it should be noted that during HTx the graft is exposed to different aggressions, such as brain death in the donor with release of catecholamines, hypothermia, ischemia-reperfusion injury or warm ischemia. Additionally, factors in the recipient may further compromise the graft, such as systemic inflammatory response syndrome (due to prior MCS or transfusions) or high PVR. In the latter case, the graft failure is rather considered a secondary graft dysfunction [1, 12].

Risk Factors

Risk factors for the development of PGD can be grouped in three main categories: donor-related, procedure-related or recipient-related. Donor factors include age, gender mismatch (female donor to male recipient) and cause of brain death. Risk factors related to the surgical procedure are weight mismatch and prolonged ischemic times. Finally, recipient-related risk factors for PGD are age, PH, requirement of inotropes, MCS or mechanical ventilatory support, previous sternotomy, among others [12].

Table 4. Risk Factors for Development of Primary Graft Dysfunction

Donor-related	**Procedure-related**	**Recipient-related**
• Age • Sex mismatch • (Female donor/male recipient) • Cause of brain death • Cardiac dysfunction • Inotropic support • Prolonged cardiac arrest • Trauma • Comorbidities* • Sepsis • Coronary artery disease • Wall motion abnormalities • Valvular heart disease • Left Ventricular hypertrophy • Illicit drug abuse**	• Ischemia time • Cardioplegic solution • Procurement team experience • Size mismatch*** • (Predicted heart mass) • Blood transfusion requirement • Emergency transplant • Retransplantation • Prolonged cardiopulmonary bypass • Non-cardiac organ donation	• Age • Weight • Mechanical support • Mechanical ventilation • Pulmonary hypertension • Amiodarone long-term use • CVP > 10 mmHg • Pretransplant anemia • (Hb < 10 g/dL) • Inotrope support • Congenital heart disease • Multiple reoperations/Retransplant • Sepsis • Multiorgan transplant • Allosensitization • Comorbidities*

*diabetes, hypertension, dyslipidemia, obesity. **alcohol, cocaine, amphetamines. ***Size mismatch: predicted left ventricular mass (g)=α x Height 0.54 (m) x Weight 0.61 (kg), where α = 6.82 for women and 8.25 for men. CVP, central venous pressure; Hb, hemoglobin. (Data from Kobashigawa J et al. Report from a consensus conference on primary graft dysfunction after cardiac transplantation. *J Heart Lung Transplant*. 2014 Apr;33(4):327-40).

Some of these risk factors were integrated and validated in a score for the prediction of PGD, the RADIAL score. This score takes into account 6 factors: RAP > 10 mm Hg, age > 60 years, diabetes, inotropic support dependence, donor age > 30 years and ischemia time > 240 minutes [22, 23]. In addition, different molecules including troponins (cTnT), tumor necrosis factor-α (TNF-α), interleukin-6 (IL-6), procalcitonin, brain natriuretic peptide (BNP) and Switch/Sucrose Non-Fermentable, a matrix-associated, actin-dependent regulator of chromatin subfamily a-like 1 (SMARCAL1) have been proposed as biomarkers for predicting PGD, especially when used in combination [18].

Although these variables are currently used in clinical practice to predict PGD, there is a need to update the information related to current risk factors for this entity. This is due in part to the increased use of VADs, the older age of candidates secondary to advances in HF treatment, and the shortage of donors, requiring longer ischemic times [24]. The main donor, recipient and surgical procedural risk factors for PGD are shown in Table 4 [12, 25].

Secondary Graft Dysfunction

Unlike PGD, in which there is no identifiable cause for graft failure, in secondary graft dysfunction (SGD) there is a discernible cause, such as rejection, PH, or surgical complications. Its incidence is declining and is reported to range from 1.6 to 8.8%, probably due to differences in diagnostic criteria [13].

Secondary Graft Dysfunction due to Pulmonary Hypertension

The most frequent cause of SGD is PH, being associated with this entity in 40 to 80% of the cases. In fact, elevated transpulmonary gradient and/or RVP are related to higher early mortality after HTx. The main mechanism for graft failure in this situation is the failure of the donor RV, not used to elevated pulmonary pressures, to adapt to the increase in afterload secondary to PH [13].

Secondary Graft Dysfunction due to Surgical Complications

SGD may also be secondary to surgical complications such as bleeding, occlusion or kinking of vascular structures or narrowed anastomosis. These complications are the second most frequent cause of SGD with incidences of up to 15%, and they all affect RV after HTx by different mechanisms, including massive transfusions due to bleeding that may cause volume overload [13].

Secondary Graft Dysfunction due to Hyperacute Rejection

As mentioned above, hyperacute rejection occurs in the immediate postoperative period and can result in graft loss. Nowadays, the incidence of hyperacute rejection is very low (less than 0.3%) and is usually secondary to the recipient's antibodies against the ABO blood antigens of the donor or the HLA of the donor heart. Anti-HLA antibodies develop when a recipient is exposed to foreign antigens through previous blood transfusions, pregnancy, and/or previous organ transplant. HLA antibody sensitization is screened using panel reactive antibodies and can range from 0% to 100% depending on the percentage of antigens that react to the candidate antibodies. Higher percentages of panel reactive antibody before HTx are associated with a higher degree of graft rejection and high early postoperative mortality. However, there are currently different strategies to decrease the risk of hyperacute rejection, such as use of ABO-compatible donors, prospective crossmatch and a restrictive approach to blood transfusions in high-risk recipients [13].

Management of Early Graft Dysfunction

Pharmacologic Treatment for Early Graft Dysfunction

The goal of treatment for early graft dysfunction is to provide hemodynamic support to allow time for the graft recovery, in the case of PGD, or for proper diagnosis and treatment of the underlying cause, in the case of SGD. The initial approach for both PGD and SGD is similar and consists of inotropes and vasopressors to maintain hemodynamic stability [4]. In the case of PGD-RV or SGD secondary to PH, inhaled nitric oxide or prostaglandins such as epoprostenol or inhaled prostacyclin may be used to assist the failing right ventricle by reducing pulmonary artery pressures and improving cardiac index. Inhaled nitric oxide is expensive and may cause methemoglobinemia or renal failure, while inhaled prostacyclin is associated with increased bleeding. Additionally, sildenafil can be used when there is PH before and/or after transplantation to decrease PVR [13].

Levosimendan can also be used in the setting of PGD to improve cardiac index and lower the dose of other inotropes. However, its onset of action is slow and it can cause hypotension secondary to vasodilation.

Inflammatory molecules may play a role in the pathogenesis of PGD. Therefore, therapies such as plasmapheresis, hemadsorption columns, ATG and anti-complement factors could be useful for removing cytokines.

However, there is insufficient data to recommend its routine use [12, 13]. Additionally, preventive measures to decrease incidence of PGD should be implemented whenever possible:

- Donor management (hormone therapy, low dose inotropes, avoid volume overload)
- Improve size matching (heart mass index)
- Improve procurement techniques
- Improve preservation (OrganCare System, additives in preservation solution)
- Decrease ischemic time
- Recipient selection
- Decrease transfusion requirements
- Gradual weaning of inotropes
- Consider using nitric oxide

When pharmacologic treatment has failed, MCS should be considered. There are no established guidelines regarding the best time to transition from pharmacologic support to MCS devices, however, early transition may be useful in preventing further hemodynamic instability and multiple organ failure [12, 18].

Mechanical Circulatory Support for Early Graft Dysfunction

Therapy with MCS is essential for the management of severe graft dysfunction, thus, after an initial treatment with vasoactive drugs, these devices should be used in refractory cases. There are different short-term MCS devices that can be used depending on the level of support needed, such as IABP, veno-arterial ECMO, temporary VADs (left, right or biventricular) with or without oxygenator or total artificial heart, among others (See Chapter 5) [13, 26].

The IABP can be rapidly placed, even bedside, and reduces afterload, improves coronary flow and increases CI. However, it only provides partial support and may be insufficient in severe cases of PGD. In these cases, veno-arterial ECMO or temporary VADs are used [27, 28]. There are different VADs, such as magnetically levitated centrifugal pumps (Centrimag) that provide up to 10 liters/min of continuous flow and can be used in the right, left or biventricular position. It is usually used in an already open chest and an oxygenator can be added to the circuit [28]. Percutaneous VADs include devices such as Impella or Tandem Heart. However, ECMO is the most common mode of support and can be placed peripherally or centrally. Peripheral cannulation does not require an open chest surgery but can lead to limb ischemia and increased afterload. Central cannulation does not have these complications, but it does increase the risk of bleeding and infection. Most of these MCS devices require anticoagulation due to the increased risk of thromboembolic complications, and the selection of a device should be made based on the patient's clinical condition and the center's experience, including discussion by a multidisciplinary heart team.

Retransplantation

When early graft dysfunction is refractory to pharmacological and non-pharmacological treatment, including MCS utilization, retransplantation may be considered.

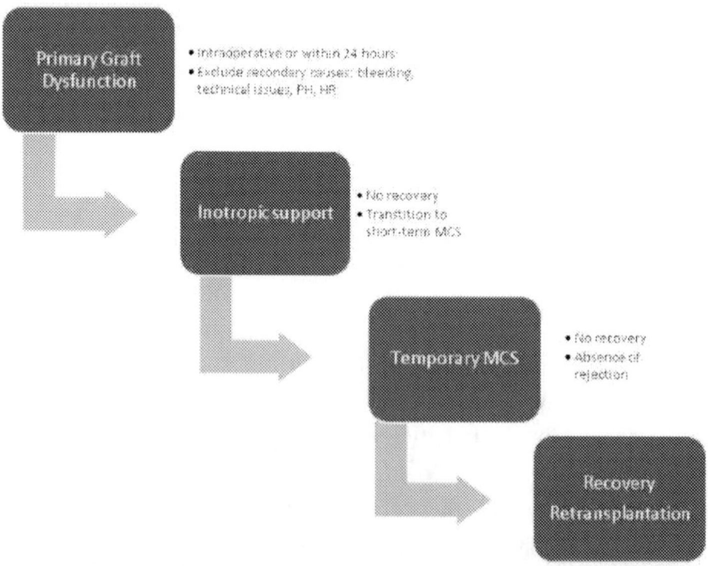

Figure 1. Primary Graft Dysfunction Management. HR, hyperacute rejection; MCS, mechanical circulatory support; PH, pulmonary hypertension. (Data from Kittleson MM et al. Cardiac Transplantation: Current Outcomes and Contemporary Controversies. *JACC Heart Fail*. 2017 Dec;5(12):857-868).

Currently, retransplantation rates range from 6 to 15%, and is performed primarily in the setting of cardiac allograft vasculopathy, and even in this setting results remain poor (See Chapter 6). Retransplantation due to early graft dysfunction may be even more challenging and is associated with several complications and worse outcomes since recipients may have multiple organ failure, coagulopathy, previous sternotomy and pulmonary congestion [1].

Figure 1 outlines a stepwise approach to managing early graft dysfunction using pharmacological therapy, device support, and ultimately considering heart retransplantation in highly selected patients.

Conclusion

Postoperative management of heart transplant patient is challenging and it has a direct impact on short- and long-term outcomes. Knowing the different complications that can follow this complex procedure is essential for a proper diagnosis and timely treatment. Early graft dysfunction remains one of the most frequent and fatal complication after HTx despite recent advances in diagnosis, classification and management. Prevention, adequate treatment with vasoactive drugs or IABP for mild to moderate cases, and rapid transition to MCS in cases of severe graft dysfunction are paramount to achieve better outcomes.

References

[1] Kittleson MM, Kobashigawa JA. Cardiac Transplantation: Current Outcomes and Contemporary Controversies. *JACC Heart Fail.* 2017 Dec;5(12):857-868.

[2] Kittleson MM. Recent advances in heart transplantation. *F1000Res.* 2018 Jul 5;7:F1000 Faculty Rev-1008.

[3] Costanzo MR, Dipchand A, Starling R, Anderson A, Chan M, Desai S, Fedson S, Fisher P, Gonzales-Stawinski G, Martinelli L, McGiffin D, Smith J, Taylor D, Meiser B, Webber S, Baran D, Carboni M, Dengler T, Feldman D, Frigerio M, Kfoury A, Kim D, Kobashigawa J, Shullo M, Stehlik J, Teuteberg J, Uber P, Zuckermann A, Hunt S, Burch M, Bhat G, Canter C, Chinnock R, Crespo-Leiro M, Delgado R, Dobbels F, Grady K, Kao W, Lamour J, Parry G, Patel J, Pini D, Towbin J, Wolfel G, Delgado D, Eisen H, Goldberg L, Hosenpud J, Johnson M, Keogh A, Lewis C, O'Connell J, Rogers J, Ross H, Russell S, Vanhaecke J; International Society of Heart and Lung Transplantation Guidelines. The International Society of

Heart and Lung Transplantation Guidelines for the care of heart transplant recipients. *J Heart Lung Transplant*. 2010 Aug;29(8):914-56.

[4] Vega E, Schroder J, Nicoara A. Postoperative management of heart transplantation patients. *Best Pract Res Clin Anaesthesiol*. 2017 Jun;31(2):201-213.

[5] Rabin J, Kaczorowski DJ. Perioperative Management of the Cardiac Transplant Recipient. *Crit Care Clin*. 2019 Jan;35(1):45-60.

[6] Barros LN, Uchoa RB, Mejia JAC, Nunes RR, Barros DASN, Rodrigues Filho F. Anesthetic protocol for right ventricular dysfunction management in heart transplantation: systematic review, development and validation. *BMC Anesthesiol*. 2021 Feb 11;21(1):46.

[7] Kansara P, Kobashigawa JA. Management of heart transplant recipients: reference for primary care physicians. *Postgrad Med*. 2012 Jul;124(4):215-24.

[8] Potena L, Zuckermann A, Barberini F, Aliabadi-Zuckermann A. Complications of Cardiac Transplantation. *Curr Cardiol Rep*. 2018 Jul 10;20(9):73.

[9] Benatti RD, Al-Kindi SG, Bacal F, Oliveira GH. Heart transplant outcomes in patients with Chagas cardiomyopathy in the United States. *Clin Transplant*. 2018 Jun;32(6): e13279.

[10] Bacal F, Silva CP, Pires PV, Mangini S, Fiorelli AI, Stolf NG, Bocchi EA. Transplantation for Chagas' disease: an overview of immunosuppression and reactivation in the last two decades. *Clin Transplant*. 2010 Mar-Apr;24(2): E29-34.

[11] Neethling E, Moreno Garijo J, Mangalam TK, Badiwala MV, Billia P, Wasowicz M, Van Rensburg A, Slinger P. Intraoperative and Early Postoperative Management of Heart Transplantation: Anesthetic Implications. *J Cardiothorac Vasc An*esth. 2020 Aug;34(8):2189-2206.

[12] Kobashigawa J, Zuckermann A, Macdonald P, Leprince P, Esmailian F, Luu M, Mancini D, Patel J, Razi R, Reichenspurner H, Russell S, Segovia J, Smedira N, Stehlik J, Wagner F; Consensus Conference participants. Report from a consensus conference on primary graft dysfunction after cardiac transplantation. *J Heart Lung Transplant*. 2014 Apr;33(4):327-40.

[13] Subramani S, Aldrich A, Dwarakanath S, Sugawara A, Hanada S. Early Graft Dysfunction Following Heart Transplant: Prevention and Management. *Semin Cardiothorac Vasc An*esth. 2020 Mar;24(1):24-33.

[14] Nicoara A, Kretzer A, Cooter M, Bartz R, Lyvers J, Patel CB, Schroder JN, McCartney SL, Podgoreanu MV, Milano CA, Swaminathan M, Stafford-Smith M. Association between primary graft dysfunction and acute kidney injury after orthotopic heart transplantation - a retrospective, observational cohort study. *Transpl Int*. 2020 Aug;33(8):887-894.

[15] Thajudeen A, Stecker EC, Shehata M, Patel J, Wang X, McAnulty JH Jr, Kobashigawa J, Chugh SS. Arrhythmias after heart transplantation: mechanisms and management. *J Am Heart Assoc*. 2012 Apr;1(2): e001461.

[16] Joglar JA, Wan EY, Chung MK, Gutierrez A, Slaughter MS, Bateson BP, Loguidice M, Drazner M, Kistler PM, Saour B, Poole JE, Murtaza G, Turagam MK, Vader J, Lakkireddy D, Birati EY, Dhingra R, Gopinathannair R. Management of Arrhythmias After Heart Transplant: Current State and Considerations for Future Research. *Circ Arrhythm Electrophysiol*. 2021 Mar;14 (3): e007954.

[17] Renedo MF, González JL, Giunta GA, Giordanino EF, Ameri AS, Mysuta MA, Ramirez DA, Favaloro LE, Favaloro RR, Absi DO, Galizio NO, Bertolotti AM. Radiofrequency ablation of supraventricular arrhythmias after orthotopic heart transplantation: Long-term follow-up of a single-center experience. *Clin Transplant*. 2021 Feb;35(2): e14165.

[18] Singh SSA, Dalzell JR, Berry C, Al-Attar N. Primary graft dysfunction after heart transplantation: a thorn amongst the roses. *Heart Fail Rev*. 2019 Sep;24(5):805-820.

[19] DePasquale EC, Ardehali A. Primary graft dysfunction in heart transplantation. *CurrOpin Organ Transplant*. 2018 Jun;23(3):286-294.

[20] D'Ancona G, Santise G, Falletta C, Pirone F, Sciacca S, Turrisi M, Biondo D, Pilato M. Primary graft failure after heart transplantation: the importance of donor pharmacological management. *Transplant Proc*. 2010 Apr;42(3):710-2.

[21] Avtaar Singh SS, Banner NR, Rushton S, Simon AR, Berry C, Al-Attar N. ISHLT Primary Graft Dysfunction Incidence, Risk Factors, and Outcome: A UK National Study. *Transplantation*. 2019 Feb;103(2):336-343.

[22] Segovia J, Cosío MD, Barceló JM, Bueno MG, Pavía PG, Burgos R, Serrano-Fiz S, García-Montero C, Castedo E, Ugarte J, Alonso-Pulpón L. RADIAL: a novel primary graft failure risk score in heart transplantation. *J Heart Lung Transplant*. 2011 Jun;30(6):644-51.

[23] CosíoCarmena MD, Gómez Bueno M, Almenar L, Delgado JF, Arizón JM, González Vilchez F, Crespo-Leiro MG, Mirabet S, Roig E, Pérez Villa F, Fernández-Yañez JF, Lambert JL, Manito N, Fuente L, Sanz Julve ML, Pascual D, Rábago G, Millán I, Alonso-Pulpón LA, Segovia J. Primary graft failure after heart transplantation: characteristics in a contemporary cohort and performance of the RADIAL risk score. *J Heart Lung Transplant*. 2013 Dec;32(12):1187-95.

[24] Beiras-Fernandez A, Kaczmarek I, Weis F. Primary graft failure after heart transplantation: urgent need for a consensus guideline. *Transplantation*. 2011 Mar 27;91(6): e31; author reply e31-2.

[25] Russo MJ, Iribarne A, Hong KN, Ramlawi B, Chen JM, Takayama H, Mancini DM, Naka Y. Factors associated with primary graft failure after heart transplantation. *Transplantation*. 2010 Aug 27;90(4):444-50.

[26] Loforte A, Fiorentino M, Murana G, Gliozzi G, Cavalli GG, Mariani C, Martin Suarez S, Pacini D. Mechanically Supported Early Graft Failure After Heart Transplantation. *Transplant Proc*. 2021 Jan-Feb;53(1):311-317.

[27] Bermudez CA, McMullan DM. Extracorporeal life support in preoperative and postoperative heart transplant management. *Ann Transl Med*. 2017 Oct;5(20):398.

[28] Marasco SF, Vale M, Pellegrino V, Preovolos A, Leet A, Kras A, Schulberg E, Bergin P, Esmore DS. Extracorporeal membrane oxygenation in primary graft failure after heart transplantation. *Ann Thorac Surg*. 2010 Nov;90(5):1541-6.

[29] Clerkin KJ, Mancini DM, Stehlik J, Cherikh WS, Lund LH. Continuous-flow mechanical circulatory support is not associated with early graft failure: An analysis of the International Society for Heart and Lung Transplantation registry. *Clin Transplant*. 2019 Dec; 33(12): e13752.

Part III: Follow-Up Care after Heart Transplantation

Chapter 10

Echocardiography in Heart Transplant Recipients

José Fabian Salmo, Diego Sánchez Luceros, Guillermo Eduardo Ganum, Juan Alberto Moukarzel, Milagros Seijo Behety and Eduardo Guevara*

Echocardiography Department, Favaloro Foundation University Hospital, Buenos Aires, Argentina

Abstract

Echocardiography is an essential non-invasive tool for daily clinical practice. In heart transplantation, echocardiography is crucial to evaluate the potential recipient, aid in peri-operative management, and assess possible complications that may develop during post-transplant follow-up. Two of these main complications are acute graft rejection and cardiac allograft vasculopathy; in both, echocardiography provides information necessary for clinical decision making. This chapter will discuss the main aspects of echocardiography in heart transplant recipients.

Keywords: heart transplantation, echocardiography, graft rejection

Introduction

The introduction of echocardiography in daily cardiology practice was contemporaneous with that of heart transplantation as a last resort for the

---

* Corresponding Author's E-mail: eguevara@ffavaloro.org.

In: Heart Transplantation
Editor: Elian Facundo Giordanino
ISBN: 978-1-68507-759-4

treatment of end-stage heart failure [1, 2]. Due to the information it provides, its low cost, wide availability, possibility of performing it at the patient's bedside and reproducibility, echocardiography is today the most widely used non-invasive diagnostic method after electrocardiography.

In heart transplantation, it is used in the pre-transplant evaluation of the recipient, as well as in the post-transplant period to aid in the diagnosis of its two most feared complications: acute rejection and cardiac allograft vasculopathy (chronic rejection) [3]. Unlike liver and kidney transplants, there are no biomarkers to determine graft dysfunction and, although endomyocardial biopsy is the gold standard for the diagnosis of acute rejection, its early detection is essential to optimize immunosuppressive treatment. Both endomyocardial biopsy and coronary angiography are expensive invasive procedures, and not without complications. Furthermore, the sensitivity of the latter for the detection of chronic rejection is limited if it is performed without intravascular ultrasound or other complementary methods. (See Chapter 12) For these reasons, transthoracic echocardiography is an invaluable tool for non-invasive detection of graft rejection. Signs that may suggest graft rejection range from pericardial effusion or increased wall thickness to graft dysfunction.

The anatomy, function, flows, tissue velocities and myocardial deformation of the graft can be analyzed to reach a presumptive diagnosis of the patient's condition. Unfortunately, the mobility of the transplanted heart in the recipient's chest, the vagal denervation with the consequent tachycardia, the fusion of E and A waves in the transmitral flow or even the competition of the atrial rhythms of the recipient and the donor, and the sometimes-irregular areas affected by rejection, threaten the inter- and intra-observer reproducibility in the follow-up of these patients. However, new echocardiographic techniques have contributed to improve the evaluation and detection of rejection in the transplanted heart: pulsed tissue Doppler and the analysis of myocardial deformation (strain) from Speckle tracking. The first allows calculating the speed at which the explored myocardial segments move, but the values obtained depend on the angle of incidence of the ultrasound beam and the traction of the neighboring segments. The second allows analyzing the deformation of the different segments of the left and right ventricle.

In addition, pharmacologic stress echocardiography may detect new segmental wall motion abnormalities secondary to cardiac allograft vasculopathy, either in the epicardial arteries or in the microcirculation.

Finally, echocardiography is used to assess complications after endomyocardial biopsy, such as cardiac perforation with pericardial effusion/tamponade or tricuspid valve chordal rupture. This chapter will address the echocardiographic evaluation of the transplant patient and its diagnostic and prognostic possibilities.

Peri-Operative Evaluation

Pre-Transplantation

In patients with heart failure, echocardiography is useful to establish the etiology, prognosis and identify factors that can modify the natural history of the disease if treated (cardiac resynchronization, correction of congenital heart disease, myocardial revascularization, valve intervention). Furthermore, in patients who are candidates for heart transplantation, echocardiography is used to evaluate pulmonary pressures and to monitor patients under mechanical circulatory support devices.

Transplantation

Echocardiography is useful to evaluate the potential donor as well as to aid in the surgical procedure. Donor evaluation should include:

- Cardiac dimensions and function
- Parietal thicknesses
- Abnormalities in motility or in the cardiac chambers
- Rule out coronary heart disease (in marginal donors, pharmacologic stress echocardiography may be useful) [4].

Intraoperative transesophageal echocardiography is important to assess the systolic function of both ventricles and the possibility of stenosis in suture areas, such as in the pulmonary veins. In addition, together with the Swan-Ganz catheter, it can detect pulmonary hypertension that may require administration of nitric oxide to prevent graft failure [5].

Post-Transplantation

In the immediate postoperative period, echocardiographic evaluation is essential to determine possible surgical complications as well as to evaluate possible graft dysfunction. In the early post-transplant period, there is no close correlation between graft dysfunction and acute rejection diagnosed by endomyocardial biopsy. This is due in part to the fact that during this critical period there can be multiple causes of graft dysfunction apart from to rejection, especially regarding the right ventricle. In addition, hyperacute graft rejection is currently less common thanks to advances in immunosuppression and detection of pre-transplant sensitization. In our experience, the determination of the tricuspid annular plane systolic excursion (TAPSE) in this context is not very useful to assess the function of the right ventricle, whereas the change in fractional area is a more reliable parameter.

Regarding wall thickness, its increase can be secondary to different causes, such as myocardial edema due to reperfusion injury, graft rejection or increased heart rate and high levels of catecholamines.

The recipient's atrial size will be determined by the surgical technique: biatrial or bicaval (See Chapter 8). In the first case, an echo-dense structure is observed in the wall of the left atrium that corresponds to the suture line [5].

The presence of pericardial effusion in the immediate postoperative period may be secondary to bleeding. However, the late appearance of pericardial effusion and its progression should raise suspicion of the possibility of rejection.

The frequency with which the echocardiographic evaluation of these patients is performed will depend on their clinical status and the protocols implemented in each center.

Acute Graft Rejection

Acute graft rejection is the leading cause of mortality during the first year after heart transplantation. Its incidence is around 20-40% and it is responsible for 12% of all deaths [6]. Echocardiography is the imaging modality of choice for evaluating these patients and provides accurate information on graft anatomy and function [7]. As mentioned above, in the immediate postoperative period, echocardiography allows the identification of surgical complications and early graft dysfunction, while in long-term follow-up, serial echocardiographic studies are useful to detect acute or chronic graft rejection. However, a drawback of this technique is that echocardiographic parameters are more variable in heart transplant patients than in the general population. This makes it difficult to define the normal morphology and function of the transplanted heart and to identify the appropriate cut-off values for the different echocardiographic parameters to detect allograft dysfunction [8]. For this reason, it is very important to have a study available for comparison during the serial follow-up studies as this is more useful than the absolute value of each measurement [9]. This baseline study should be at least 6 months after heart transplantation, because in the earlier period the adaptation of the new heart to the thoracic space, its different positioning in the chest compared with the native heart, and the presence of confounders such as early allograft dysfunction, pericardial effusion, and other comorbidities may affect the recorded echocardiographic parameters and decrease the sensitivity of echocardiography to detect graft rejection during follow-up [10].

During the first month after heart transplantation, the left ventricle has an increased mass and wall thickness, probably due to inflammatory cell infiltration and graft edema [11]. This thickness usually decreases after 3 months, probably secondary to liquid reabsorption. In contrast, during long-term follow-up an increase in left ventricular mass and wall thickness secondary to graft rejection causing myocardial inflammation that induces cellular edema may be observed. However, several reports demonstrate low sensitivity of this parameter due to wall thickness fluctuation related to scattered acute rejection cellular edema pattern combined with the anti-inflammatory effect of immunosuppressive therapy [12, 13]. In addition, left ventricular ejection fraction (LVEF) is not an early indicator of graft dysfunction and its sensitivity for acute graft rejection is low [14]. Although, when a heart transplant recipient does present with acute left ventricular dysfunction, the first presumptive diagnosis should be graft rejection (Figure 1).

Changes in diastolic function are a more sensitive but less specific marker of acute graft rejection than reduced LVEF [15, 16]. These changes are probably caused by myocardial edema or by early fibrosis that stiffens the myocardium. Mitral inflow Doppler indices have been extensively investigated in this context.

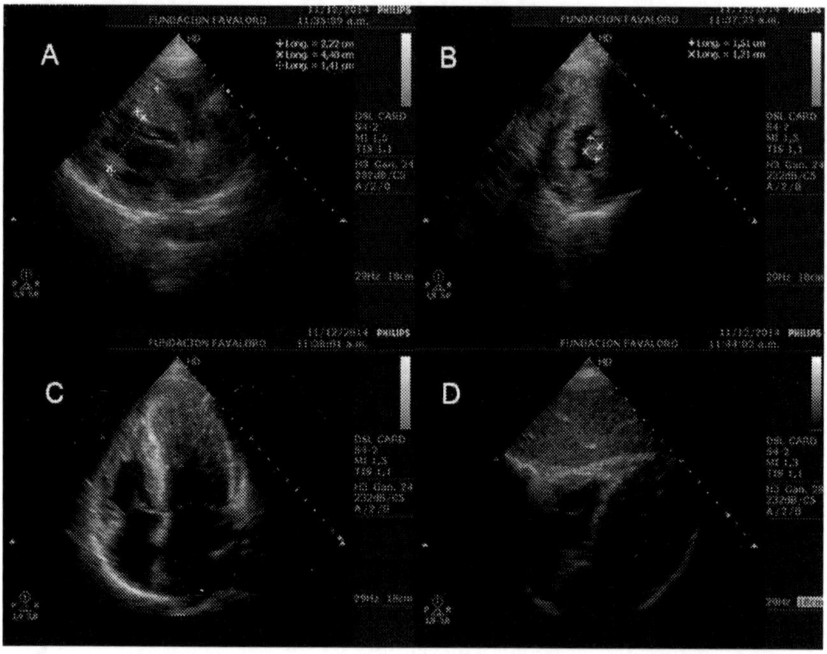

Figure 1. 43-year-old patient with acute graft rejection. A. Left ventricle with increased wall thickness. B. Papillary muscle with increased thickness. C. Right ventricle free wall with increased thickness.

E wave, A wave, E/A ratio, deceleration time, isovolumetric relaxation time failed to demonstrate any significant correlation between variations in LV filling parameters and proven graft rejection [9]. Left ventricular filling is affected by many variables, including preload conditions, compliance and contractility, end-systolic volume, atrial dynamics and morphology, and heart rate. Diastolic function can be affected for multiple reasons and is therefore not specific to rejection. However, it is recommended to continue evaluating diastolic parameters because the diagnosis of rejection becomes increasingly accurate when additional echocardiographic parameters are impaired (Figure 2) [17].

Tissue Doppler imaging parameters are generally useful to improve the accuracy of diastolic function assessment. However, in heart transplant patients, the role of myocardial velocities should be interpreted with caution because they may be affected by increased translational motion of the transplanted heart [18].

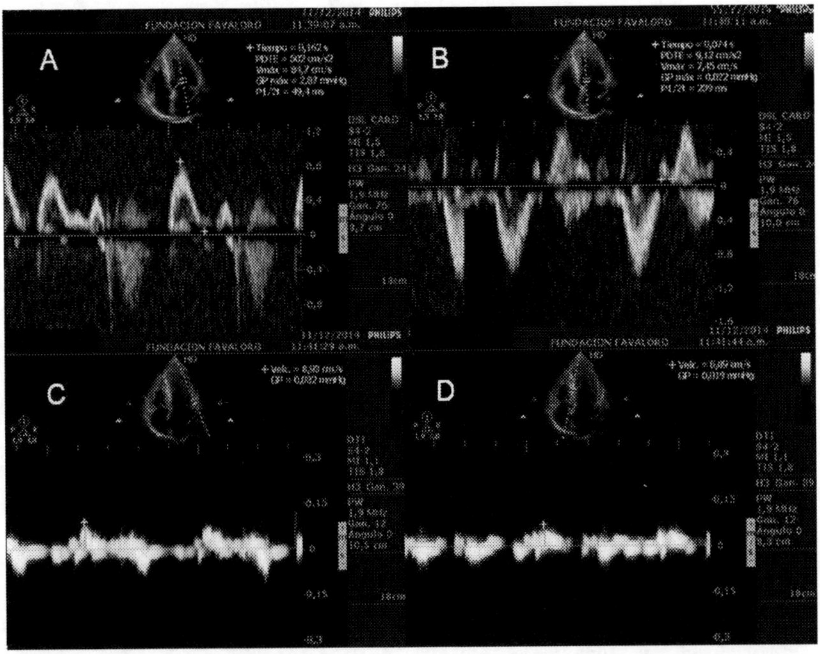

Figure 2. Pseudo-normal diastolic pattern. A. E/A ratio = 2. B. Short isovolumetric relaxation time. C. and D. Reduction of tissue Doppler imaging waves velocities.

In these patients, left ventricular e' and s' wave velocities tend to be low in the first few weeks after transplantation and gradually increase thereafter. There is a strong association between reduced e' wave velocity and graft rejection episodes in some reports [19, 20]. Therefore, due to the high specificity of tissue Doppler imaging parameters, severe rejection could be safely excluded in the presence of a mitral annular wave velocity >8.7 cm/s or < 10% reduction in diastolic mitral annular motion velocities [21].

A study by Sun et al. found that pericardial effusion, isovolumetric relaxation time <90 milliseconds, mitral inflow E/A ratio >1.7, diameter of inferior vena cava, and duration of pulmonary vein atrial reversal were independently associated with rejection. Because the odds ratios were similar for all 5 predictors, a simplified model was developed based on the sum of the number of abnormal predictors present (0 to 5). The probability of rejection increased from 15.9%, in the absence of any predictor, to 39.7%, 52.0% and 71.1%, if 1, 2 or 3 predictors were present, respectively (Table 1) [22].

Table 1. Accuracy of different echocardiography techniques to detect acute graft rejection

	Patients/ Prevalence AGR	**Method (parameters cut-off value)**	**Gold standard (EMB grade)**	**Sensitivity (%)**	**Specificity (%)**	**NPV**
Puleo et al.	121 (13%)	PW-TDI(e′ of inferior wall <16 cm/s)	Grade ≥3A	76	88	96
Mankad et al.	78 (18%)	Color TDI (combined peak MV systolic and peak diastolic velocity <135 mm/s) (posterior wall tissue Doppler diastolic time-gradient integral <0.26)	Grade ≥1B	93 91	71 61	98 97
Stengel et al.	94 (20%)	PW-TDI (Aa of lateral MV annulus <8.7 cm/s)	Grade ≥3A	82	53	82
Dandel et al.	408 (39.9%)	Sm reduction >10%	Clinical relevant	88.3	94	93
Sun et al.	223 (37%) 183 (27%) 264 (29%)	2D and standard Doppler (≥2 among: PE, IVRT < 90 ms E/A >1.7). Post-OHT ≤6 months. Post-OHT >6 months PW-TDI (Aa of septal/lateral MV annulus <0.9 cm/s)	Grade ≥ 1B	57 60 67	54 93 49	68 86 78

Aa, peak late diastolic velocity; AGR, acute graft rejection; DTI, tissue Doppler Imaging; EMB, endomyocardial biopsy; IVRT, isovolumetric relaxation time; MV, mitral valve; NPV, negative predictive value; OHT, orthotropic heart transplantation; PE, pericardial effusion; PW, pulse wave; Sm, peak radial systolic velocity. (Data from Badano LP et al. European Association of Cardiovascular Imaging/Cardiovascular Imaging Department of the Brazilian Society of Cardiology recommendations for the use of cardiac imaging to assess and follow patients after heart transplantation. *Eur Heart J Cardiovasc Imaging*. 2015 Sep;16(9):919-48.)

Similarly, when peak systolic wave Doppler (s′ wave) is combined with peak diastolic e′ wave velocity (evaluated at lateral mitral annulus) the peak - to-peak mitral annular velocity is obtained. Values equal to or greater than 135 mm/s have a sensitivity of 93%, a specificity of 71% and a negative predictive value of 98% in excluding acute graft rejection [23].

Myocardial deformation imaging is especially useful for monitoring allograft function because strain and strain rate data are independent of overall cardiac motion which is usually more pronounced in heart transplant patients [24]. It also has the ability to discriminate between active and passive myocardial motion [25, 26]. Two-dimensional transthoracic speckle-tracking echocardiography is a non-invasive modality that has shown utility in undifferentiated left ventricular hypertrophy, cardio-oncology, aortic stenosis, and ischemic heart disease (Figure 3).

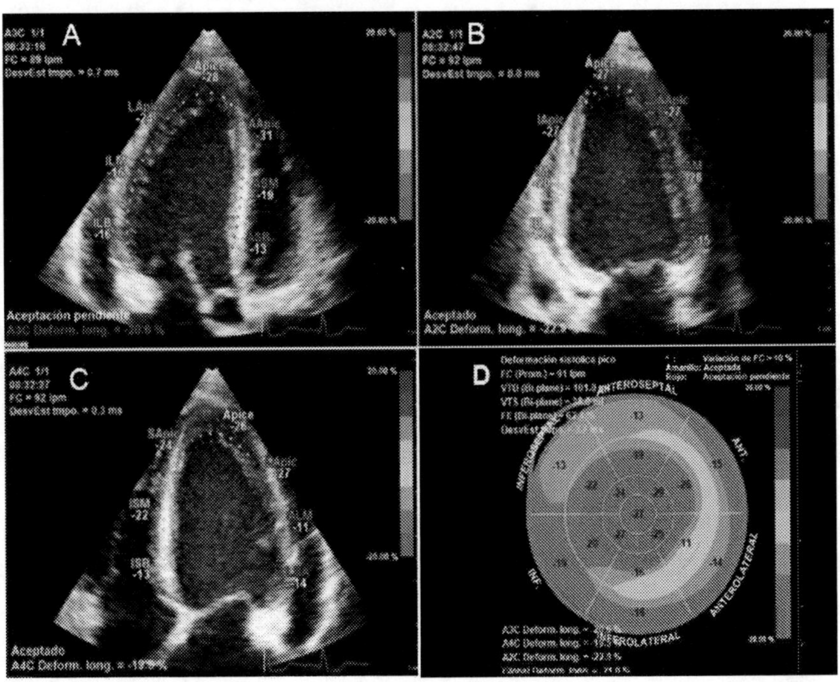

Figure 3. 2D Strain-Speckle Tracking, left ventricular global longitudinal strain on three conventional apical views. A. Apical long axis. B. Two-chamber. C. Four-chamber. D. Left ventricular segmental values of longitudinal strain displayed as numbers and parametric coloring on a bull's eye display.

It has been theorized that it may have a role as an alternative non-invasive imaging tool in screening heart transplant recipients for subclinical rejection [27-30]. Specifically, left ventricular global longitudinal strain assessed by speckle-tracking echocardiography allows detection of subclinical ventricular dysfunction, allowing prompt interventions [31-36]. A recent meta-analysis revealed an overall sensitivity and specificity for left ventricular global longitudinal strain in detecting acute rejection of 78% and 68%, respectively [24]. These results may support its use as a non-invasive imaging modality in routine surveillance of post-heart transplant rejection.

To summarize, a thorough baseline echocardiographic study should be obtained at 6 months from heart transplantation with careful quantification of cardiac chambers size, right ventricular systolic function, systolic and diastolic parameters of left ventricular function, and pulmonary artery pressure. Subsequent echocardiographic studies should be interpreted in comparison with the data obtained from this reference study. An echocardiographic study that shows no change from the baseline study, has a high negative predictive value for graft rejection. However, there is no single systolic or diastolic parameter that can be reliably used to diagnose rejection. Instead, when several parameters are abnormal, the probability of rejection increases. This is why careful revision of images of the present and baseline study (side-by-side) is highly recommended [10, 37].

Cardiac Allograft Vasculopathy

Cardiac allograft vasculopathy (CAV) is an obliterative and diffuse form of vasculopathy that can be considered a late complication of heart transplantation. According to the registry of the International Society for Heart and Lung Transplantation (ISHLT), the prevalence is 7.6% at the first year, 29.2% at 5 years and 47.2% at 10 years, and is a limiting factor in survival [38]. From the pathophysiological point of view, CAV is a different disease from coronary atherosclerosis, it is a concentric myointimal thickening of the distal epicardial arteries and small vessels that is characterized by endothelial injury, proliferation of vascular cells, fibrosis and remodeling, all triggered by immune and non-immune factors. Given the denervation of the cardiac allograft, CAV can occur silently, even in those cases where progression is rapid, especially in the early stages of the disease.

Angiography remains the gold standard for diagnosis, particularly when combined with intravascular ultrasound or optical coherence tomography, and is used to annually evaluate heart transplant patients, even in the absence of left ventricular dysfunction or symptoms [39]. CAV is currently classified according to the ISHLT criteria, which are based on angiographic findings and evidence of graft dysfunction (See Chapter 12) [40]. However, angiography is an invasive method with potential complications, such as contrast-induced nephropathy and procedure-related vascular injury. In addition, heart transplant recipients are a fragile population, often with renal dysfunction, due to pre-transplantation cardiorenal syndromes and nephrotoxic immunosuppressive regimens [41]. Non-invasive imaging methods, including echocardiography, are trying to achieve comparable accuracy to angiography in detecting CAV and could represent an alternative to angiography in those patients who have contraindications to it.

Unlike its usefulness in detecting acute graft rejection, resting echocardiography has low sensitivity and specificity for detecting CAV, particularly in mild forms. However, some indirect parameters may lead to suspicion of this entity: LVEF impairment, wall motion abnormalities, diastolic dysfunction, and tissue Doppler and myocardial deformation abnormalities, especially left ventricular global longitudinal strain [42].

Left Ventricular Ejection Fraction

LVEF is often at the upper normal limit and is generally preserved, even in advanced forms of CAV, making it unsuitable as an early marker of disease. In one study, patients with severe forms of CAV were characterized by lower LVEF values and a higher prevalence of grade 2 and 3 diastolic dysfunction compared to less severe forms of the disease (52% vs. 62%, $p< 0.05$, and 75% vs. 11%, $p< 0.05$ respectively) [43]. As a general concept, in the first years after heart transplantation, the reduction in LVEF is usually related to graft rejection, while in later stages it may be due to progression of CAV.

Diastolic Dysfunction

The diastolic function of the transplanted heart usually presents a bimodal course. In the very early phase, relevant alterations can be observed, even in the absence of acute rejection or CAV, and may be related to peri-operative inflammation or reperfusion injury. These changes usually fade after the first month. In a later phase, worsening of diastolic function is usually due to rejection or development and/or progression of CAV. This bimodal pattern was not fully considered in the current ISHLT classification of CAV, as a restrictive filling pattern is used in the CAV 3 category regardless of the time of observation [40].

Abnormalities in Wall Motion

The appearance of new regional wall motion abnormalities should make us suspect the presence or progression of CAV. In a prospective study in heart transplant patients, only the appearance of new wall motion abnormalities had a high specificity (69 to 100%) for the diagnosis of CAV [39]. However, these findings also have their limitations, as they can sometimes develop in the absence of CAV or acute rejection, usually in a diffuse pattern, especially several years after heart transplantation.

Tissue Doppler Imaging

Tissue Doppler imaging is used to measure the velocity of myocardial motion at the level of the basal septum and the lateral mitral ring. Compared to wall motion abnormalities, it constitutes an early detector of ventricular dysfunction and, indirectly, of the detection of CAV. Different studies have evaluated this method for the diagnosis of CAV, with different results according to the gold standard technique used for comparison. A series of heart transplant patients without wall motion abnormalities, found that a septal s' wave ≤10cm/s had a sensitivity of 90% for the identification of patients with angiographically and/or by IVUS detectable CAV, however, when considering the detection of focal stenosis >50% in main epicardial coronary arteries, even lower s' septal values (≤9 cm/s) reached only a sensitivity of 51% [44, 45]. These apparently misleading differences of the s' wave could be due to changes in left ventricle afterload, time since transplantation and differences in translational movement of the allograft (especially in the biatrial technique), as they affect the velocities of movement of the wall, varying greatly from patient to patient and thus influencing Tissue Doppler imaging parameters [45].

Left Ventricular Global Longitudinal Strain

Regarding deformation parameters, the left ventricular global longitudinal strain is less dependent on heart rate and loading conditions than LVEF and other diastolic indices. Endomyocardial fibers are predominantly longitudinally oriented and represent the most susceptible to ischemia, either macrovascular or microvascular (Figure 3). For the detection of CAV, the global value (left ventricular global longitudinal strain) is more important than the regional one. Several studies have shown a correlation between a reduced absolute value of global longitudinal strain and the presence of CAV and coronary microvascular dysfunction, especially when combined with tissue Doppler imaging. A study by Clemmensen et al. in 178 heart transplant patients with a prevalence of CAV of 38.8%, found a significant correlation between the degree of CAV (CAV 0 to 3) and the reduction in global longitudinal strain, even with preserved LVEF [46]. Another small study of 34 heart transplant patients (12 with CAV) excluding grade 3 CAV, found that layer-specific left ventricular global longitudinal strain as well as endocardial-epicardial longitudinal strain gradient predicted CAV. Strain values were significantly reduced in the presence of CAV in each myocardial layer, but in particular in the endocardial-epicardial gradient (- 4.15 ± 1.6 vs. - 1.7 ± 0.4% $p < .0001$) which was highly predictive of CAV (area under the receiver operating characteristic curve [AUC] 0.97). Among diastolic parameters, E wave deceleration time and mean E/e' ratio were also positively associated with CAV [47].

Stress Echocardiography

The latest ISHLT guidelines recommend dobutamine or treadmill stress echocardiography for the evaluation of CAV in patients who cannot undergo invasive testing, such as patients with impaired renal function (Recommendation Class IIa, Level of Evidence B) [40].

In the general population, of the functional tests evocative of ischemia, the exercise stress echocardiography by semisupine bicycle or treadmill is the most widely used. However, due to denervation and alterations in the chronotropic response of heart transplant patients, physical exercise would not be adequate for the detection of myocardial ischemia. Therefore, pharmacological stress echocardiography is preferred in this population.

However, a small study comparing exercise stress testing with dobutamine pharmacological stress, highlighted that exercise may still represent a more efficient stressor compared to dobutamine in transplant patients who prefer and are able to perform an exercise stress test [48].

Dobutamine Stress Echocardiography

Regarding pharmacological agents, dobutamine stress echocardiography is the most used. Unfortunately, the target heart rate (85% of the maximum rate expected for the patient's age) may not be easily achieved in some patients, even if the test is sensitized with the additional use of atropine.

Nevertheless, the role of dobutamine stress echocardiography in the diagnosis of CAV is controversial, especially in its early stages. Different studies report different results depending on the method used for CAV detection (intravascular ultrasound, angiography or both) and the grade of CAV. A recent meta-analysis that included 749 heart transplant patients confirmed a limited sensitivity (60.2%) of this technique in detecting CAV, despite a higher specificity (85.7%) [49, 50]. Perhaps more important is the prognostic value of the test, a positive test was predictive of cardiac events or death at a 4-year follow-up, while a negative test has a low risk of events [51].

An alternative method to improve sensitivity can be quantitative analysis using strain parameters. A prospective study of 42 patients concluded that a peak systolic strain rate <0.5/s had a sensitivity of 88% for detecting CAV, including diffuse irregularities, and thus could added to standard dobutamine stress echocardiography as a non-invasive method to detect CAV (Figure 4) [52].

Dipyridamole Stress Echocardiography

Another option for pharmacological stress echocardiography is the use of dipyridamole. Although some studies demonstrated good sensitivity and specificity of dipyridamole stress echocardiology in the detection of CAV, dobutamine stress echocardiography still represents the first option.

Dipyridamole stress echocardiography can be used to non-invasively assess coronary flow reserve (the vasodilation of the coronary circulation in the face of increased oxygen demand). This is done by evaluating the stress/rest ratio of the diastolic peak flow of the anterior descending artery taken in its mid-distal portion, adding an integrated evaluation of epicardial artery stenosis and microcirculation to the visual evaluation of wall motion. In normal hearts, a value less than or equal to 2 is considered abnormal. In heart transplant patients, one study reported that coronary flow reserve ≤2.7 showed good accuracy for detecting CAV (87% specificity and 82% sensitivity) [53]. In addition, a value equal to or less than 2.9 correlated with a maximum intimal thickness ≥0.5 mm assessed by intravascular ultrasound, with a sensitivity of 80%, a specificity of 100%, and a negative predictive value of 89% [54].

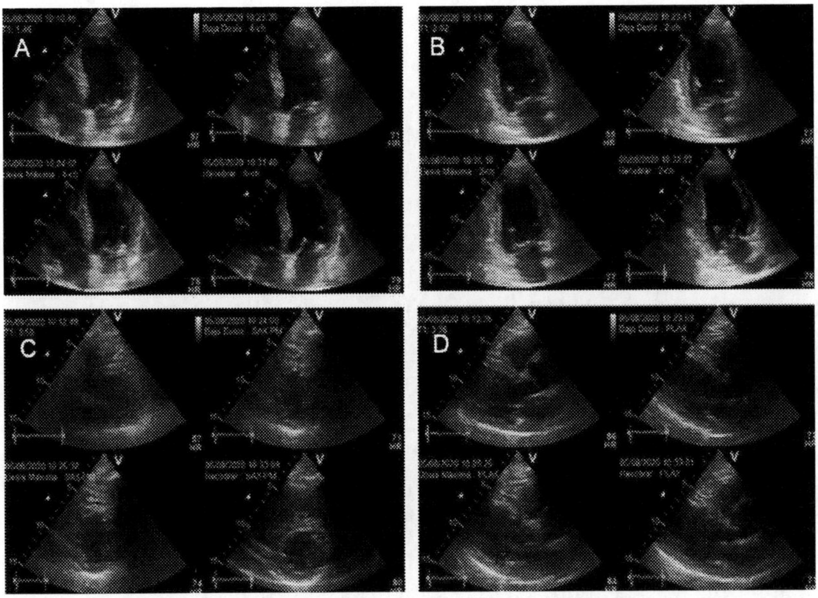

Figure 4. Dobutamine Stress Echocardiography. Images are compared at baseline, low dose, peak dose and recovery. A. Apical four chambers. B. Apical two chambers. C. Parasternal short axis. D. Parasternal long axis.

Dipyridamole can also be combined with dobutamine stress echocardiography, integrating coronary flow reserve with the parameters commonly assessed. A 5-year follow-up study shows that annual coronary flow reserve measurements together with dobutamine stress echocardiography can be used to detect CAV with high sensitivity (77.8%) and specificity (87.2%). which makes it possible to identify patients who would benefit from an invasive study [55].

Contrast Use in Stress Echocardiography

Myocardial perfusion studies by echocardiography with specific ultrasonic contrast allow better definition of the endocardial borders to evaluate wall motion disorders, improving sensitivity. However, this is a time-consuming procedure that requires specific software and is not widely used [10].

Conclusion

Follow-up of heart transplant patients is challenging as they can present with multiple complications, including acute graft rejection and cardiac allograft vasculopathy. The gold standard techniques for diagnosing these entities are invasive and potentially hazardous. In contrast, echocardiography is a useful non-invasive method for the initial evaluation and follow-up of these patients. Different modalities such as strain, tissue Doppler imaging, and stress testing, are increasingly being used in this setting with good results. Dobutamine stress echocardiography could be a suitable alternative to routine coronary angiography to assess CAV in centers with adequate experience. Furthermore, coronary flow reserve and/or contrast infusion can be combined with this technique to improve its accuracy. Global longitudinal strain may aid in the detection of subclinical graft dysfunction, regardless of etiology, by comparing changes that occur during serial evaluations, and could be used in association with endomyocardial biopsy to characterize and monitor rejection. Therefore, knowledge about the usefulness and versatility of these tools is crucial for the correct approach to heart transplant patients.

References

[1] Feigenbaum H, Waldhausen JA, Hyde LP: Ultrasound diagnosis of pericardial effusion. *JAMA.* 1965 Mar 1;191:711-4.

[2] Barnard CN. Human heart transplantation. *Can Med Assoc J.* 1969 Jan 18;100(3):91-104.

[3] Hornick P, Rose M. Chronic rejection in the heart. *Methods Mol Biol.* 2006;333:131-44.

[4] Leone O, Gherardi S, Targa L, Pasanisi E, Mikus P, Tanganelli P, Maccherini M, Arpesella G, Picano E, Bombardini T. Stress echocardiography as a gatekeeper to donation in aged marginal donor hearts: anatomic and pathologic correlations of abnormal stress echocardiography results. J Heart Lung Transplant. 2009 Nov;28(11):1141-9.

[5] Johnson MR. Echocardiographic evaluation of the cardiac transplant recipient. What is normal? *Chest.* 1993 Jul;104(1):3-5. doi: 10.1378/chest.104.1.3. PMID: 8325095.

[6] Stehlik J, Edwards LB, Kucheryavaya AY, Aurora P, Christie JD, Kirk R, Dobbels F, Rahmel AO, Hertz MI. The Registry of the International Society for Heart and Lung Transplantation: twenty-seventh official adult heart transplant report--2010. *J Heart Lung Transplant.* 2010 Oct;29(10):1089-103.

[7] Costanzo MR, Dipchand A, Starling R, Anderson A, Chan M, Desai S, Fedson S, Fisher P, Gonzales-Stawinski G, Martinelli L, McGiffin D, Smith J, Taylor D, Meiser B, Webber S, Baran D, Carboni M, Dengler T, Feldman D, Frigerio M, Kfoury A, Kim D, Kobashigawa J, Shullo M, Stehlik J, Teuteberg J, Uber P, Zuckermann A, Hunt S, Burch M, Bhat G, Canter C, Chinnock R, Crespo-Leiro M, Delgado R, Dobbels F, Grady K, Kao W, Lamour J, Parry G, Patel J, Pini D, Towbin J, Wolfel G, Delgado D, Eisen H, Goldberg L, Hosenpud J, Johnson M, Keogh A, Lewis C, O'Connell J, Rogers J, Ross H, Russell S, Vanhaecke J; International Society of Heart and Lung Transplantation Guidelines. The International Society of Heart and Lung Transplantation Guidelines for the care of heart transplant recipients. *J Heart Lung Transplant.* 2010 Aug;29(8):914-56.

[8] Valantine HA, Hatle LK, Appleton CP, Gibbons R, Popp RL. Variability of Doppler echocardiographic indexes of left ventricular filling in transplant recipients and in normal subjects. *J Am Soc Echocardiogr.* 1990 Jul-Aug;3(4):276-84.

[9] Gorcsan J 3rd, Snow FR, Paulsen W, Arrowood JA, Thompson JA, Nixon JV. Echocardiographic profile of the transplanted human heart in clinically well recipients. *J Heart Lung Transplant.* 1992 Jan-Feb;11(1 Pt 1):80-9.

[10] Badano LP, Miglioranza MH, Edvardsen T, Colafranceschi AS, Muraru D, Bacal F, Nieman K, Zoppellaro G, Marcondes Braga FG, Binder T, Habib G, Lancellotti P; Document reviewers. European Association of Cardiovascular Imaging/Cardiovascular Imaging Department of the Brazilian Society of Cardiology recommendations for the use of cardiac imaging to assess and follow patients after heart transplantation. *Eur Heart J Cardiovasc Imaging.* 2015 Sep;16(9):919-48.

[11] Goland S, Siegel RJ, Burton K, De Robertis MA, Rafique A, Schwarz E, Zivari K, Mirocha J, Trento A, Czer LS. Changes in left and right ventricular function of donor hearts during the first year after heart transplantation. *Heart.* 2011 Oct;97(20):1681-6.

[12] Angermann CE, Nassau K, Stempfle HU, Krüger TM, Drewello R, Junge R, Uberfuhr P, Weiss M, Theisen K. Recognition of acute cardiac allograft rejection from serial integrated backscatter analyses in human orthotopic heart transplant recipients. Comparison with conventional echocardiography. *Circulation.* 1997 Jan 7;95(1):140-50.

[13] Ciliberto GR, Mascarello M, Gronda E, Bonacina E, Anjos MC, Danzi G, Colombo P, Frigerio M, Alberti A, De Vita C. Acute rejection after heart transplantation: noninvasive echocardiographic evaluation. *J Am Coll Cardiol.* 1994 Apr;23(5):1156-61.

[14] Streeter RP, Nichols K, Bergmann SR. Stability of right and left ventricular ejection fractions and volumes after heart transplantation. *J Heart Lung Transplant.* 2005 Jul;24(7):815-8.

[15] Valantine HA, Appleton CP, Hatle LK, Hunt SA, Billingham ME, Shumway NE, Stinson EB, Popp RL. A hemodynamic and Doppler echocardiographic study of ventricular function in long-term cardiac allograft recipients. Etiology and prognosis of restrictive-constrictive physiology. *Circulation.* 1989 Jan;79(1):66-75.

[16] Yun KL, Niczyporuk MA, Daughters GT 2nd, Ingels NB Jr, Stinson EB, Alderman EL, Hansen DE, Miller DC. Alterations in left ventricular diastolic twist mechanics during acute human cardiac allograft rejection. *Circulation.* 1991 Mar;83(3):962-73.

[17] Ross HJ, Gullestad L, Hunt SA, Tovey DA, Puryear JB, McMillan A, Stinson EB, Valantine HA. Early Doppler echocardiographic dysfunction is associated with an increased mortality after orthotopic cardiac transplantation. *Circulation.* 1996 Nov 1;94(9 Suppl):II289-93.

[18] Aranda JM Jr, Weston MW, Puleo JA, Fontanet HL. Effect of loading conditions on myocardial relaxation velocities determined by Doppler tissue imaging in heart transplant recipients. *J Heart Lung Transplant.* 1998 Jul;17(7):693-7.

[19] Puleo JA, Aranda JM, Weston MW, Cintrón G, French M, Clark L, Fontanet HL. Noninvasive detection of allograft rejection in heart transplant recipients by use of Doppler tissue imaging. *J Heart Lung Transplant.* 1998 Feb;17(2):176-84.

[20] Dandel M, Hummel M, Müller J, Wellnhofer E, Meyer R, Solowjowa N, Ewert R, Hetzer R. Reliability of tissue Doppler wall motion monitoring after heart transplantation for replacement of invasive routine screenings by optimally timed cardiac biopsies and catheterizations. *Circulation.* 2001 Sep 18;104(12 Suppl 1):I184-91.

[21] Stengel SM, Allemann Y, Zimmerli M, Lipp E, Kucher N, Mohacsi P, Seiler C. Doppler tissue imaging for assessing left ventricular diastolic dysfunction in heart transplant rejection. *Heart.* 2001 Oct;86(4):432-7.

[22] Sun JP, Abdalla IA, Asher CR, Greenberg NL, Popović ZB, Taylor DO, Starling RC, Thomas JD, Garcia MJ. Non-invasive evaluation of orthotopic heart transplant rejection by echocardiography. *J Heart Lung Transplant.* 2005 Feb;24(2):160-5.

[23] Mankad S, Murali S, Kormos RL, Mandarino WA, Gorcsan J 3rd. Evaluation of the potential role of color-coded tissue Doppler echocardiography in the detection of allograft rejection in heart transplant recipients. *Am Heart J.* 1999 Oct;138(4 Pt 1):721-30.

[24] Dandel M, Hetzer R. Echocardiographic strain and strain rate imaging--clinical applications. *Int J Cardiol.* 2009 Feb 6;132(1):11-24.

[25] Gorcsan J 3rd, Tanaka H. Echocardiographic assessment of myocardial strain. *J Am Coll Cardiol.* 2011 Sep 27;58(14):1401-13.

[26] Dandel M, Knosalla C, Lehmkuhl H, Hetzer R. Non-Doppler two-dimensional strain imaging-clinical applications. *J Am Soc Echocardiogr.* 2007 Aug;20(8):1019.

[27] Elkaryoni A, Altibi AM, Khan MS, Okasha O, Ellakany K, Hassan A, Singh A, Qarajeh R, Mehta S, Nanda NC. Global longitudinal strain assessment of the left ventricle by speckle tracking echocardiography detects acute cellular rejection in orthotopic heart transplant recipients: A systematic review and meta-analysis. *Echocardiography.* 2020 Feb;37(2):302-309.

[28] Sera F, Kato TS, Farr M, Russo C, Jin Z, Marboe CC, Di Tullio MR, Mancini D, Homma S. Left ventricular longitudinal strain by speckle-tracking echocardiography is associated with treatment-requiring cardiac allograft rejection. *J Card Fail.* 2014 May;20(5):359-64.

[29] Du GQ, Hsiung MC, Wu Y, Qu SH, Wei J, Yin WH, Tian JW. Three-Dimensional Speckle-Tracking Echocardiographic Monitoring of Acute Rejection in Heart Transplant Recipients. *J Ultrasound Med.* 2016 Jun;35(6):1167-76.

[30] Ruiz Ortiz M, Peña ML, Mesa D, Delgado M, Romo E, Santisteban M, Puentes M, López Granados A, Castillo JC, Arizón JM, de Lezo JS. Impact of asymptomatic acute cellular rejection on left ventricle myocardial function evaluated by means of two-dimensional speckle tracking echocardiography in heart transplant recipients. *Echocardiography.* 2015 Feb;32(2):229-37.

[31] Mingo-Santos S, Moñivas-Palomero V, Garcia-Lunar I, Mitroi CD, Goirigolzarri-Artaza J, Rivero B, Oteo JF, Castedo E, González-Mirelis J, Cavero MA, Gómez-Bueno M, Segovia J, Alonso-Pulpón L. Usefulness of Two-Dimensional Strain Parameters to Diagnose Acute Rejection after Heart Transplantation. *J Am Soc Echocardiogr.* 2015 Oct;28(10):1149-56.

[32] Clemmensen TS, Løgstrup BB, Eiskjær H, Poulsen SH. Serial changes in longitudinal graft function and implications of acute cellular graft rejections during the first year after heart transplantation. *Eur Heart J Cardiovasc Imaging.* 2016 Feb;17(2):184-93.

[33] Clemmensen TS, Løgstrup BB, Eiskjær H, Poulsen SH. Changes in longitudinal myocardial deformation during acute cardiac rejection: the clinical role of two-dimensional speckle-tracking echocardiography. *J Am Soc Echocardiogr.* 2015 Mar;28(3):330-9.

[34] Ambardekar AV, Alluri N, Patel AC, Lindenfeld J, Dorosz JL. Myocardial strain and strain rate from speckle-tracking echocardiography are unable to differentiate asymptomatic biopsy-proven cellular rejection in the first year after cardiac transplantation. *J Am Soc Echocardiogr.* 2015 Apr;28(4):478-85.

[35] Podrouzkova H, Bedanova H, Tretina M, Korinek J, Stepanova R, Hruskova J, Nemec P, Konecny T, Orban M. Decrease in longitudinal strain in heart transplant recipients is associated with rejection. *Biomed Pap Med Fac Univ Palacky Olomouc Czech Repub.* 2015 Dec;159(4):601-6.

[36] Antończyk K, Niklewski T, Antończyk R, Zakliczyński M, Zembala M, Kukulski T. Speckle-Tracking Echocardiography for Monitoring Acute Rejection in Transplanted Heart. *Transplant Proc.* 2018 Sep;50(7):2090-2094.

[37] Sade LE, Hazirolan T, Kozan H, Ozdemir H, Hayran M, Eroglu S, Pirat B, Sezgin A, Muderrisoglu H. T1 Mapping by Cardiac Magnetic Resonance and Multidimensional Speckle-Tracking Strain by Echocardiography for the Detection of Acute Cellular Rejection in Cardiac Allograft Recipients. *JACC Cardiovasc Imaging.* 2019 Aug;12(8 Pt 2):1601-1614.

[38] Khush KK, Cherikh WS, Chambers DC, Goldfarb S, Hayes D Jr,, Kucheryavaya AY, Levvey BJ, Meiser B, Rossano JW, Stehlik J; International Society for Heart and Lung Transplantation. The International Thoracic Organ Transplant Registry

of the International Society for Heart and Lung Transplantation: Thirty-fifth Adult Heart Transplantation Report-2018; Focus Theme: Multiorgan Transplantation. *J Heart Lung Transplant*. 2018 Oct;37(10):1155-1168.

[39] Thorn EM, de Filippi CR. Echocardiography in the cardiac transplant recipient. *Heart Fail Clin.* 2007 Jan;3(1):51-67.

[40] Mehra MR, Crespo-Leiro MG, Dipchand A, Ensminger SM, Hiemann NE, Kobashigawa JA, Madsen J, Parameshwar J, Starling RC, Uber PA. International Society for Heart and Lung Transplantation working formulation of a standardized nomenclature for cardiac allograft vasculopathy-2010. *J Heart Lung Transplant.* 2010 Jul;29(7):717-27.

[41] González-Vílchez F, Vázquez de Prada JA. Chronic renal insufficiency in heart transplant recipients: risk factors and management options. *Drugs.* 2014 Sep;74(13):1481-94.

[42] Sciaccaluga C, Ghionzoli N, Mandoli GE, Sisti N, D'Ascenzi F, Focardi M, Bernazzali S, Vergaro G, Emdin M, Valente S, Cameli M. The role of non-invasive imaging modalities in cardiac allograft vasculopathy: an updated focus on current evidences. *Heart Fail Rev.* 2021 Aug 12.

[43] Daud A, Xu D, Revelo MP, Shah Z, Drakos SG, Dranow E, Stoddard G, Kfoury AG, Hammond MEH, Nativi-Nicolau J, Alharethi R, Miller DV, Gilbert EM, Wever-Pinzon O, McKellar SH, Afshar K, Khan F, Fang JC, Selzman CH, Stehlik J. Microvascular Loss and Diastolic Dysfunction in Severe Symptomatic Cardiac Allograft Vasculopathy. *Circ Heart Fail.* 2018 Aug;11(8):e004759.

[44] Störk S, Behr TM, Birk M, Uberfuhr P, Klauss V, Spes CH, Angermann CE. Assessment of cardiac allograft vasculopathy late after heart transplantation: when is coronary angiography necessary? *J Heart Lung Transplant.* 2006 Sep; 25(9): 1103-8.

[45] Dandel M, Hetzer R. Post-transplant surveillance for acute rejection and allograft vasculopathy by echocardiography: Usefulness of myocardial velocity and deformation imaging. *J Heart Lung Transplant.* 2017 Feb;36(2):117-131.

[46] Clemmensen TS, Løgstrup BB, Eiskjær H, Poulsen SH. Evaluation of longitudinal myocardial deformation by 2-dimensional speckle-tracking echocardiography in heart transplant recipients: relation to coronary allograft vasculopathy. *J Heart Lung Transplant.* 2015 Feb;34(2):195-203.

[47] Sciaccaluga C, Mandoli GE, Sisti N, Natali MB, Ibrahim A, Menci D, D'Errico A, Donati G, Benfari G, Valente S, Bernazzali S, Maccherini M, Mondillo S, Cameli M, Focardi M. Detection of cardiac allograft vasculopathy by multi-layer left ventricular longitudinal strain in heart transplant recipients. *Int J Cardiovasc Imaging.* 2021 May;37(5):1621-1628.

[48] Gebska MA, Williford NN, Schadler AJ, Laxson C, Alvarez P, Briasoulis A, Cadaret LM, Yumul-Non IKT, Kerber RE, Weiss RM. Pharmacological vs Exercise Stress Echocardiography for Detection of Cardiac Allograft Vasculopathy. *Mayo Clin Proc Innov Qual Outcomes.* 2020 Jan 8;4(1):65-75.

[49] Elkaryoni A, Abu-Sheasha G, Altibi AM, Hassan A, Ellakany K, Nanda NC. Diagnostic accuracy of dobutamine stress echocardiography in the detection of

cardiac allograft vasculopathy in heart transplant recipients: A systematic review and meta-analysis study. *Echocardiography.* 2019 Mar;36(3):528-536.

[50] Derumeaux G, Redonnet M, Mouton-Schleifer D, Bessou JP, Cribier A, Saoudi N, Koning R, Soyer R, Letac B. Dobutamine stress echocardiography in orthotopic heart transplant recipients. VACOMED Research Group. *J Am Coll Cardiol.* 1995 Jun;25(7):1665-72.

[51] Bacal F, Moreira L, Souza G, Rodrigues AC, Fiorelli A, Stolf N, Bocchi E, Bellotti G, Ramires JA. Dobutamine stress echocardiography predicts cardiac events or death in asymptomatic patients long-term after heart transplantation: 4-year prospective evaluation. *J Heart Lung Transplant.* 2004 Nov;23(11):1238-44.

[52] Eroglu E, D'hooge J, Sutherland GR, Marciniak A, Thijs D, Droogne W, Herbots L, Van Cleemput J, Claus P, Bijnens B, Vanhaecke J, Rademakers F. Quantitative dobutamine stress echocardiography for the early detection of cardiac allograft vasculopathy in heart transplant recipients. *Heart.* 2008 Feb;94(2):e3.

[53] Tona F, Caforio AL, Montisci R, Angelini A, Ruscazio M, Gambino A, Ramondo A, Thiene G, Gerosa G, Iliceto S. Coronary flow reserve by contrast-enhanced echocardiography: a new noninvasive diagnostic tool for cardiac allograft vasculopathy. *Am J Transplant.* 2006 May;6(5 Pt 1):998-1003.

[54] Tona F, Osto E, Tarantini G, Gambino A, Cavallin F, Feltrin G, Montisci R, Caforio AL, Gerosa G, Iliceto S. Coronary flow reserve by transthoracic echocardiography predicts epicardial intimal thickening in cardiac allograft vasculopathy. *Am J Transplant.* 2010 Jul;10(7):1668-76.

[55] Sade LE, Eroğlu S, Yüce D, Bircan A, Pirat B, Sezgin A, Aydınalp A, Müderrisoğlu H. Follow-up of heart transplant recipients with serial echocardiographic coronary flow reserve and dobutamine stress echocardiography to detect cardiac allograft vasculopathy. *J Am Soc Echocardiogr.* 2014 May;27(5):531-9.

Chapter 11

Cardiac Allograft Rejection: Diagnosis and Treatment

Elian Facundo Giordanino[1,*], Karin Padros[2] and Carlos Vigliano[3]

[1]Heart Failure and Heart Transplantation, Favaloro Foundation University Hospital, Buenos Aires, Argentina

[2]Histocompatibility, PRICAI-Favaloro Foundation University Hospital, Buenos Aires, Argentina

[3]Pathology department, Favaloro Foundation University Hospital, Buenos Aires, Argentina

Abstract

Heart transplantation remains the gold standard treatment for advanced heart failure. However, despite great advances in this therapy, graft rejection continues to be one of the most delicate complications to address to ensure survival. In order to overcome this problem, adequate diagnosis, monitoring, classification and treatment of different types of graft rejection are of enormous importance.

Keywords: heart transplantation, antibodies, graft rejection

Introduction

Heart transplantation remains the gold standard treatment for advanced heart failure [1]. However, graft rejection continues to be one of the most delicate complications to address to ensure survival. The first human heart transplant was performed on December 3, 1967 by Dr. Christiaan Barnard at the Groote Schuur Hospital, in Cape Town, South Africa. The recipient was a

---

* Corresponding Author's E-mail: efgiordanino@ffavaloro.org.

54-year-old male patient with end-stage ischemic cardiomyopathy, Louis Washkansky, who survived 18 days after transplantation [2]. After that, different attempts were made to achieve better results, but the outcome was always the same: some patients survived the surgery, but died within the first few weeks. At first it was thought that the short survival was due to surgical complications, but later it was understood that one of the main problems was graft rejection. In the 1970s, heart transplantation was being abandoned as a procedure due to poor results and few operations were performed around the world. It was not until 1980, with the introduction of cyclosporine, that this technique was reconsidered and the era of heart transplantation began around the world. Therefore, since the beginnings of heart transplantation, adequate immunosuppression is essential to achieve good results. Nevertheless, although there have been some advances in the management of immunosuppressive therapy in heart transplantation, graft rejection continues to be one of the main causes of death, not only in the early stages after heart transplantation (acute humoral and cellular rejection), but also in the later stages in the form of cardiac allograft vasculopathy (chronic rejection).

Regarding the current impact of cardiac allograft rejection on survival, the thirty-sixth adult heart transplantation report of the International Thoracic Organ Transplant Registry of the International Society for Heart and Lung Transplantation (ISHLT) describes that approximately 10% of deaths in the first 3 years after heart transplantation are due to acute rejection and approximately another 10% in the late stage due to cardiac allograft vasculopathy (chronic rejection) [3]. These numbers would probably be bigger if we took into account that many "graft failures" in the early period are, in fact, undiagnosed graft rejections (Figure 1).

As it was mentioned above, there are different types of rejection and they can be divided according to their time of onset in hiperacute, acute and chronic and according to their immune mechanism in cellular, humoral or antibody mediated rejection (AMR) and mixed rejection. Hiperacute rejection is rare nowadays due to the advances in the detection of preformed antibodies against human leukocyte antigen (HLA) before heart transplantation and due to improvements in the immunosuppressive regimens in the early postoperative period as described in Chapter 9. Chronic rejection in heart transplantation takes the form of cardiac allograft vasculopathy and will be discussed in Chapter 12.

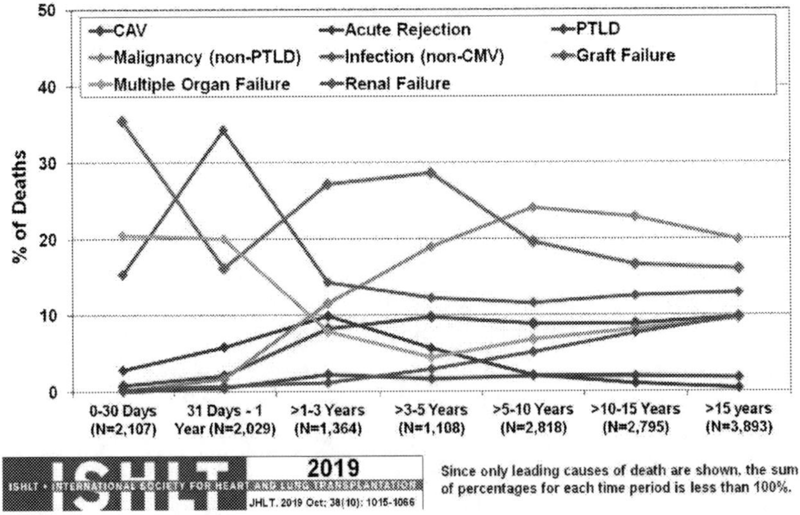

Figure 1. Relative incidence of leading causes of death in adult heart transplant recipients (January 2010 - June 2018). CAV, cardiac allograft vasculopathy; PTLD, post-transplant lymphoproliferative disorders; CMV, Cytomegalovirus. (Data from ISHLT. 2019. *Adult Heart Transplantation Statistics*. Accessed 20 Dec 2021. https://ishltregistries.org/registries/slides.asp).

Despite maintaining an adequate immunosuppressive therapy in heart transplant recipients, cardiac allograft rejection is still prevalent and not only increases the death rates of these patients but also causes major comorbidities. On the other hand, treatment of rejection is not without consequences, since it predisposes to infections and malignancies [4]. Therefore, it is crucial to promptly and adequately detect cardiac allograft rejection and to treat it accordingly.

Diagnosis and Classification of Cardiac Allograft Rejection

The main obstacle to organ transplantation from one individual to another of the same species (allograft) is the immunological rejection of the transplanted tissue. Rejection is a complex phenomenon involving cell-mediated hypersensitivity reactions and antibodies that destroy the graft. The main antigenic differences between a donor and recipient that result in rejection of transplants are differences in HLA alleles [5].

Following transplantation, the recipient's T-cells recognize donor antigens from the graft by direct and indirect allorecognition pathways. In the direct pathway, host T-cells directly recognize allogeneic (donor) HLA molecules that are expressed on graft cells. In the indirect pathway, host CD4+ T-cells recognize donor HLA molecules after they are taken up, processed, and presented by the host's own antigen presenting cells [6]. B-cells also recognize antigens in the graft, including HLA and other antigens that differ between donor and recipient. Activation of these B-cells typically requires T-cell collaboration [7]. Therefore, the pathogenesis of acute cardiac allograft rejection involves cell-mediated and antibody-mediated immunologic mechanisms of action.

Acute Cellular Rejection

This type of rejection Is most commonly seen within the initial months after transplantation. Classic cellular rejection is characterized by interstitial lymphocytic inflammation with associated cardiomyocyte damage with a histology resembling myocarditis. CD8+ T-cells and an inflammatory reaction in the graft triggered by cytokines secreted by activated CD4+ T cells are a major component of the reaction. The inflammatory response generates an increase in vascular permeability and an accumulation of mononuclear cells (lymphocytes and macrophages) and occasionally eosinophils. Myocyte damage in milder rejection is often characterized by myocytolysis, without signs of coagulation necrosis. The presence of cardiomyocyte injury is frequently accompanied by invasion of inflammatory cells at the perimeter, resulting in irregular cardiomyocyte borders, partial or complete replacement, or distortion of normal myocardial architecture [8].

Antibody-Mediated Rejection

Since Hammond's work and over the past 30 years, the understanding of AMR has evolved to become a recognized clinical complication in the management of heart transplant recipients [9, 10].

AMR occurs under conditions of recipient presensitization to donor antigens or due to anti-donor antibodies produced after transplantation. In recipients not previously sensitized to donor antigens, exposure to HLA class I and class II antigens form the donor graft may elicit antibodies production.

Antibodies formed by the recipient may cause injury by several mechanisms, including complement-dependent cytotoxicity, inflammation, and antibody-dependent cell-mediated cytotoxicity. The initial target of these antibodies in rejection seems to be the graft vasculature, eventually producing allograft dysfunction and failure, acceleration of cardiac allograft vasculopathy, and, thus, decreased survival [11].

Cardiac Allograft Vasculopathy (Chronic Vascular Rejection)

Cardiac allograft vasculopathy is the single most important long-term limitation to heart transplant survival. It is a late, progressive, diffusely stenosing intimal proliferation of the coronary arteries that leads to ischemic injury [12].

Within 5 years of transplantation, 50% of patients develop significant cardiac allograft vasculopathy, and virtually all patients have lesions within 10 years. The pathogenesis of this entity involves immunological responses that induce local production of growth factors that promote recruitment and proliferation of intimal smooth muscle cell together with extracellular matrix synthesis. Cardiac allograft vasculopathy is a particularly vexing problem because it can lead to silent myocardial infarction as recipients have denervated hearts and do not experience angina. It can also lead to progressive heart failure or sudden cardiac death (See Chapter 12) [13].

Endomyocardial Biopsy

Endomyocardial biopsy (EMB) is the gold standard for monitoring rejection in heart transplant patients, with high diagnostic sensitivity and specificity for acute cellular rejection [14]. Other non-invasive tests that help diagnose graft rejection are discussed in Chapter 10. Endomyocardial tissue samples from the right interventricular septum are obtained through a bioptome introduced from the jugular or femoral vein [15, 16]. All patients are followed up with surveillance biopsies according to the protocols of each center (See Chapter 14). For pathology examination and diagnosis, tissue samples are fixed in 10% buffered formaldehyde and embedded in Histowax. Four to 5 μm sections of each endomyocardial biopsy are then routinely stained with Hematoxylin-eosin.

Histologic Diagnosis and Grading of Acute Cellular Rejection

In 1990, the ISHLT proposed an international grading system for cardiac allograft biopsies [17]. It should be noted that this grading system was defined in biopsies from patients generally receiving triple-drug immunosupressive therapy with steroids, cyclosporine and azathioprine. Since then, immunosuppressive regimens and the incidence of rejection have changed, and the histology of rejection may have changed as well. In the follow-up revision of the 2004 ISHLT nomenclature and diagnostic criteria, detailed histopathologic features and immunopathologic criteria were proposed (Table 1) [18].

Table 1. Acute cellular rejection classification

2004	**1990**	
Grade		
0	0	No rejection
1R	1A	Focal perivascular or interstitial infiltrate without myocyte damage
	1B	Diffuse infiltrate without myocyte damage
	2	One focus of infiltrate with myocyte damage
2R	3A	Multifocal infiltrate with myocyte damage
3R	3B	Diffuse infiltrate with myocyte damage
	4	Diffuse polymorphous infiltrate with extensive myocyte damage, edema, hemorrhage and/or vasculitis

(Data from Stewart S et al. Revision of the 1990 working formulation for the standardization of nomenclature in the diagnosis of heart rejection. *J Heart Lung Transplant*. 2005 Nov;24(11):1710-20.)

Grade 0 R (no rejection)

In Grade 0 R there is no evidence of mononuclear (lymphocytes/macrophages) inflammation or myocyte damage (Figure 2A)

Grade 1 R (mild, low-grade rejection)

Mild or low-grade rejection may manifest in one of two ways: (1) Perivascular and/or interstitial mononuclear cells (lymphocytes/histiocytes) are present. In general, these cells respect myocyte borders, do not invade adjacent myocytes, and do not distort the normal architecture (Figure 2B). A focus of mononuclear cells with associated myocyte damage may be present (Figure 2C).

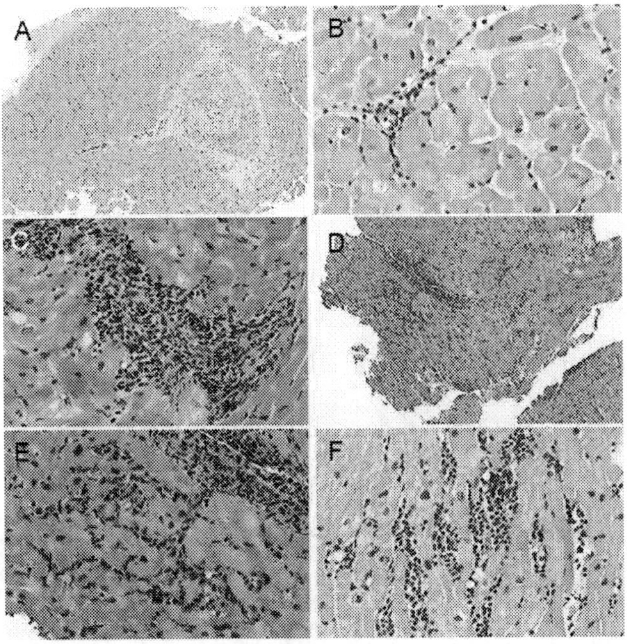

Figure 2. Acute cellular rejection. A. Grade 0 B. Grade 1R C. Grade 1R (Grade 2 ISHLT 1990) D. and E. Grade 2R. F. Grade 3R.

Grade 2 R (moderate, intermediate-grade rejection)

In Grade 2 R two or more foci of mononuclear cells (lymphocytes/macrophages) are present with associated myocyte damage. Eosinophils may also be present. The foci may be distributed in one or more than one biopsy fragment (Figure 2D and E).

Grade 3 R (severe, high-grade rejection)

A diffuse inflammatory process, either predominantly lymphocytes and macrophages or a polymorphous infiltrate, is present, involving multiple biopsy fragments. In most cases, the majority of biopsy fragments are involved, although the intensity of the infiltrate may vary between pieces. Multiple areas of associated cardiomyocyte damage are present. In the most severe forms of cellular (and humoral) rejection, edema, interstitial hemorrhage and vasculitis may be present (Figure 2F).

Acute Antibody-Mediated (Humoral) Rejection

The morphologic findings demonstrated on routine hematoxylin and eosin-stained tissue sections include endothelial cell enlargement or swelling and accumulations of macrophages within the lumens of capillaries and small vessels of the myocardial interstitium (Figure 3A and B).

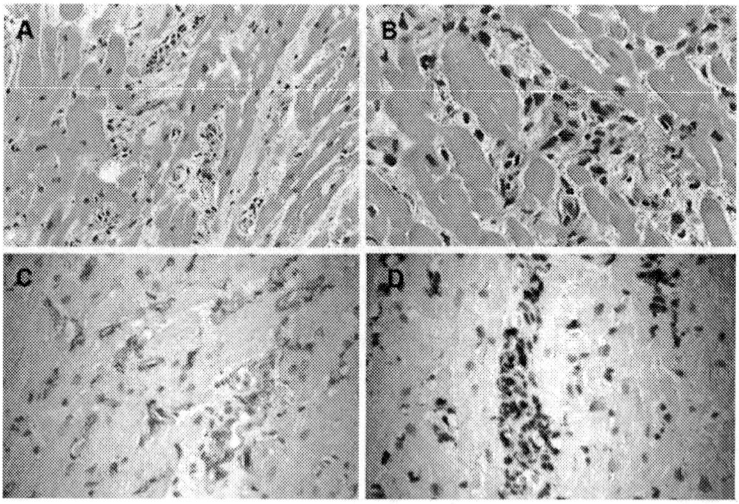

Figure 3. Antibody-mediated rejection. A. and B. Hematoxylin-eosin staining C. C4d immunohistochemistry staining D. CD68 immunohistochemistry staining.

The immunopathologic features of AMR are based on immune-histochemical evaluation of formalin-fixed, paraffin-embedded EMB [19]. Determination of C4d staining is evaluated only in interstitial capillaries and is considered positive when there is a multifocal/diffuse distribution of more than 50% (Figure 3C). The presence of more than 10% of the sample of intravascular macrophages by CD68 staining is considered positive (Figure 3D).

Pathologic grading and reporting of cardiac AMR according the 2013 ISHLT consensus are shown in Table 2 [20].

Mixed cellular and AMR rejection is defined as the presence of cellular infiltrates of cellular rejection and the histopathologic and/or immunopathologic characteristics of AMR in the EMB specimen. Each EMB sample should be evaluated and graded separately for cellular rejection and AMR according to the established ISHLT criteria [18, 20].

Table 2. Antibody-mediated rejection classification

Grade	Definition	Description
pAMR 0	No AMR	H and I studies negative
pAMR 1 (H+)	H AMR alone	H findings present
pAMR 1 (I+)	I AMR alone	I findings present
pAMR 2	Pathologic AMR	H and I findings both present
pAMR 3	Severe pathologic AMR	Interstitial hemorrhage, capillary fragmentation, mixed inflammatory infiltrates, endothelial cell pyknosis or karyorrhexis, and marked edema. I findings are also present

AMR, antibody-mediated rejection; H, histologic; I, immunopathologic. (Data from Berry GJ et al. The 2013 International Society for Heart and Lung Transplantation Working Formulation for the standardization of nomenclature in the pathologic diagnosis of antibody-mediated rejection in heart transplantation. *J Heart Lung Transplant*. 2013 Dec;32(12):1147-62.)

Anti-HLA Antibodies

Even though patient selection and immunosuppressive treatment has greatly improved in time, every transplant is at risk of graft loss. The presence of donor-specific alloantibodies (DSA), either existing at the time of transplantation or arising *de novo* after transplantation, is a risk factor for antibody mediated rejection (AMR) and potentially allograft loss in almost all types of organ transplants [21-23]. Ideally, all DSA should be avoided, although this is not always achieved. Instead, the transplant team must estimate the risk of AMR in each situation.

The goal of this overview is to present general recommendations to study the pre- and post-transplant alloantibody status in candidates for heart transplant using solid phase assays and crossmatch (XM) testing.

Patients awaiting heart transplantation who carry antibodies against human leukocyte antigens are disadvantaged because they must wait longer for an organ from an appropriate matched donor and they also have an increased risk of rejection. The number of sensitized patients in waiting lists has been increasing, probably due to the use of mechanical circulatory support devices. Patients with panel reactive antibody (PRA) of more than 10% have been shown to be at risk for earlier rejection as well as worse survival [24, 25]. Besides, patients who are not pre-sensitized can produce DSA after transplantation, which is associated with worse outcomes. In the post-heart transplant setting, there is large evidence proving the detrimental effects of DSA on outcomes such as rejection, cardiac allograft vasculopathy (CAV), and survival [26-28]. DSA can bind HLA on heart allograft endothelial cells and induce cytotoxicity by activating complement system as well as through other effector mechanisms, increasing risk of AMR, CAV and decreasing survival.

Antibody screening has become the most frequent pretransplant evaluation aiming to identify recipients at risk of graft rejection [29]. Antigens corresponding with antibodies detected pre-transplant should be listed as not acceptable and candidates should not receive organs from donors expressing these antigens. There is, however, some concern in defining the anti-HLA antibodies that are clinically relevant. If we restrict the pool of acceptable donors because of the presence of irrelevant antibodies, that could unfairly lead to longer times on waitlists, increasing the risk of death. Low-level DSA detected on solid-phase tests are postulated to be less dangerous than higher level DSA, and then, they should not always be viewed as an obstacle to transplantation. In fact, studies in kidney and heart transplantation show acceptable outcomes for recipients transplanted with low-level DSA [30]. Numerous factors must be considered to decide whether there is an immunologic barrier to transplantation.

In this section we describe different methods for detecting DSA to assess pre-transplant risk and post-transplant monitoring. There are several HLA antibody screening methods, with varying sensitivities, specificities, and clinical usefulness. They can be used pre-transplant to assess for sensitization and risk of AMR, post-transplant for DSA monitoring, and for monitoring the efficacy of desensitization therapy.

Detecting Donor-Specific Antibodies and Crossmatching

In the earliest era of solid organ transplantation, cross matching based on complement dependent cytotoxicity (CDC) was used for detecting cytotoxic DSAs. Although clinically relevant, CDC crossmatch lacks specificity, has low sensitivity, and requires viable donor lymphocytes. Furthermore, an acceptable correlation between CDC results and clinical outcomes has not been well described. Then, tests more sensitive than CDC, such as flow cytometry crossmatch (FXCM) and solid phase assays using purified HLA antigens, have been developed (Table 3).

Table 3. Methods for detecting donor-specific antibodies and crossmatching

Method	Target	Antibody specificity	Sensitivity	Effects of medications	Comments
CDC	Lymphocytes (donor)	Donor-specific complement-binding Ab	Low Only complement binding Ab	Influenced by cytotoxic Ab (ATG, rituximab)	Prevention of HAR or early AMR
FCXM	Lymphocytes (donor)	Donor-specific complement-binding/ nonbinding Ab	High Both complement binding and nonbinding Ab	Influenced by Ab therapies (high-dose IVIG, ATG, rituximab)	Prevention of HAR or early AMR
SP LUMINEX PHENOTYPE	Purified HLA antigens	Known HLA Ab	High Both complement binding and nonbinding Ab	Influenced by Ab therapies (high-dose IVIG)	Detection and specification of HLA Ab
SP LUMINEX SINGLE ANTIGEN	Purified HLA antigens	Known HLA Ab Non-HLA Ab	High Both complement binding and nonbinding Ab	Influenced by Ab therapies (high-dose IVIG)	Comprehensive specification of HLA Ab

Ab, antibodies; AMR, antibody mediated rejection; ATG, Antithymocyte globulin; CDC, complement-dependent cytotoxicity; FCXM, flow cytometry crossmatching; HAR, hyperacute rejection; HLA, human leukocyte antigens; IVIG, intravenous immunoglobulin; SP, solid-phase. (Data from Tait BD et al. Consensus guidelines on the testing and clinical management issues associated with HLA and non-HLA antibodies in transplantation. Transplantation. 2013 Jan 15;95(1):19-47 and Nunoda S. Impact of pretransplant antibodies on outcomes after heart transplantation. *Curr Opin Organ Transplant*. 2019 Jun;24(3):220-226.).

Cell Based Assays

CDC cross matching was developed by Terasaki and colleagues in the 1960s [31]. The assay involves reacting patient serum with donor T and B lymphocytes, adding rabbit complement, and visualizing cell damage caused by the antigen-antibody reactions. A cytotoxic reaction suggests the presence of complement-fixing DSA against donor HLA. Although highly clinically relevant, the CDC assay is nonspecific because it cannot distinguish between anti HLA Class I or Class II antibodies and has low sensitivity. Furthermore, CDC crossmatch requires viable donor lymphocytes, a condition that is not always accessible in heart transplantation.

Nowadays, crossmatching is often performed by flow cytometry. This method, first described in 1983, involves reacting patient serum with donor lymphocytes and adding a fluorescent-labeled anti human immunoglobulin secondary antibody to label the antibodies bound to lymphocytes, and finally running them through a flow cytometer [32]. The level of fluorescence detected is proportional to the amount of antibody bound to the cell. Markers with different fluorochromes are also added to separate T and B cell reactivity. This is important because class I anti HLA antibodies bind both T and B cells, whereas antibodies against class II antigens usually bind only B cells. This assay is more sensitive than CDC for detecting DSA, and has been proven useful in identifying patients with weak DSA who are at increased risk of AMR and graft rejection [33-35]. This method also reduces the subjectivity and inter-observer variability associated with CDC-XM because it is reported as a mean channel shift rather than a positive or negative result based on visual interpretation. Negative CDC crossmatches suggest that the DSA titer is low or of a type that does not activate the complement system. Positive T Cell flow crossmatch suggests that there is a DSA to a class I antigen while positive B cell crossmatch may be due to the same class I antibody or due to other antibodies directed against either class I or II (Table 4).

Flow cytometry assays are difficult to standardize due to variability among cytometers, fluorochromes, antiglobulin reagents, and variations in cell-to-serum ratios. The flow cytometry B-cell XM is associated with high background antibody binding, which may be reduced by incubation of target lymphocytes with Pronase. However, Pronase treatment may affect HLA expression and lead to false-positive T-cell XM [36]. Each center must therefore validate FCXM result thresholds with respect to its clinical risk.

Table 4. Flow cytometry crossmatch interpretation

T CELL	B CELL	XM INTERPRETATION
NEGATIVE	NEGATIVE	NEGATIVE
POSITIVE	POSITIVE	POSITIVE
NEGATIVE	WEAK POSITIVE	POSSIBLE WEAK CLASS I OR CLASS II
NEGATIVE	POSITIVE	PROBABLY CLASS II
POSITIVE	NEGATIVE	NON-HLA SPECIFIC
WEAK POSITIVE	WEAK POSITIVE	POSSIBLE WEAK CLASS I

HLA, human leukocyte antigens; XM, crossmatch.

The XM is considered the final test to determine the safety to decide transplantation. Nowadays, sensitive single antigen beads (SAB) assays have made the virtual crossmatch possible. When SAB testing is completely negative in a patient who has not had a sensitizing event, XM testing is not probably useful to AMR risk assessment. The XM result is most important when there is SAB positivity.

In order to confirm the presence of anti-HLA antibodies as the cause of the positive flow cytometry crossmatch antibody specificity should be determined by Luminex testing. This will also provide some information regarding the antibody levels.

Solid Phase Based Assays

Advances in screening for HLA antibodies have yielded solid-phase, multiplex testing platforms with better sensitivity and specificity than traditional cell-based assays. Currently, these tests are performed mainly by Luminex. The main advantages of this technology are the high specificity and sensitivity, semi-quantitation, and multiplexing capability. Commercial kits come in three formats according to their targets: (i) screening assays, where antigens are pooled from multiple cell lines, (ii) phenotype beads, carrying panels of individual class I or class II phenotypes, (iii) single antigen beads or SAB, consisting of panels of HLA class I or class II antigens, where each bead population is coated with multiple copies of a single recombinant antigen (Figure 4). Screening assays are used for detecting HLA class I or II antibodies and monitoring changes in antibody levels. Phenotype beads are used to determine how broadly sensitized a patient is before transplant, giving the percentage of panel reactive antibodies. SAB tests are used for assessing antibody specificity and level.

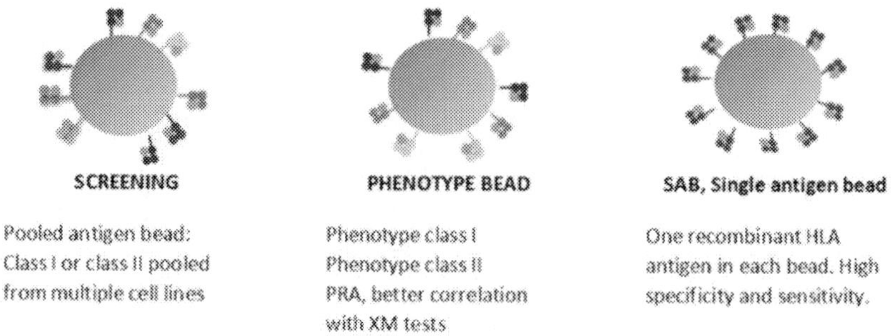

Figure 4. Solid phase-based assays. HLA, human leukocyte antigens; PRA, panel reactive antibody; SAB, single antigen beads; XM, crossmatch.

To estimate the antibody level, the mean fluorescence intensity (MFI) of the reporter signal is used. However, its value is only a semi-quantitative measure of strength, distinct from antibody titer [37]. Conventional solid-phase assays do not discriminate between complement-fixing and non-complement-fixing antibodies. Therefore, the MFI intensity may not always correlate with the antibodies' cytotoxic capacity since not all the antibodies at high concentration may be detrimental to graft function. Several studies have suggested that assessing antibodies for the ability to bind the Complement protein C1q can help differentiate pathogenic from non-pathogenic DSA [38, 28]. Complement activation is an important mechanism by which DSA leads to allograft damage. Commercially available modified SAB tests have been developed to specifically detect C1q and C3d binding, which represents the presence of DSA of a complement-fixing subtype of IgG at enough level to bind complement. Some groups routinely use these tests to distinguish the most deleterious DSA, although it is not yet universally performed.

Knowledge of antibodies specificity can be used in virtual crossmatch to avoid transplantation with organs from donors carrying the HLA reactive antigens. In this way, when patients are sensitized before heart transplant the use of this approach is recommended to identify the specificity of anti-HLA antibodies at high levels in the recipient to prevent the acceptance of organs with those specific antigens. Although the threshold of antibody binding strength that absolutely might rule out transplantation is still unknown, levels between 1000 and 5000 MFI are commonly set as an upper limit to accept a heart donor [29]. At present, it is strongly recommended to define the immunological risk of patients waiting for heart transplantation with SAB technology (Luminex) because of its high sensitivity and specificity for the detection of anti-HLA antibodies [39]. The transplant team, together with their histocompatibility consultant, should define the HLA antigens to be avoided in the donor because of anti-HLA antibodies specific to those antigens present in the patient serum. Finally, they can consider additional assays like C1q or C3d to estimate the immunological risk of the recipient.

Circulating antibodies need to be periodically monitored while awaiting heart transplantation. Furthermore, this is very important in the post-transplantation setting, to detect *de novo* DSA since circulating DSAs in heart transplant recipients have been associated with graft survival, development of AMR and CAV [40]. There is evidence that *de novo* DSAs (mainly anti-HLA class II DQ) are linked to increased graft loss and mortality. Appearance of DSAs during the first year and later has shown to have a negative impact on long term outcome [41, 42].

DSA monitoring by SAB tests after heart transplant provides a relatively early diagnostic marker of rejection before the allograft becomes damaged. The presence of *de novo* DSAs has been found to be a good diagnostic indicator and predictor of antibody-mediated rejection, CAV and acute allograft dysfunction, with a particularly prominent effect observed when antibodies target HLA-DQ antigens, the most commonly formed DSA [43-45].

In conclusion, since the development of lymphocyte cytotoxicity tests in the 1960s by Terasaki et al. antibodies have been known to affect post-transplant outcomes. The solid-phase assay (Luminex platform) which involves fixing purified HLA antigens onto microbeads, allows identification of specific anti-HLA antibodies in the pre- and post-transplant stages. Anti-HLA antibodies should be periodically monitored in patients that are in organ waiting lists and after transplantation in order to detect the production of *de novo* DSA.

Treatment of Cardiac Allograft Rejection

The treatment of graft rejection depends on the type of rejection (cellular, AMR or mixed rejection), the clinical status of the patient and the functional compromise of the graft. There are different drugs and procedures that are used to treat graft rejection and, although there are some general principles and guidelines on different treatment regimens, there is no universal consensus on the best treatment in each setting, and different schemes are used in different institutions [4]. This is mainly due to the lack of randomized trials to assess the usefulness of one regimen over the others.

When evaluating a patient with suspected rejection it is important to assess whether immunosuppressive therapy was being taken correctly. If this is the case, in addition to treating the acute episode, baseline oral immunosuppression should be increased in order to avoid future graft rejections. In the event that immunosuppressive therapy is not being taken correctly, the decision to increase baseline immunosuppression should be made on an individual basis and the patient should be carefully re-educated on correct medication intake. Additionally, if the patient is on cyclosporine, it should be switched to tacrolimus and if they are on azathioprine, it should be switched to mycophenolate, whenever possible.

It is also important to note that in all endomyocardial biopsies with acute cellular rejection, immunohistochemical staining should be performed to rule out concomitant AMR. Additionally, approximately 7-10 days after the adequate treatment of the acute event, an endomyocardial biopsy should be performed to control that the patient no longer has graft rejection.

Acute Cellular Rejection

Most of the time, grade 1R acute cellular rejection grade 1R (2004 ISHLT classification) should be treated only by increasing baseline oral immunosuppression in case it was being taken correctly, however, there are some particular situations that may require further treatment options. If the endomyocardial biopsy shows one focus of infiltrate with associated myocyte damage (Grade 2 of the 1990 ISHLT classification) and the patient has undergone transplantation in the last 6 months, an oral bolus of steroids (such as prednisone) with progressive tapering could be considered. Furthermore, if the patient has symptoms of heart failure or reduced ejection fraction on echocardiographic assessment, intravenous bolus of corticosteroids should be used, such as methylprednisolone at a dose of 1 gram per three days (750 milligrams if low body mass index) [46]. Additionally, careful surveillance should be implemented, since in these cases in which there is clinical or echocardiographic compromise it should be taken into account that the endomyocardial biopsy could be underdiagnosing a grade 2R rejection if the histological involvement is patched, because only a few samples are taken during the procedure.

In the event of grade 2R acute cellular rejection, 1 gram of an intravenous bolus of methylprednisolone for three days is preferred. In some centers, if the patient has undergone transplantation more than 6 months before acute rejection, there is no clinical or echocardiographic compromise, and strict surveillance can be performed, the treatment could be limited to oral corticosteroids and increased baseline oral immunosuppression, especially in the case of a history of recurrent infections or malignancy [46, 47].

In the case of 3R acute cellular rejection there is general consensus that 1 gram of an intravenous bolus of methylprednisolone for three days is the preferred treatment. Furthermore, anti-thymocyte globulin (ATG) or other more aggressive therapies could be considered in the case of severe echocardiographic compromise or severe heart failure [47].

Finally, it is important to highlight that if the patient has severe hemodynamic compromise, independently of the result of the endomyocardial biopsy, or even if the result is not yet available, methylprednisolone, ATG, plasmapheresis and intravenous immune globulin (IVIG) should be used to avoid further deterioration.

Antibody Mediated Rejection

There are different options to treat AMR and there is no general consensus of the combination of these therapies for each grade of AMR. Therefore, when treating AMR, it is important to consider the advantages and disadvantages of each of these strategies [48, 4]. Additionally, since these regimens cause severe immunosuppression, concomitant antimicrobial prophylaxis should be considered.

Anti-Thymocyte Globulin

ATG are polyclonal antibodies against the T-cell lymphocyte (or "thymocyte"). Although it has primarily anti-T cell effects, it can also inhibit the interaction of CD4+ helper T cells with B cells, thereby decreasing B-cell activation. The standard dose for this indication is 1-1.5 milligram per Kilogram per day for 3 to 5 days [4]. Thrombocytopenia and lymphocytopenia may occur, so platelet and lymphocyte counts should be monitored. The CD3 count can be useful for tailoring ATG therapy, as there is some evidence that if CD3s are below 50 cells/milliliter after a dose of ATG, the following dose can be skipped and still be considered as a day of effective treatment [49].

Plasmapheresis

Plasmapheresis removes circulating antibodies, mainly through plasma exchange, and is frequently used to treat AMR. It can be used from 1 to 5 sessions per week for 1 to 4 weeks. As it only removes antibodies without acting on the B-cells that produce them, it is used in combination with other therapies to prevent antibody rebound. It also removes other proteins from plasma, such as coagulation factors, which can predispose to bleeding [48, 4]. When used in combination with ATG, plasmapheresis should be performed prior to administration of ATG in order to avoid possible removal of the latter.

Intravenous Immunoglobulin

IVIG is a polyclonal preparation of pooled IgG antibodies. Its main effect can be attributed to the blockade of Fc-γ receptors, inhibition of the complement system, neutralization of autoantibodies and cytokines, and downregulation of the B-cell receptor. The usual dose is 1 gram per kilogram per day for 2 days, but there are other protocols [4]. It is generally used after completion of treatment with ATG and plasmapheresis and infectious complications are uncommon, but it can cause volume overload and reversible kidney injury [48].

Rituximab

Rituximab is a chimeric murine-human monoclonal antibody against the cell-marker CD20, which is present on B-cell lymphocytes. It is generally not used as default therapy for AMR, but rather for refractory AMR or when there is a high level of pathogenic DSA to prevent further compromise or recurrence [4].

Treatment Schemes

There is no universal treatment scheme for AMR, but one possible protocol that we use in our center includes treatment with 5 days of plasmapheresis and ATG (tailored by CD3/lymphocyte counts) concomitantly with 1 gram of an intravenous bolus of methylprednisolone for three days. After these initial 5 days, IVIG 1 gram per kilogram per day for 2 days. If there are also DSAs that persist after this treatment, Rituximab is considered. The aggressiveness of treatment depends on the clinical and echocardiographic status of the patient, the grade of AMR (AMR 1 or AMR ≥ 2) and the presence or absence of DSA [4, 48].

Mixed Rejection and Recurrent Rejection

Mixed rejection occurs when there is concomitant acute cellular rejection and AMR. Patients often have symptoms and even hemodynamic compromise; therefore, a combination of therapies is used. In general, treatment is similar to AMR $\geq$ 2, with corticosteroids, plasmapheresis, ATG, IVIG, with or without rituximab, but pharmacological or mechanical circulatory support may be necessary in severe cases.

In case of recurrent acute cellular rejection or corticosteroid-resistant rejection, ATG should be considered in conjunction with a significant increase in baseline oral immunosuppression.

Conclusion

Cardiac allograft rejection remains a major concern in the heart transplant recipient due to its prevalence and high morbidity and mortality despite current immunosuppression regimens. Proper diagnosis, classification and surveillance are of utmost importance to promptly detect and treat these patients. Although there are some general principles in the treatment of this condition, specific interventions should be evaluated on an individual basis.

References

[1] McDonagh TA, Metra M, Adamo M, Gardner RS, Baumbach A, Böhm M, Burri H, Butler J, Čelutkienė J, Chioncel O, Cleland JGF, Coats AJS, Crespo-Leiro MG, Farmakis D, Gilard M, Heymans S, Hoes AW, Jaarsma T, Jankowska EA, Lainscak M, Lam CSP, Lyon AR, McMurray JJV, Mebazaa A, Mindham R, Muneretto C, Francesco Piepoli M, Price S, Rosano GMC, Ruschitzka F, Kathrine Skibelund A; ESC Scientific Document Group. 2021 ESC Guidelines for the diagnosis and treatment of acute and chronic heart failure. *Eur Heart J*. 2021 Sep 21;42(36):3599-3726.

[2] Stolf NAG. History of Heart Transplantation: a Hard and Glorious Journey. *Braz J Cardiovasc Surg*. 2017 Sep-Oct;32(5):423-427.

[3] Khush KK, Cherikh WS, Chambers DC, Harhay MO, Hayes D Jr, Hsich E, Meiser B, Potena L, Robinson A, Rossano JW, Sadavarte A, Singh TP, Zuckermann A, Stehlik J; International Society for Heart and Lung Transplantation. The International Thoracic Organ Transplant Registry of the International Society for Heart and Lung Transplantation: Thirty-sixth adult heart transplantation report -

2019; focus theme: Donor and recipient size match. *J Heart Lung Transplant.* 2019 Oct;38(10):1056-1066.

[4] Colvin MM, Cook JL, Chang P, Francis G, Hsu DT, Kiernan MS, Kobashigawa JA, Lindenfeld J, Masri SC, Miller D, O'Connell J, Rodriguez ER, Rosengard B, Self S, White-Williams C, Zeevi A; American Heart Association Heart Failure and Transplantation Committee of the Council on Clinical Cardiology; American Heart Association Heart Failure and Transplantation Committee of the Council on Cardiopulmonary Critical Care, Perioperative and Resuscitation; American Heart Association Heart Failure and Transplantation Committee of the Council on Cardiovascular Disease in the Young; American Heart Association Heart Failure and Transplantation Committee of the Council on Clinical Cardiology, Council on Cardiovascular and Stroke Nursing; American Heart Association Heart Failure and Transplantation Committee of the Council on Cardiovascular Radiology and Intervention; American Heart Association Heart Failure and Transplantation Committee of the Council on Cardiovascular Surgery and Anesthesia. Antibody-mediated rejection in cardiac transplantation: emerging knowledge in diagnosis and management: a scientific statement from the American Heart Association. *Circulation.* 2015 May 5;131(18):1608-39.

[5] Gras S, Kjer-Nielsen L, Chen Z, Rossjohn J, McCluskey J. The structural bases of direct T-cell allorecognition: implications for T-cell-mediated transplant rejection. *Immunol Cell Biol.* 2011 Mar;89(3):388-95.

[6] Siu JHY, Surendrakumar V, Richards JA, Pettigrew GJ. T cell Allorecognition Pathways in Solid Organ Transplantation. *Front Immunol.* 2018 Nov 5;9:2548.

[7] Chong AS. B cells as antigen-presenting cells in transplantation rejection and tolerance. *Cell Immunol.* 2020 Mar;349:104061.

[8] Laguens RP, Meckert PM, Martino JS, Perrone S, Favaloro R. Identification of programmed cell death (apoptosis) in situ by means of specific labeling of nuclear DNA fragments in heart biopsy samples during acute rejection episodes. *J Heart Lung Transplant.* 1996 Sep;15(9):911-8.

[9] Hammond EH, Yowell RL, Nunoda S, Menlove RL, Renlund DG, Bristow MR, Gay WA Jr, Jones KW, O'Connell JB. Vascular (humoral) rejection in heart transplantation: pathologic observations and clinical implications. *J Heart Transplant.* 1989 Nov-Dec;8(6):430-43.

[10] Manfredini V, Leone O, Agostini V, Potena L. Antibody-mediated rejection in heart transplantation: new developments and old uncertainties. *Curr Opin Organ Transplant.* 2017 Jun;22(3):207-214.

[11] Su JA, Baxter-Lowe LA, Kantor PF, Szmuszkovicz JR, Menteer J. The clinical impact of donor-specific antibodies on antibody-mediated rejection and long-term prognosis after heart transplantation. *Curr Opin Organ Transplant.* 2019 Jun;24(3):245-251.

[12] Mehra MR, Crespo-Leiro MG, Dipchand A, Ensminger SM, Hiemann NE, Kobashigawa JA, Madsen J, Parameshwar J, Starling RC, Uber PA. International Society for Heart and Lung Transplantation working formulation of a standardized nomenclature for cardiac allograft vasculopathy-2010. *J Heart Lung Transplant.* 2010 Jul;29(7):717-27.

[13] Nikolova AP, Kobashigawa JA. Cardiac Allograft Vasculopathy: The Enduring Enemy of Cardiac Transplantation. *Transplantation.* 2019 Jul;103(7):1338-1348.

[14] Zerbe TR, Arena V. Diagnostic reliability of endomyocardial biopsy for assessment of cardiac allograft rejection. *Hum Pathol.* 1988 Nov;19(11):1307-14.

[15] Sakakibara S, Konno S. Endomyocardial biopsy. *Jpn Heart J.* 1962 Nov;3:537-43.

[16] Caves PK, Stinson EB, Graham AF, Billingham ME, Grehl TM, Shumway NE. Percutaneous transvenous endomyocardial biopsy. JAMA. 1973;225:288–291.

[17] Billingham ME, Cary NR, Hammond ME, Kemnitz J, Marboe C, McCallister HA, Snovar DC, Winters GL, Zerbe A. A working formulation for the standardization of nomenclature in the diagnosis of heart and lung rejection: Heart Rejection Study Group. The International Society for Heart Transplantation. *J Heart Transplant.* 1990 Nov-Dec;9(6):587-93.

[18] Stewart S, Winters GL, Fishbein MC, Tazelaar HD, Kobashigawa J, Abrams J, Andersen CB, Angelini A, Berry GJ, Burke MM, Demetris AJ, Hammond E, Itescu S, Marboe CC, McManus B, Reed EF, Reinsmoen NL, Rodriguez ER, Rose AG, Rose M, Suciu-Focia N, Zeevi A, Billingham ME. Revision of the 1990 working formulation for the standardization of nomenclature in the diagnosis of heart rejection. *J Heart Lung Transplant.* 2005 Nov;24(11):1710-20.

[19] Tan CD, Baldwin WM 3rd, Rodriguez ER. Update on cardiac transplantation pathology. *Arch Pathol Lab Med.* 2007 Aug;131(8):1169-91.

[20] Berry GJ, Burke MM, Andersen C, Bruneval P, Fedrigo M, Fishbein MC, GoddardM, Hammond EH, Leone O, Marboe C, Miller D, Neil D, Rassl D, Revelo MP, Rice A, Rene Rodriguez E, Stewart S, Tan CD, Winters GL, West L, Mehra MR, Angelini A. The 2013 International Society for Heart and Lung Transplantation Working Formulation for the standardization of nomenclature in the pathologic diagnosis of antibody-mediated rejection in heart transplantation. *J Heart Lung Transplant.* 2013 Dec;32(12):1147-62.

[21] Hidalgo LG, Campbell PM, Sis B, Einecke G, Mengel M, Chang J, Sellares J, Reeve J, Halloran PF. De novo donor-specific antibody at the time of kidney transplant biopsy associates with microvascular pathology and late graft failure. *Am J Transplant.* 2009 Nov;9(11):2532-41.

[22] Hodges AM, Lyster H, McDermott A, Rice AJ, Smith JD, Rose ML, Banner NR. Late antibody-mediated rejection after heart transplantation following the development of de novo donor-specific human leukocyte antigen antibody. *Transplantation.* 2012 Mar 27;93(6):650-6.

[23] Taner T, Stegall MD, Heimbach JK. Antibody-mediated rejection in liver transplantation: current controversies and future directions. *Liver Transpl.* 2014 May;20(5):514-27.

[24] Suciu-Foca N, Reed E, Marboe C, Harris P, Yu PX, Sun YK, Ho E, Rose E, Reemtsma K, King DW. The role of anti-HLA antibodies in heart transplantation. *Transplantation.* 1991 Mar;51(3):716-24.

[25] Michaels PJ, Espejo ML, Kobashigawa J, Alejos JC, Burch C, Takemoto S, Reed EF, Fishbein MC. Humoral rejection in cardiac transplantation: risk factors,

hemodynamic consequences, and relationship to transplant coronary artery disease. *J Heart Lung Transplant*. 2003 Jan;22(1):58-69.

[26] Smith JD, Banner NR, Hamour IM, Ozawa M, Goh A, Robinson D, Terasaki PI, Rose ML. De novo donor HLA-specific antibodies after heart transplantation are an independent predictor of poor patient survival. *Am J Transplant*. 2011 Feb;11(2):312-9.

[27] Tambur AR, Pamboukian SV, Costanzo MR, Herrera ND, Dunlap S, Montpetit M, Heroux A. The presence of HLA-directed antibodies after heart transplantation is associated with poor allograft outcome. *Transplantation.* 2005 Oct 27;80(8):1019-25.

[28] Zeevi A, Lunz J, Feingold B, Shullo M, Bermudez C, Teuteberg J, Webber S. Persistent strong anti-HLA antibody at high titer is complement binding and associated with increased risk of antibody-mediated rejection in heart transplant recipients. *J Heart Lung Transplant*. 2013 Jan;32(1):98-105.

[29] Kobashigawa J, Colvin M, Potena L, Dragun D, Crespo-Leiro MG, Delgado JF, Olymbios M, Parameshwar J, Patel J, Reed E, Reinsmoen N, Rodriguez ER, Ross H, Starling RC, Tyan D, Urschel S, Zuckermann A. The management of antibodies in heart transplantation: An ISHLT consensus document. *J Heart Lung Transplant.* 2018 May;37(5):537-547.

[30] Schinstock CA, Gandhi M, Cheungpasitporn W, Mitema D, Prieto M, Dean P, Cornell L, Cosio F, Stegall M. Kidney Transplant With Low Levels of DSA or Low Positive B-Flow Crossmatch: An Underappreciated Option for Highly Sensitized Transplant Candidates. *Transplantation.* 2017 Oct;101(10):2429-2439.

[31] Patel R, Terasaki PI. Significance of the positive crossmatch test in kidney transplantation. N Engl J Med. 1969 Apr 3;280(14):735-9.

[32] Garovoy MRRM, Bigos M, Perkins H, Colombe BFN, Salvatierra O. Flow cytometry análisis: A high technology crossmatch technique facilitating transplantation. *Transplant. Proc*. 1983;XV:1939.

[33] Bryan CF, Baier KA, Nelson PW, Luger AM, Martinez J, Pierce GE, Ross G, Shield CF 3rd, Warady BA, Aeder MI, Helling TS, Muruve N. Long-term graft survival is improved in cadaveric renal retransplantation by flow cytometric crossmatching. *Transplantation.* 1998 Dec 27;66(12):1827-32.

[34] Limaye S, O'Kelly P, Harmon G, O'Neill D, Dorman AM, Walshe J, Donohoe J, Little D, Conlon PJ, Keogan MT. Improved graft survival in highly sensitized patients undergoing renal transplantation after the introduction of a clinically validated flow cytometry crossmatch. *Transplantation.* 2009 Apr 15;87(7):1052-6.

[35] Couzi L, Araujo C, Guidicelli G, Bachelet T, Moreau K, Morel D, Robert G, Wallerand H, Moreau JF, Taupin JL, Merville P. Interpretation of positive flow cytometric crossmatch in the era of the single-antigen bead assay. *Transplantation.* 2011 Mar 15;91(5):527-35.

[36] Hetrick SJ, Schillinger KP, Zachary AA, Jackson AM. Impact of pronase on flow cytometric crossmatch outcome. *Hum Immunol*. 2011 Apr;72(4):330-6.

[37] Tambur AR, Herrera ND, Haarberg KM, Cusick MF, Gordon RA, Leventhal JR, Friedewald JJ, Glotz D. Assessing Antibody Strength: Comparison of MFI, C1q, and Titer Information. *Am J Transplant.* 2015 Sep;15(9):2421-30.

[38] Loupy A, Lefaucheur C, Vernerey D, Prugger C, Duong van Huyen JP, Mooney N, Suberbielle C, Frémeaux-Bacchi V, Méjean A, Desgrandchamps F, Anglicheau D, Nochy D, Charron D, Empana JP, Delahousse M, Legendre C, Glotz D, Hill GS, Zeevi A, Jouven X. Complement-binding anti-HLA antibodies and kidney-allograft survival. *N Engl J Med*. 2013 Sep 26;369(13):1215-26.

[39] Pajaro OE, George JF. On solid-phase antibody assays. *J Heart Lung Transplant.* 2010 Nov;29(11):1207-9.

[40] Mangiola M, Marrari M, Feingold B, Zeevi A. Significance of Anti-HLA Antibodies on Adult and Pediatric Heart Allograft Outcomes. *Front Immunol.* 2017 Jan 27;8:4.

[41] Tran A, Fixler D, Huang R, Meza T, Lacelle C, Das BB. Donor-specific HLA alloantibodies: Impact on cardiac allograft vasculopathy, rejection, and survival after pediatric heart transplantation. *J Heart Lung Transplant.* 2016 Jan;35(1):87-91.

[42] Fine NM, Daly RC, Shankar N, Park SJ, Kushwaha SS, Gandhi MJ, Pereira NL. The role of donor-specific antibodies in acute cardiac allograft dysfunction in the absence of cellular rejection. *Transplantation*. 2014 Jul 27;98(2):229-38.

[43] Ho EK, Vlad G, Vasilescu ER, de la Torre L, Colovai AI, Burke E, Deng M, Schwartz J, Marboe C, Mancini D, Opelz G, Suciu-Foca N. Pre- and posttransplantation allosensitization in heart allograft recipients: major impact of de novo alloantibody production on allograft survival. *Hum Immunol.* 2011 Jan;72(1):5-10.

[44] Ware AL, Malmberg E, Delgado JC, Hammond ME, Miller DV, Stehlik J, Kfoury A, Revelo MP, Eckhauser A, Everitt MD. The use of circulating donor specific antibodies to predict biopsy diagnosis of antibody-mediated rejection and to provide prognostic value after heart transplantation in children. *J Heart Lung Transplant.* 2016 Feb;35(2):179-85.

[45] Omrani O, Alawwami M, Buraiki J, Selimovic N. Donor-specific HLA-DQ antibodies may contribute to poor graft outcome after heart transplantation. *Ann Saudi Med.* 2018 Mar-Apr;38(2):97-104.

[46] Patel JK, Kittleson M, Kobashigawa JA. Cardiac allograft rejection. *Surgeon.* 2011 Jun;9(3):160-7.

[47] Costanzo MR, Dipchand A, Starling R, Anderson A, Chan M, Desai S, Fedson S, Fisher P, Gonzales-Stawinski G, Martinelli L, McGiffin D, Smith J, Taylor D, Meiser B, Webber S, Baran D, Carboni M, Dengler T, Feldman D, Frigerio M, Kfoury A, Kim D, Kobashigawa J, Shullo M, Stehlik J, Teuteberg J, Uber P, Zuckermann A, Hunt S, Burch M, Bhat G, Canter C, Chinnock R, Crespo-Leiro M, Delgado R, Dobbels F, Grady K, Kao W, Lamour J, Parry G, Patel J, Pini D, Towbin J, Wolfel G, Delgado D, Eisen H, Goldberg L, Hosenpud J, Johnson M, Keogh A, Lewis C, O'Connell J, Rogers J, Ross H, Russell S, Vanhaecke J; International Society of Heart and Lung Transplantation Guidelines. The International Society of Heart and Lung Transplantation Guidelines for the care of heart transplant recipients. *J Heart Lung Transplant.* 2010 Aug;29(8):914-56.

[48] Levine MH, Abt PL. Treatment options and strategies for antibody mediated rejection after renal transplantation. *Semin Immunol.* 2012 Apr;24(2):136-42.

[49] Krasinskas AM, Kreisel D, Acker MA, Bavaria JE, Pochettino A, Kotloff RM, Arcasoy S, Blumenthal N, Kamoun M, Moore JS, Rosengard BR. CD3 monitoring of antithymocyte globulin therapy in thoracic organ transplantation. *Transplantation.* 2002 Apr 27;73(8):1339-41.

Chapter 12

Diagnosis and Follow-Up of Cardiac Allograft Vasculopathy

Elian Facundo Giordanino*
Heart Failure and Heart Transplantation, Favaloro Foundation University Hospital, Buenos Aires, Argentina

Abstract

Long-term survival of heart transplantation is limited by chronic rejection in the form of cardiac allograft vasculopathy. Despite improvements in the field of immunosuppressive therapy, this entity continues to be the main cause of death in the late stages after heart transplantation. Therefore, it is important to understand its underlying mechanisms, diagnostic methods, classification, prognosis and potential treatments.

Keywords: heart transplantation, graft rejection, coronary vessels

Introduction

Heart transplantation is the treatment of choice for end-stage heart failure. Although it is truly a life-saving option that allows patients with a poor short-term survival to significantly increase their life expectancy, there might be complications that limit long-term results. When the first heart transplants were performed, the main limitation was acute graft rejection. The recipient's

* Corresponding Author's E-mail: elianfg@gmail.com.

In: Heart Transplantation
Editor: Elian Facundo Giordanino
ISBN: 978-1-68507-759-4

immune system recognized several antigens of the foreign organ eliciting a strong response that ended in a graft dysfunction not compatible with life. This was subsequently overcome with the advances in immunosuppressive therapy and the introduction of cyclosporine, which allowed good short- and medium-term results (See Chapter 11) [1]. However, the donor's heart is still a foreign body for the recipient that activates the immune response, and although acute rejection may be prevented or even treated with immunosuppressive therapy, chronic rejection in the form of cardiac allograft vasculopathy (CAV) may still occur and limit long-term survival. In fact, this is still one of the major problems in heart transplantation. The thirty-sixth adult heart transplantation report of the International Thoracic Organ Transplant Registry of the International Society for Heart and Lung Transplantation (ISHLT) states that approximately 10% of deaths in the late stage of heart transplantation are due to CAV [2]. Therefore, prevention, early detection, proper classification and prognosis estimation, and treatment of CAV are essential in the care of heart transplant recipients. This report also describes an increasing incidence of CAV of approximately 50% at 10 years. However, these numbers may also be secondary to improvements in diagnostic methods that allow earlier detection.

Pathogenesis and Risk Factors

The development of CAV involves multiple and complex mechanisms, some of them not yet fully understood. However, these mechanisms may be basically grouped into two categories: immunological and non-immunological.

Immunological mechanisms are the most important as CAV is ultimately a form of chronic rejection. The endothelial cells of the coronary arteries of the transplanted graft express class I human leukocyte antigen (HLA) molecules that are recognized by CD8+ T-cells. This leads to endothelial damage and the production of cytokines that subsequently activate endothelial cells and these cells express HLA class II molecules that interact with CD4+ T-cells. In addition, the local production of chemoquines recruits pro-inflammatory cells from the vessel wall and trigger the expression of adhesion molecules on the endothelial cells [3]. All of this impaired immune response to vascular injury causes smooth muscle proliferation, lipid deposition and accumulation of inflammatory cells, leading to intimal hyperplasia and fibrosis that progressively narrows the lumen of the vessel (Figure 1) [4, 5]. In contrast to atherosclerotic vascular disease that is secondary to an eccentric and focal lipid deposition and plaque inflammation, CAV is a more uniform immunological reaction. Therefore, CAV lesions are diffuse, concentric, affect epicardial and intramural arteries and even veins.

Non-immunological mechanisms include cardiovascular risk factors such as age, male sex, smoking, dyslipidemia, diabetes mellitus, body mass index, and hypertension. Similarly, donor-related factors such as age, male sex, coronary artery disease, and history of smoking also increase the risk of CAV. Finally, ischemia-reperfusion injury during transplantation and sudden intracranial hemorrhage as the donor's mode of death are also associated with CAV. All these factors result in endothelial injury and inflammation that trigger and exacerbate the immunological mechanisms [3, 4]. In fact, direct graft injury by phenomena such as previous rejection episodes, especially antibody mediated rejection, and the presence of donor specific antibodies are also associated with increased risk of CAV.

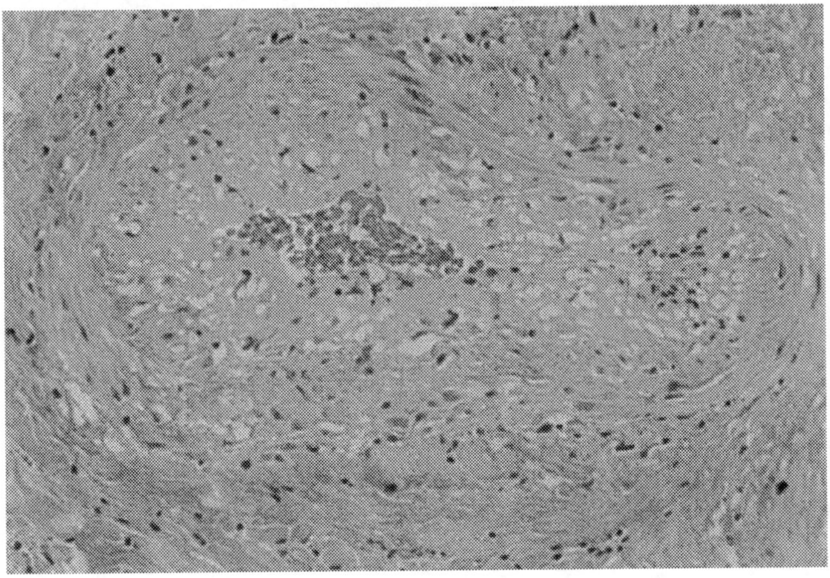

Figure 1. Intimal thickening of an epicardial coronary artery in a patient with cardiac allograft vasculopathy.

Despite the general acceptance of these underlying mechanisms, there is now evidence that immunological and non-immunological factors are more complex and that the pathogenesis of CAV may include innate immune response and cytomegalovirus (CMV) infection [5].

Diagnosis and Clinical Presentation

One of the difficulties in diagnosing CAV is that heart transplant recipients may not experience chest pain, since the transplanted graft is denervated. However, it should be noted that, in some cases, chest pain may indeed be experienced in patients with some degree of renervation, but is usually atypical. Additionally, they might present with other non-specific symptoms such as fatigue, nausea or abdominal pain. If graft dysfunction or restrictive physiology is present, patient may experience heart failure symptoms, with sudden death, arrhythmia or silent myocardial infarction also being possible forms of presentation due to the absence of prior symptoms. Finally, patients are often completely asymptomatic, therefore regular CAV screening is mandatory in this population (See Chapter 14) [5].

There are different imaging techniques that are useful for the evaluation of CAV. In general, non-invasive methods such as echocardiography, single-photon emission computed tomography or even computed tomography can help in diagnosis, but the gold standard technique is still coronary angiography (See Chapter 10). However, coronary angiography cannot visualize beyond the arterial lumen, and CAV lesions are usually diffuse and concentric, so other methods that allow evaluation of the vessel wall may be more sensitive.

Intravascular ultrasound (IVUS) is a technique that combines ultrasound technology with invasive angiographic evaluation. It consists of a special catheter with a miniature ultrasound probe that allows the visualization not only of the lumen but also of the surrounding vessel wall. It detects early intimal thickening with high sensitivity, and has been used in this context with good results. Some of the advantages of IVUS are deep tissue penetrance with direct evaluation of the arterial wall. This allows lumen area and plaque size to be quantified, and intimal thickness measurement allows early identification of CAV, even in the absence of detectable lesions by coronary angiography. The first studies with IVUS in the context of CAV were performed in 1992 by St Goar et al., and found that 1-year after heart transplantation, 70% of patients had at least minimal intimal thickening but angiographically normal coronary arteries [6]. Subsequently, it has been described that the prevalence of CAV 1-year after heart transplantation can be approximately 60% if evaluated with IVUS in contrast to less than 20% when assessed with coronary angiography (Figure 2) [7, 8]. The evaluation of CAV with IVUS is characterized in the Stanford Classification into four classes according to the intimal thickness and degree of vessel circumference affected [6].

- Class I (minimal): intimal thickness < 0.3mm
- Class II (mild): intimal thickness < 0.3mm but more than 180° of the circumference affected
- Class III (moderate): intimal thickness 0.3 - 0.5mm or more than 0.5mm but less than 180° of the circumference affected.
- Class IV (severe): intimal thickness 0.5 – 1mm and more than 180° of the circumference affected or an intimal thickness greater than 1mm.

There are some limitations in the information provided by IVUS, mainly due to the limited data it provides regarding the composition of the vessel wall. Therefore, other methods have also been evaluated in the setting of CAV.

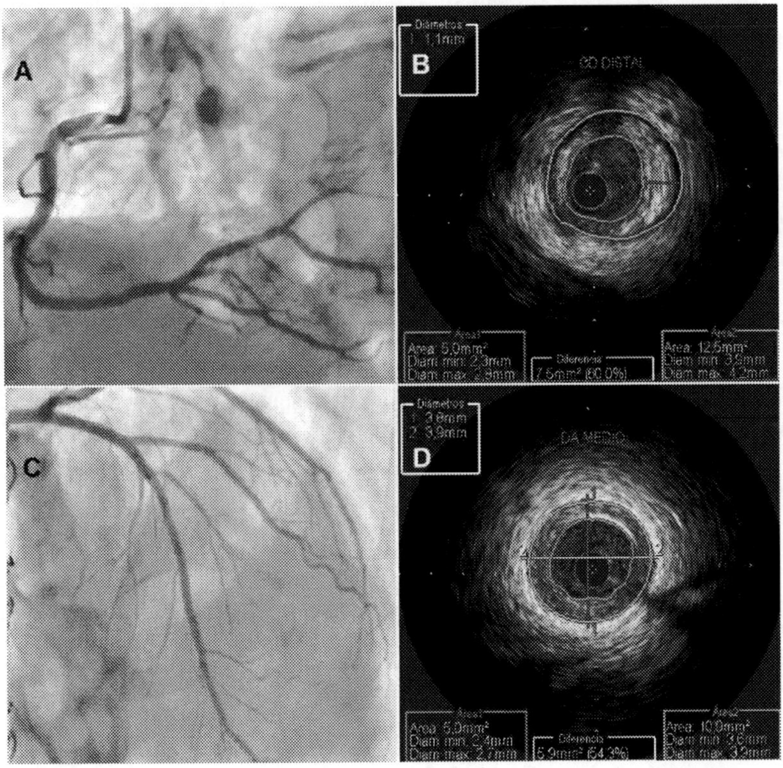

Figure 2. Coronary angiography and intravascular ultrasound. A. and B. Right coronary artery with mild lesion by angiography but moderate by ultrasound. C. and D. Left anterior descending artery with mild lesion by angiography but moderate by ultrasound.

Optical coherence tomography (OCT) is a method that uses long-wavelength, near-infrared light, to provide cross-sectional images with higher resolution than IVUS. Therefore, it can differentiate among the variety of vascular wall components, such as the intima–media interface, and characterize tissues providing a "virtual histology" analysis of the vessel. Although it has not consistently shown a clinical benefit in diagnosis of CAV compared to IVUS, the utilization of OCT provided interesting insight in the pathophysiology of this entity.

A study by Cassar et al., prospectively analyzed 53 heart transplant recipients using IVUS and OCT and found that OCT identified different morphological components of CAV that were thought to be exclusive of atherosclerotic vascular disease such as calcifications and the presence of lipid pool [9]. However, there are some limitations to OCT. Although it has higher resolution, vessel wall penetration is lower, making lesions thicker than 1.5mm difficult to assess. Therefore, it is not a good diagnostic technique for long-term follow-up of patients with advanced disease. Furthermore, it requires more contrast volume than coronary angiography with IVUS, which can be a drawback in heart transplant patients who are more prone to renal dysfunction due to concomitant medication and comorbidities [8].

Classification

Until 2010, the definitions of cardiac allograft vasculopathy were diverse, and there were no universal international standards for the nomenclature of this syndrome. In 2010, the ISHLT endorsed the 'International Society for Heart and Lung Transplantation working formulation of a standardized nomenclature for cardiac allograft vasculopathy' that established a definition and classification of this entity. This classification is based on the number and type of affected vessels, the angiographic severity of the lesions, and the systolic and diastolic impact on the graft. There are four degrees of severity depending on the combination of these variables. In ISHLT CAV_0 there are no detectable lesions on angiography. In ISHLT CAV_1 (mild) there is stenosis of left main less than 50%, or primary vessel with maximum lesion of less than 70%, or any branch stenosis less than 70%. In ISHLT CAV_2 (moderate) there is stenosis of left main less than 50% but with a single primary vessel stenosis of at least 70% or isolated stenosis of at least 70% in branches of 2 systems. Finally, in ISHLT CAV_3 (severe) there is left main stenosis of at least 50%, or two or more primary vessels with a stenosis of at least 70%, or isolated branch stenosis of at least 70% in all 3 systems. Additionally, in this category are included the ISHLT CAV_1 or CAV_2 when there is allograft dysfunction (defined as a left ventricular of less than 45% usually in the presence of regional wall motion abnormalities) or evidence of significant restrictive physiology (Table 1) [10].

This classification is not only useful for proper grading and diagnosis, but it also correlates with prognosis. In a study by Van Keer et al, they analyzed 501 heart transplant patients with a follow-up of up to 20 years. The prevalence of CAV was 59% at 20 years, and they found that, compared to patients without CAV, patients with ISHLT CAV_1 did not have a worse prognosis, but patients with ISHLT CAV_2 and ISHLT CAV_3 had a higher risk of death or retransplantation (hazard ratio 1.86, $p = 0.03$ and 5.71 $p < 0.001$, respectively) [11].

Prevention and Treatment

The cornerstone of CAV prevention is to focus exhaustively on the adequate management of modifiable risk factors and to use preventive medication with an acceptable benefit/risk ratio. If we take into account that traditional cardiovascular risk factors such as hypertension, diabetes or dyslipidemia are important in the development of CAV, it is imperative to treat them accordingly. Furthermore, the majority of these cardiovascular risk factors are exacerbated by the adverse effects of immunosuppressive therapy, thus, strict follow-up with periodic clinical and biochemical evaluations is essential for their early detection.

Multidisciplinary approach is also relevant, for instance, heart transplant patients with diabetes should be evaluated together with the diabetologist in order to offer them the best possible treatment. However, when different medications are used to treat conditions such as hypertension, diabetes or dyslipidemia it is important to consider interactions with immunosuppressive therapies or risk of nephrotoxicity. Another modifiable risk factor is rejection; therefore, careful surveillance and prompt treatment of acute graft rejection episodes also contributes to lowering the risk of future development of CAV. This includes adequate screening and treatment of donor specific antibodies (See Chapter 11). Finally, CMV infection is also associated with CAV, so careful screening of CMV DNA by polymerase chain reaction tests and proper antiviral treatment in case of reactivation also contribute to the prevention of CAV (See Chapter 13) [5].

Table 1. Recommended nomenclature for cardiac allograft vasculopathy

ISHLT CAV_0 (Not significant)
No angiographic lesion.
ISHLT CAV_1 (Mild)
LM < 50% Primary vessel < 70% Any branch < 70% (including diffuse narrowing) (Without allograft dysfunction)
ISHLT CAV_2 (Moderate)
LM < 50% Single primary vessel ≥ 70% Isolated branch stenosis ≥ 70% in branches of 2 systems (Without allograft dysfunction)
ISHLT CAV_3 (Severe)
LM ≥ 50% two or more primary vessels ≥ 70% Isolated branch stenosis > 70% in all 3 systems ISHLT CAV1 or CAV2 with allograft dysfunction
Definitions Allograft dysfunction: LVEF ≤ 45% usually with regional wall motion abnormalities; or significant restrictive physiology (common but not specific) Primary Vessel: proximal and Middle 33% of the left anterior descending artery, the left circumflex, the ramus and the dominant or co-dominant right coronary artery with the posterior descending and posterolateral branches. Secondary Branch Vessel: distal 33% of the primary vessels or any segment within a large septal perforator, diagonals and obtuse marginal branches or any portion of a non-dominant right coronary artery.

CAV, cardiac allograft vasculopathy; ISHLT, International Society for Heart and Lung Transplantation; LM, left main; LVEF, left ventricular ejection fraction. (Data form Mehra MR et al. International Society for Heart and Lung Transplantation working formulation of a standardized nomenclature for cardiac allograft vasculopathy-2010. *J Heart Lung Transplant*. 2010 Jul;29(7):717-27.)

Apart from treating these modifiable risk factors, there are some specific therapies that may be beneficial in the prevention of CAV and in slowing the progression of the disease.

Aspirin

Heart transplant patients have increased platelet aggregation and reactivity [12]. Since platelets are key in the process of inflammation, endothelial injury and thrombosis, all of which participate in the pathogenesis of CAV, inhibition of platelet aggregation is a useful strategy. Different studies have shown the benefit of aspirin in the prevention of CAV. A meta-analysis of 1911 patients showed that aspirin may reduce the development of CAV but with low certainty evidence since most data come from small single-center observational studies. However, when the two studies that performed propensity-weighted analyses are considered, the effect in the prevention of CAV is more evident [13]. Although its use is recommended in this setting, randomized controlled trials are needed to further evaluate the true benefit of aspirin in the prevention and treatment of CAV.

Statins

As mentioned above, dyslipidemia is an important risk factor for the development of CAV, therefore, the use of statins in this setting may be beneficial. Furthermore, statins also have immunomodulatory effects that enhance their benefit for CAV prevention. There are different randomized controlled trials that showed a significant reduction in the incidence of CAV and even improved survival [14, 15]. Thus, statin therapy is recommended for all patients to prevent and treat CAV.

Immunosuppressive Therapy

Improvements in immunosuppressive schemes have led to better management not only of acute graft rejection but also of chronic rejection. In this sense, there is evidence that, in addition to reducing mortality, mycophenolate mofetil is better than azathioprine in preventing CAV progression. In a randomized controlled trial that assigned 289 heart transplant recipients to receive mycophenolate mofetil and 289 to receive azathioprine, mortality and change in mean maximal intimal thickness were lower in the mycophenolate mofetil group [16].

Furthermore, mammalian target of rapamycin (mTOR) inhibitors, such as sirolimus and everolimus, may have a more direct effect in the management of CAV. These drugs inhibit the proliferation of fibroblasts and smooth muscle cells, which are essential for coronary intimal hyperplasia in CAV. A meta-analysis by Jennings et al., identified 14 trials that used mTOR inhibitors in heart transplant recipients and found that change in mean maximal intimal thickness was significantly reduced in patients with mTOR (-0.04 [-0.07 to -0.02]) compared to calcineurin inhibitor and mycophenolate mofetil. Additionally, CMV infection and renal function deterioration was also reduced with mTOR. However, this was at the expense of a higher incidence of acute graft rejection and d drug discontinuation due to adverse effects, with no differences in mortality [17]. Therefore, mTOR are useful for the prevention and treatment of CAV, but they cannot be routinely recommended as first-line immunosuppressive regimens. Instead, in the setting of CAV, they may be used in those patients in whom CAV is early detected in order to prevent progression.

Revascularization

Revascularization of lesions secondary to CAV in heart transplant recipients is still a matter an ongoing debate. As mentioned above, stenosis due to CAV is morphologically and pathophysiologicaly different from that secondary to atherosclerotic vascular disease. Therefore, revascularization strategies for atherosclerotic vascular disease are not necessarily useful in CAV. In addition, symptoms are usually absent in the latter, and cannot be used to decide revascularization. In this context, decision should be made on an individual basis according to the morphology of the lesion, graft function, symptoms and comorbidities. In general, focal lesion may be amenable to percutaneous coronary intervention, however, rates of restenosis are high.

A systematic review by Dasari et al., analyzed 312 patients with CAV who were treated with percutaneous coronary intervention using either drug eluting stents or bare metal stents. They found that drug eluting stent reduced the risk of in stent restenosis compared to bare metal stents, with no differences in mortality and major adverse cardiac events [18].

Coronary artery bypass surgery might also be considered; however, it is limited by the diffuse morphology of lesions in CAV with poor distal vessel targets. In addition, patients often have increased operative risk due to comorbidities [5]. A meta-analysis by Luc et al., analyzed the revascularization strategy for CAV in 1520 heart transplant patients. Patients that underwent coronary artery bypass surgery had a higher early mortality than those that underwent percutaneous coronary intervention (36.4% vs. 4.3%, respectively $p < 0.001$) and higher overall mortality (42.3% vs. PCI 21.4%, $p < 0.05$) [19]. Therefore, decision regarding revascularization with coronary artery bypass surgery should be performed in a case-by-case basis and only in selected patients.

Alternatively, heart retransplantation can be considered in some situations (See Chapter 6). However, it has poorer outcomes than heart transplantation for other etiologies, and the shortage of donors and often comorbidities of the receptor in this setting also limits its usage. Currently, it should be reserved for selected patients with ISHLT CAV_3 with graft dysfunction.

Conclusion

After many years, heart transplantation remains the gold standard treatment for advanced heart failure. However, despite many advances in the field of immunosuppressive therapy, graft rejection continues to be the main limiting factor for prolonged survival. Specifically, chronic rejection in the form of CAV in one of the most frequent causes of death in the late stages after heart transplantation. There are still gaps in understanding of the underlying mechanisms, however, advances in diagnostic methods, classification, and treatment options may be the initial path towards improved long-term outcomes in this particular entity.

References

[1] Stolf N A G. History of Heart Transplantation: a Hard and Glorious Journey. *Braz. J. Cardiovasc. Surg.* 2017 Sep-Oct;32(5):423-427.

[2] Khush K K, Cherikh W S, Chambers D C, Harhay M O, Hayes D Jr, Hsich E, Meiser B, Potena L, Robinson A, Rossano J W, Sadavarte A, Singh TP, Zuckermann A, Stehlik J; International Society for Heart and Lung Transplantation. The International Thoracic Organ Transplant Registry of the International Society for Heart and Lung Transplantation: Thirty-sixth adult heart transplantation report - 2019; focus theme: Donor and recipient size match. *J. Heart Lung Transplant.* 2019 Oct;38(10):1056-1066.

[3] Skorić B, Čikeš M, Ljubas Maček J, Baričević Ž, Škorak I, Gašparović H, Biočina B, Miličić D. Cardiac allograft vasculopathy: diagnosis, therapy, and prognosis. *Croat. Med. J.* 2014 Dec;55(6):562-76.

[4] Lee F, Nair V, Chih S. Cardiac allograft vasculopathy: Insights on pathogenesis and therapy. *Clin. Transplant.* 2020 Mar;34(3):e13794.

[5] Pober J S, Chih S, Kobashigawa J, Madsen J C, Tellides G. Cardiac allograft vasculopathy: current review and future research directions. *Cardiovasc. Res.* 2021 Nov 22;117(13):2624-2638.

[6] St Goar F G, Pinto F J, Alderman E L, Valantine H A, Schroeder J S, Gao S Z, Stinson EB, Popp RL. Intracoronary ultrasound in cardiac transplant recipients. In vivo evidence of "angiographically silent" intimal thickening. *Circulation.* 1992 Mar;85(3):979-87.

[7] Kapadia S R, Ziada K M, L'Allier P L, Crowe T D, Rincon G, Hobbs R E, Bott-Silverman C, Young JB, Nissen SE, Tuzcu EM. Intravascular ultrasound imaging after cardiac transplantation: advantage of multi-vessel imaging. *J. Heart Lung Transplant*. 2000 Feb;19(2):167-72.

[8] Dyrbuś M, Gąsior M, Szyguła-Jurkiewicz B, Przybyłowski P. The role of optical coherence tomography and other intravascular imaging modalities in cardiac allograft vasculopathy. *Postepy Kardiol. Interwencyjnej*. 2020 Mar;16(1):19-29.

[9] Cassar A, Matsuo Y, Herrmann J, Li J, Lennon R J, Gulati R, Lerman L O, Kushwaha SS, Lerman A. Coronary atherosclerosis with vulnerable plaque and complicated lesions in transplant recipients: new insight into cardiac allograft vasculopathy by optical coherence tomography. *Eur. Heart J.* 2013 Sep;34 (33):2610-7.

[10] Mehra M R, Crespo-Leiro M G, Dipchand A, Ensminger S M, Hiemann N E, Kobashigawa J A, Madsen J, Parameshwar J, Starling R C, Uber P A. International Society for Heart and Lung Transplantation working formulation of a standardized nomenclature for cardiac allograft vasculopathy-2010. *J. Heart Lung Transplant.* 2010 Jul;29(7):717-27.

[11] Van Keer J M, Van Aelst L N L, Rega F, Droogne W, Voros G, Meyns B, Vanhaecke J, Emonds MP, Janssens S, Naesens M, Van Cleemput J. Long-term outcome of cardiac allograft vasculopathy: Importance of the International Society for Heart and Lung Transplantation angiographic grading scale. *J. Heart Lung Transplant.* 2019 Nov;38(11):1189-1196.

[12] Hognestad A, Michelsen A, Brosstad F, Damås J K, Holm T, Simonsen S, Kjekshus J K, Aukrust P, Andreassen AK. Platelet activation in heart transplant recipients. *Clin. Transplant.* 2004 Apr;18(2):142-7.

[13] Aleksova N, Brahmbhatt D H, Kiamanesh O, Petropoulos J A, Chang Y, Guyatt G, Chih S, Ross H J. The effect of antiplatelet therapy on survival and cardiac allograft vasculopathy following heart transplantation: A systematic review and meta-analysis. *Clin. Transplant.* 2021 Jan;35(1):e14125.

[14] Kobashigawa J A, Moriguchi J D, Laks H, Wener L, Hage A, Hamilton M A, Cogert G, Marquez A, Vassilakis M E, Patel J, Yeatman L. Ten-year follow-up of a randomized trial of pravastatin in heart transplant patients. *J. Heart Lung Transplant.* 2005 Nov;24(11):1736-40.

[15] See V Y Jr, DeNofrio D, Goldberg L, Chang G, Sasseen B, Kolansky D M, Pickering F, Kao A, Loh E, Wilensky RL. Effect of atorvastatin on postcardiac transplant increase in low-density lipoprotein cholesterol reduces development of intimal hyperplasia and progression of endothelial dysfunction. *Am. J. Cardiol.* 2003 Jul. 1;92(1):11-5.

[16] Eisen H J, Kobashigawa J, Keogh A, Bourge R, Renlund D, Mentzer R, Alderman E, Valantine H, Dureau G, Mancini D, Mamelok R, Gordon R, Wang W, Mehra M, Constanzo MR, Hummel M, Johnson J; Mycophenolate Mofetil Cardiac Study Investigators. Three-year results of a randomized, double-blind, controlled trial of mycophenolate mofetil versus azathioprine in cardiac transplant recipients. *J. Heart Lung Transplant.* 2005 May;24(5):517-25.

[17] Jennings D L, Lange N, Shullo M, Latif F, Restaino S, Topkara V K, Takeda K, Takayama H, Naka Y, Farr M, Colombo P, Baker W L. Outcomes associated with mammalian target of rapamycin (mTOR) inhibitors in heart transplant recipients: A meta-analysis. *Int. J. Cardiol.* 2018 Aug 15;265:71-76.

[18] Dasari T W, Hennebry T A, Hanna E B, Saucedo J F. Drug eluting versus bare metal stents in cardiac allograft vasculopathy: a systematic review of literature. *Catheter. Cardiovasc. Interv.* 2011 Jun 1;77(7):962-9.

[19] Luc J G Y, Choi J H, Rizvi S A, Phan K, Moncho Escrivà E, Patel S, Reeves G R, Boyle A J, Entwistle J W, Morris R J, Massey H T, Tchantchaleishvili V. Percutaneous coronary intervention versus coronary artery bypass grafting in heart transplant recipients with coronary allograft vasculopathy: a systematic review and meta-analysis of 1,520 patients. *Ann. Cardiothorac. Surg.* 2018 Jan;7(1):19-30.

Chapter 13

Infectious Diseases in Heart Transplantation

Sergio Daniel Andino Di Masi[1], Rocío Emilia Gago[2], Patricia Lourdes Giorgio[3], Melisa Belén Martínez Rios[4], Natalia Rosana Pujato[5,*] and Silvina Villamandos[6]

[1]Favaloro Foundation University Hospital, Buenos Aires, Argentina
[2]Austral University Hospital, Buenos Aires, Argentina
[3]British Hospital, Buenos Aires, Argentina
[4]Mendoza Central Hospital, Mendoza, Argentina
[5]ITAC Institute of Transplantation and High Complexity, Buenos Aires, Argentina
[6]Juana F. Cabral. Corrientes Cardiology Institute, Corrientes, Argentina

Abstract

Infectious complications are frequent in heart transplantation, but are no longer the leading cause of death. Bacterial infections are the most common, particularly as early post-transplant complications. The overall incidence of fungal infections has decreased in recent years but pulmonary aspergillosis remains the most common and is associated with high mortality. Late infections (particularly viral infections) are still a threat to long-term graft survival in these patients, such as cytomegalovirus, which is one of the most important pathogens in heart transplantation. Toxoplasmosis, a particularly serious entity in this population, has decreased with the use of routine prophylaxis in seronegative recipients. This chapter will delve into these points of interest and other aspects of heart transplant infections.

Keywords: heart transplantation, infections, antibiotic prophylaxis

---

* Corresponding Author's E-mail: nataliapujato@gmail.com.

In: Heart Transplantation
Editor: Elian Facundo Giordanino
ISBN: 978-1-68507-759-4

Introduction

Since the first transplants to date, significant reductions in risk factors for infection and complications have been achieved in heart transplant recipients. This is in part due to better management of immunosuppression, advances in diagnostic methods, the introduction of antimicrobial prophylaxis, and new antibiotic treatments.

According to a Stanford University Medical Center publication, between 2008-2017 the rate of cardiac post-transplant infection episodes was 2.15 per patient, predominantly due to bacteria (1.34 per patient), followed by viruses (0.65 per patient) and fungi (0.02 per patient) [1].

Infections in the early post-transplant period include surgical site infections, hospital acquired infections or infections transmitted by the allograft. Later, reactivation of latent infections (e.g., Cytomegalovirus) or infections acquired in the community are more frequent.

The evaluation of donors and recipients prior to transplantation (clinical examination, epidemiological exposure and laboratory tests), aims to identify infections that may exclude donor organ or tissue donation, as well as to establish strategies for the prevention of post-transplant infections (vaccines or prophylaxis).

Pre-Transplant Evaluation

Baseline screening is proposed in most transplant programs for the detection of infections in donors and recipients. In addition, supplementary tests should be carried out according to epidemiological exposure such as country of birth, travels or respiratory contacts. It should be kept in mind, that despite the high sensitivity and specificity of the currently used tests, errors in determinations due to false positives and false negatives can still be detected.

The recommended screening for donor and recipient should include serological or molecular test for Human Immunodeficiency Virus (HIV) 1 and 2, Hepatitis B (HBV), Hepatitis C (HCV), Syphilis, Cytomegalovirus (CMV), Epstein Barr virus (EBV), Toxoplasmosis, Chagas (in endemic areas), Human T-cell lymphotropic virus (HTLV) 1 and 2 (in endemic areas) and Tuberculosis [2, 3]. At the time of transplantation, most guidelines recommend obtaining donor blood cultures, preservation fluid culture, bronchoalveolar fluid culture (in lung or heart-lung transplants), and rectal and nasal surveillance swab culture for the detection of multidrug resistant bacteria in recipients. Additional screening tests in outbreaks or epidemics should be used (e.g., Influenza, Coronavirus disease [COVID-19], Dengue, Epidemic encephalitis).

High-Risk Donors

Risk stratification is successfully accomplished by careful review of the donor's medical and social history [4]. High-risk donors are understood to be donors with active infection at the time of donation and high-risk profiles for HIV, HCV, and HBV based on their medical history. Currently, this definition has been changing according to the diagnostic methods available in each country. In the United States, Organ Procurement and Transplantation Network (OPTN) 2020 removed any specific label (i.e., "increased risk donor") to describe donors with risk factors for acute HIV, HBV, and HCV infection" [5]. Instead, behaviors such as risk factors for transmission of HIV, HBV and HCV have been used for stratification (Table 1) [6, 7].

Table 1. Donor with increased risk of transmitting human immunodeficiency virus, hepatitis B virus, and hepatitis C virus

High-risk sexual contacts • People who have had sex with a person known or suspected to have HIV, HBV or HCV infection in the preceding 12 months. • Men who have had sex with another man in the preceding 12 months. • Women who have had sex with a man with a history of sex with another man in the preceding 12 months. • Persons who have had sex in exchange for money or drugs in the preceding 12 months. • Persons who have had sex with a person who injected drugs intravenously, intramuscularly, or subcutaneously for non-medical reasons in the preceding 12 months.
Birth to a mother infected with HIV, HBV or HCV (for infants' donors ≤ 2 years of age).
Persons who have injected drugs intravenously, intramuscularly, or subcutaneously for non-medical reasons in the last 12 months
Inmates of a correctional facility (e.g., jail, prison) for > 3 days in the preceding 12 months.
Persons who have or have been treated for syphilis, gonorrhea, chlamydia, or genital ulcers in the preceding 12 months
Persons who have been on hemodialysis in the preceding 12 months (HCV risk only).

HIV, Human Immunodeficiency Virus; HBV, Hepatitis B Virus; HCV, Hepatitis C Virus (Data from Wolfe CR et al. Donor-derived infections: Guidelines from the American Society of Transplantation Infectious Diseases Community of Practice. *Clin Transplant*. 2019 Sep; 33(9):e13547).

In countries where nucleic acid testing is available, risk criteria can be reduced to the 30 days before organ procurement due to its high sensitivity and specificity [8].

Relevant Infections in Heart Transplantation

Viral Infections

Cytomegalovirus

CMV is a ubiquitous β-herpesvirus that infects the majority of humans. CMV seroprevalence rate in adults is 50%-80%, although this rate varies depending on age, geography, and socioeconomic status [9].

Primary CMV infection may be asymptomatic or manifest as a self-limited febrile illness in immunocompetent individuals. After primary infection, CMV persists as a latent virus, which then serves as a reservoir for reactivation and transmission to susceptible individuals, such as solid organ transplant recipients [10].

CMV is a major cause of morbidity and mortality after transplantation; it has direct effects and several indirect effects due to its ability to modulate the immune system, and it is associated with increased risk of other infectious complications such as bacteremia, invasive fungal diseases, EBV-mediated post-transplant lymphoproliferative disorders, acute rejection and chronic allograft injury (bronchiolitis obliterans in lung recipients and coronary allograft vasculopathy in heart recipients) [9]. Without a prevention strategy, CMV infection and disease typically occur within the first 3-6 months after transplantation; however, its appearance may be later in patients who received prophylaxis [9].

The factors related to a higher risk are: serological status of the donor and recipient, type and intensity of immunosuppressive drugs, rejection, and type of transplant (Table 2) [9].

It is important to distinguish between CMV infection and disease. CMV infection is the presence of CMV replication in tissue, blood, or other bodily fluids regardless of symptomatology. CMV disease is the infection that is accompanied by clinical signs and symptoms (CMV syndrome and end-organ CMV disease) [11].

The laboratory methods for CMV detection are molecular tests; pp65 antigenemia assay (less sensitive); histopathology (the gold standard for the definitive diagnosis of end-organ CMV diseases); viral culture (poor sensitivity and slow turn-around time); CMV serology (not recommended in immunocompromised patients); and cellular immunity assays that measure nonspecific immunity (CD4+T-cells and mitogen T-cell responses) and CMV-specific immunity (interferon-gamma release assay, enzyme-linked immunosorbent spot assay, intracellular cytokine staining for interferon-gamma and major histocompatibility complex multimer-based assay). The latter are emerging as clinical tools for risk stratification and management in transplantation [12, 13].

Table 2. Risk of Cytomegalovirus infection

High Risk	**Serostatus**	**(D + / R -)**
	Immunosuppressors	Anti-thymocyte globulins, alemtuzumab
	Graft rejection	Especially when treated with lymphocyte - depleting antibodies.
	Type of transplant	Lung-heart recipients
Moderate risk	**Serostatus**	**(D -/ R +)**
Lower risk	**Serostatus**	**(D- / R-)**
	Immunosuppression	mTOR inhibitors
	Type of transplant	Heart recipients

D+, Donor CMV seropositive; D-, Donor CMV seronegative; R+, Receptor CMV seropositive; R-, Receptor CMV seronegative. (Data from Razonable RR et al. Cytomegalovirus in solid organ transplant recipients-Guidelines of the American Society of Transplantation Infectious Diseases Community of Practice. *Clin Transplant*. 2019 Sep; 33(9):e13512).

The two major strategies for CMV disease prevention after heart transplantation are antiviral prophylaxis and preemptive therapy. In CMV donor seropositive/receptor seronegative, antiviral prophylaxis is strongly recommended and duration is 3-6 months for heart recipients and 6-12 months for heart-lung recipients. When prophylaxis is chosen for CMV receptor seropositive, the suggested duration is 3 months for heart recipients and 6 to 12 months for heart-lung recipients. Antiviral drugs are valganciclovir and ganciclovir. Currently, there are limited data to support prophylaxis in solid transplantation with letermovir. The use of CMV-specific T-cell immune measures to guide the duration of antiviral prophylaxis has been suggested, but this remains investigational. Preemptive therapy consists of weekly monitoring CMV DNA or pp65 antigenemia for at least for 12 weeks after transplantation, and the administration of antivirals when there is evidence of replication [9, 14].

Regarding its treatment, first line drugs for CMV disease are ganciclovir or valganciclovir [9]. Foscarnet and cidofovir are regarded as second-line agents due to the high risk of nephrotoxicity and are considered for resistant CMV. Letermovir has been used off-label in some cases of CMV disease, but to date it is not approved for treatment [15].

Herpes Simplex Virus and Varicella Zoster Virus

The seroprevalence for herpes simplex virus (HSV) 1 and 2 in the adult population is around 59.7% and 21.2% respectively. Most HSV infections in adults are due to reactivation of latent endogenous virus, although primary infection transmitted through the graft has been described [16]. In seronegative patients, the most frequent form of transmission is by contact.

The most common presentation of HSV is orolabial, genital, or perineal. Invasive or disseminated disease can present in the form of esophagitis, fulminant hepatitis, or pneumonitis, and usually appears late after transplantation. Pneumonitis is more common in heart or lung recipients (Figure 1). Fever, leukopenia, and hepatitis are frequent manifestations of disseminated disease. In the absence of prophylaxis, most cases occur in the first month after transplantation, with an incidence of approximately 30%. In transplant recipients, the incidence of symptomatic HSV during the first year after transplantation was 3% in patients who received antiviral prophylaxis versus 9.8% in those who did not. Female gender, HSV seropositivity, rejection episodes, and preemptive strategy for CMV (without routine prophylaxis) are associated with increased risk of symptomatic HSV. In contrast, transplant recipients taking antiviral medications to prevent CMV replication (i.e., ganciclovir and valganciclovir) prevent most HSV replication. HSV-specific prophylaxis (acyclovir) should be considered for all HSV-1 and HSV-2 seropositive organ recipients not receiving antiviral medication to prevent CMV replication. Most serious HSV illnesses occur within the first month after transplantation, so antiviral prophylaxis should continue for at least a month. Resumption of prophylaxis may be considered for patients being treated for rejection (especially with agents that reduce T-cells such as anti-thymocyte globulin) [16].

The seroprevalence of varicella zoster virus (VZV) in the adult population is around 90%. Post-transplant disease is usually due to reactivation of latent virus. It is a common infectious complication in adult transplant recipients with an incidence of about 8% -11% during the first 4 years after transplantation. Donor-derived infection is rare. Heart and lung transplant patients have higher rates of VZV compared with other transplant recipients, possibly related to deeper immunosuppression. The distribution is usually dermatomal or generalized, and tends to occur after the third month after transplantation. Visceral complications can occur, including pneumonitis, hepatitis, and encephalitis.

VZV primary infection occurs in seronegative patients and is more severe, with visceral and cutaneous involvement, which leads to higher morbidity and mortality. Contagion comes from community exposure. The diagnosis is often clinical by the typical skin lesions of HSV and VZV. Atypical or visceral presentations require verification with rapid laboratory tests by polymerase chain reaction (PCR) or direct fluorescent-antibody assays in tissues or fluids. The use of oral acyclovir prevents HSV and VZV disease, which usually occurs when this drug is stopped. Presumably, famciclovir and valacyclovir should be equally effective.

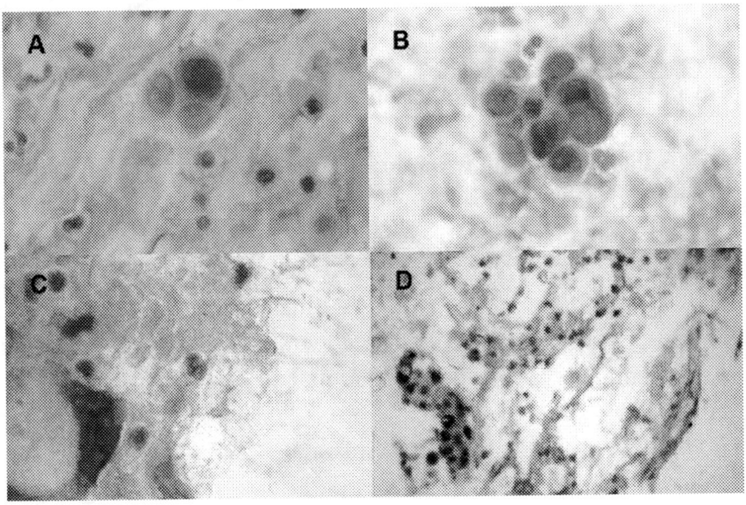

Figure 1. Herpes simplex virus pneumonitis. A-C. Multinucleated and mononuclear cells with intranuclear inclusions. D. Immunohistochemistry for herpes simplex virus 1.

In VZV seronegative recipients, varicella vaccine (live attenuated VZV, Oka strain) should be administered prior to heart transplantation to prevent primary varicella infection after it. As it is a live vaccine, a minimum of 4-6 weeks must elapse from the administration of the vaccine to transplantation and its administration is not recommended in post-transplant patients. Inactivated VZV vaccine is promising in these hosts. It is also recommended to vaccinate seronegative relatives. Options for post-exposure prophylaxis include passive immunoprophylaxis and/or antiviral therapy. Immunoglobulin prophylaxis should be administered as soon as possible and within 10 days of exposure. Prophylaxis with oral antiviral drug (e.g., acyclovir) should be used in patients past the window period [17]. Intravenous acyclovir should be used for the treatment of disseminated HSV and VZV disease. Disease limited to orolabial involvement in HSV or one dermatome in VZV, can be treated with oral acyclovir, famciclovir, or valaciclovir. Acyclovir resistance is rare and may respond to foscarnet.

Epstein Barr Virus

EBV infection is universally distributed. After infection, the virus remains latent for life. It is estimated that 50% of the population under 18 years old and 90% of the adult population have positive serology; therefore, if antibodies are not available in adult donors, they should be assumed to be positive.

There are different consequences of EBV infection. In transplant patients, they range from uncomplicated infectious mononucleosis to organ-specific diseases or malignancies. Knowing the EBV serological status of the donor and the recipient is mandatory in order to identify risk groups, determine the need for post-transplant EBV viral load monitoring, and carry out preventive interventions.

Primary infection occurs in EBV-mismatched patients (donor seropositive/recipient seronegative). The allograft carries B-cells with latent virus. Viral shedding through the oropharynx occurs around the sixth week after transplantation. The rapid increase in and the high levels of viral load are related to the later onset of post-transplant lympho-proliferative disorder (PTLD). Common manifestations are infectious mononucleosis, organ specific diseases (hepatitis, pneumonitis, enteritis) and hematologic diseases (cytopenia, hemophagocytic lymph histiocytosis or macrophage activation syndrome). Diagnosis is by detection of EBV in blood using PCR.

Reactivation/infection events are often observed within 2 to 3 months after transplantation.

The most serious manifestation of EBV is PTLD. Overall mortality for PTLD often exceeds 50% and is most often of recipient origin. However, it must be considered that if PTLD is limited to the graft and occurs early after transplantation, it may be donor derived [18-20]. The incidence of PTLD also depends on the type of organ allograft. Heart transplantation is of moderate risk (3-12%). High risk factors are [21]:

- EBV donor/recipient mismatch (10-fold increased risk for EBV disease and PTLD)
- Pediatric recipients
- Immunosuppressants (anti-T lymphocyte agents and tacrolimus)
- CMV infection
- Acute rejection

The diagnosis of PTLD is made by pathological anatomy. Cellular phenotype (B, T, or NK cells) should also be studied, clonality determined, and tissue markers of EBV infection sought. EBV is integrated into the B-cell genome in more than 90% of early post-transplant PTLD cases [22].

The most widely accepted prevention strategies in high-risk patients are EBV viral load surveillance (weekly to fortnightly, during the first year after transplantation) and preemptive interventions (reduction of immunosuppression associated or not to antiviral drugs -ganciclovir/ valganciclovir- or intravenous immunoglobulin [IVIG]) [22]. The use of antiviral agents, IVIG, and immunotherapy is not recommended as universal prophylaxis for early prevention of PTLD [22, 23].

PTLD treatment is based on decreasing immunosuppression. Escalation with other therapies is considered according to clinical response and histopathologic features of PTLD, and includes rituximab (anti-CD20 monoclonal antibody) and conventional chemotherapy.

Herpes Virus 6

Herpesvirus 6 (HHV-6) is a lymphotropic virus. Seroprevalence reaches up to 95% in adults and remains latent in different cells of the immune system. Post-transplant HHV-6 infection is more likely due to virus reactivation, but can also be transmitted through the allograft.

The clinical manifestation is an acute viral syndrome similar to CMV. Rarely, it can cause pneumonitis, encephalitis, gastroduodenitis, hepatitis or allograft dysfunction. Furthermore, HHV-6 can act as an immunomodulatory virus that could facilitate superinfection with fungi or other opportunistic agents [24].

Quantification of HHV-6 DNA, either in whole blood, plasma or serum with real-time PCR, is currently the most widely used method for diagnosing active infection. The results are not standardized and there are no clear cut-off points to differentiate asymptomatic viral replication from clinical disease [25.

The American Society of Transplantation (AST) guidelines do not recommend antiviral prophylaxis or preemptive therapy for HHV-6, but when the disease is confirmed, ganciclovir and foscarnet are considered the first-line drugs for treatment [24-26].

Hepatitis B Virus

HBV prevalence in patients with heart or lung disease is similar to that in the general population. Vaccination is recommended in those candidates with negative serologies, but response to vaccines in patients with advanced heart failure may be lower than expected [27]. It is recommended to evaluate serological response with Hepatitis B surface antibody (HBsAb) [28].

In candidates in whom HBV surface antigen (HBsAg) is positive, additional studies including hepatitis B e-antigen and antibody, viral load, liver enzymes, and abdominal ultrasonography should be performed. Patient should be referred to a specialist for HBV treatment, monitoring and surveillance of hepatocellular carcinoma. Due to the high risk of reactivation of the disease in recipients with chronic HBV hepatitis, it is recommended to start treatment with antivirals and continue it indefinitely [28].

The management strategy is unclear when the non-hepatic solid organ transplant candidate presents markers of previous HBV infection (negative HBsAg with positive HBV core antibody [HBcAb] and/or positive HBsAb). The risk of reactivation in these cases is low, around 5%, and could occur during the first year after transplantation or when there are periods of maximum immunosuppression [28-30]. However, universal antiviral prophylaxis is not recommended in these cases. Monitoring of HBsAg and viral load should be considered for at least the first year after transplantation or in the event of increased immunosuppression. Likewise, antiviral prophylaxis could be considered in patients with an assumed higher risk of reactivation (e.g., use of lymphocyte depleting agents, B-cell depleting agents, positive HBcAb with negative HBsAb or the presence of detectable viral load) [28, 29]. The risk of HBV transmission through the non-hepatic organ donor with positive HBsAg is considered high. It is recommended to use prophylaxis with antivirals indefinitely and consider the use of specific anti-HBV immunoglobulin for the first 6-12 months in recipients with HBsAb <100 IU/mL [28-31]. On the other hand, the risk of transmission from a non-hepatic organ donor with only HBcAb positive is significantly lower and antiviral prophylaxis is recommended only in recipients without demonstrated immunity, not in those recipients who are already immunized. Liver enzyme monitoring, HBsAg and quarterly viral load during the first year after transplantation could also be considered. The use of specific anti-HBV immunoglobulin is not recommended [28, 30].

Hepatitis C Virus

The prevalence of HCV in thoracic transplant recipients is similar to the general population, around 2% [28]. Direct-acting antivirals have high success rate and safety profile, which is why they have been implemented as HCV treatment in transplant recipients [32]. Untreated HCV infection in heart recipients has been associated with increased mortality, liver failure, and accelerated coronary allograft vasculopathy compared with recipients without HCV infection [32].

Detection of HCV viral load by PCR is recommended to confirm active infection, at the time of evaluation of the transplant candidate. Likewise, the degree of liver fibrosis should be evaluated in candidates with chronic HCV infection, either with liver biopsy or with non-invasive methods, in order to focus therapeutic strategies [28]. The timing of treatment, before or after transplantation, must be individualized.

To date, there are no documented cases of HCV transmission from HCV antibody-positive but PCR-negative donor organs, so these organs can be used safely [28, 33, 34]. Recipients of increased risk donors should be follow-up with HCV viral load for 1–3 months [28]. On the other hand, the use of organs from donors with a positive HCV viral load has increased in recent years, also in heart transplantation. Survival rates, as well as rejection rates, malignancies and complications of recipients of viremic donors treated with direct-acting antivirals are similar to those of recipients of non-viremic donors. According to recommendations of the AST, HCV-viremic donors can be considered for HCV-negative recipients in the framework of clinical trials or protocols with informed consent and with an established post-transplant treatment plan. The Infectious Diseases Society of America recommends starting treatment preventively, ideally within the first 7 days, while the AST suggests that it can be started at the time of transplantation or immediately after detection of HCV viremia [32-34].

Human T-cell Lymphotropic Virus Type 1

HTLV-1 is an RNA virus with a low incidence of infection worldwide. It is endemic to the Caribbean, some regions of South America (Brazil, Peru, Ecuador and Venezuela), West Africa, Asia (mainly Japan), and Oceania. On the contrary, the HTLV-2 virus is not clearly related to human disease [35].

HTLV-1 carriers have a 5-10% higher risk of developing adult T-cell leukemia / lymphoma throughout their lives. To a lesser extent, it can produce severe neurological involvement such as HTLV-1 associated myelopathy, called tropical spastic paraparesis, or other inflammatory disorders (e.g., Sjogren's syndrome, uveitis, interstitial pneumonitis) [35].

The effect of immunosuppression on the natural history of HTLV-1 infection remains uncertain. HTLV-1-related disease in recipients of organs from seropositive donors has been recently described [25]. These reports emphasize the need to screen donors and recipients in HTLV-1 endemic regions. The screening method is enzyme-linked immunosorbent assay and the confirmatory tests are Western Blot, PCR or "line immunoassay" [35].

HTLV-1 infection of the donor or recipient is not an absolute contraindication to proceed with transplantation. However, a post-transplant follow-up, with serological tests and molecular techniques is recommended on a quarterly basis during the first year and semi-annually during the following year. Additionally, the strategy of monitoring viral load could be useful in guiding changes in immunosuppression [35]. There is currently no antiretroviral treatment that has been shown to be effective for asymptomatic HTLV-1 infection.

Human Immunodeficiency Virus

The introduction of antiretroviral treatment (ART) decreased mortality, as well as the frequency of opportunistic diseases in HIV-infected patients. The actual longer survival, secondary to the control of viral load and CD4+ cells, allows patients with other chronic diseases (liver, kidney, heart) to progress to organ failure, whose only treatment would be transplantation.

Good outcomes have been reported on kidney and liver transplants recipients under ART. There is less experience in heart transplant. The first report was from Calabrese et al. in 2003 in the United States. Since then, success has been reported in various experiences in small cases series [36-40]. In a recent publication, Koval et al. in a multicenter, retrospective study of 29 HIV infected thoracic transplant recipients reported that the 1-year survival rate was similar to HIV-negative recipients from The International Society for Heart and Lung Transplantation. Post-transplant infections in heart transplant recipients occurred in 39% at 1 year, similar to HIV-negative patients [41]. Chen Chao et al. in 2019 published a series of 35 HIV-positive heart transplants. Comparing a registry of HIV-negative heart transplants, no significant differences in survival or overall graft survival were found at 5-year follow-up [42].

Patients typically experience transient decreases in the CD4+ T-cell counts following transplantation, but these do not appear to impact long-term risk of infection [43]. Management of HIV recipients is the same as that of HIV-negative patients. Controls, prophylaxis and routine immunizations for post-transplant patients and for HIV patients should be combined. However, interactions between ART and immunosuppressants should be taken into account. Protease inhibitors increase the levels of cyclosporin A, tacrolimus, and rapamycin. Efavirenz and nevirapine decrease corticosteroid levels and efavirenz decreases cyclosporin A and tacrolimus levels. Atazanavir is the protease inhibitor with the fewest interactions. Raltegravir and Dolutegravir have the best profile for combining with immunosuppressants. Intensive monitoring of immunosuppressant levels is also essential [44].

There is consensus that HIV infection in candidates is not a contraindication to receiving a solid organ transplant. Based on the available data, it is accepted to include HIV-positive patients for kidney and liver transplantation, but in some countries, there are still no recommendations for intrathoracic organs (See Chapter 6). The selection criteria suggested by the AST are listed in Table 3 [43].

Table 3. Selection criteria for human immunodeficiency virus positive heart transplant candidates

Meet center-specific inclusion criteria.
CD4 count ≥200 cells / μL during 3 month prior to transplantation.
Undetectable HIV viral load while receiving antiretroviral therapy.
Documented adherence with a stable antiretroviral regimen.
Absence of active opportunistic infection and malignancy
Absence of chronic wasting or severe malnutrition.
Appropriate follow-up with providers experienced in the management of HIV.
Easy access to immunosuppressive medication therapeutic drug monitoring.

HIV, Human Immunodeficiency Virus. (Data from Blumberg EA, et al. Human immunodeficiency virus in solid organ transplantation. *Am J Transplant.* 2013 Mar; 13 Suppl 4:169-78).

Regarding the use of organs from HIV-positive donors, transplant centers should consult the regulatory framework of each country and should obtain specific informed consent that includes a discussion of the risks related to disease transmission [8].

Polyomavirus BK

Polyomavirus BK (BKV) is a DNA virus with worldwide distribution with a high prevalence in the general population. After an asymptomatic primary infection, the virus remains latent in the urinary tract, more specifically in renal tubular epithelial cells [25].

In recent years, cases of BKV nephropathy have been observed in native kidneys of non-renal solid organ transplant patients, such as heart, lung, and liver, with the potential to cause chronic kidney failure [46]. BKV-related micropapillary urothelial carcinoma have also been described in non-kidney transplants such as heart transplants [47]. Risk factors for reactivation are age, male sex, donor/recipient mismatch, rejection, and the use of corticosteroids.

The gold standard for diagnosis is renal biopsy. It should be considered when renal dysfunction has no recognizable cause or when the viremia detected by PCR is greater than 10,000 copies/mL, even without impaired renal function [48]. There is no standardized treatment for BKV infection, it is mainly focused on reducing immunosuppression. The use of different agents such as cidofovir, leflunomide, fluoroquinolones, or switching to mTOR inhibitors could be considered [25, 46, 48, 49].

Coronavirus 2019

COVID-19 is a disease caused by Severe Acute Respiratory Syndrome Coronavirus 2 (SARS-CoV-2) and is considered the most important pandemic of the 21st century. Since the first reports from Wuhan, China, COVID-19 has rapidly spread throughout the world. By December 2021, an estimated 270 million people have been infected with SARS-CoV-2 worldwide, with more than 5 million deaths [50]. Current evidence suggests that heart and lung recipients may have a worse outcome than non-transplant patients, with a mortality rate of 30% [51].

The clinical manifestations of COVID-19 range from mild and non-specific symptoms to severe pneumonia requiring mechanical ventilation or multiple organ failure. The clinical presentation of heart transplant patients with COVID-19 is similar to that reported in other types of transplants. Mortality is directly related to age and other comorbidities that increase cardiovascular risk, such as high blood pressure, diabetes, chronic kidney disease, chronic lung disease, and obesity [52].

In a multicenter study conducted in Germany, 21 heart transplants with COVID-19 were evaluated. Overall mortality was 33%, mostly associated with left ventricular dysfunction, arrhythmias, thromboembolic events and markedly elevated cardiac biomarkers [53]. In another descriptive multicenter study with 99 heart transplant recipients, atypical presentations were observed: 43% did not develop fever, 49% had cough, while in 46% gastrointestinal symptoms predominated. Two-thirds of the patients required hospitalization and a quarter had severe disease, defined as the need for mechanical ventilation, renal replacement therapy, and use of vasoactive drugs [54]. Finally, Latif et al. conducted a retrospective study of 28 adult heart transplant recipients with COVID-19 and found out that mortality was 25% [55].

The severity of the disease depends not only on viral invasion and proliferation, but also on the intense immune response determined by the cytokine storm that leads to myocardial injury and death [55]. Left ventricular dysfunction, elevated pulmonary arterial pressures, and tricuspid pulmonary valve regurgitation are seen particularly in patients with a severe course of disease and high mortality. This could be a result of mechanical ventilation but it could also be related to the thromboembolic complications of COVID-19. In severe forms of the disease, sepsis increases pro-inflammatory cytokines and promotes activation of the coagulation cascade. This can be reflected in elevated D-dimer levels that worsen the prognosis of patients. Concomitantly, COVID-19 patients that present with elevated cardiac biomarkers such as high-sensitivity cardiac troponin T and natriuretic peptides have more severe disease. This could be related to direct viral myocardial injury, myocardial injury secondary to pro-inflammatory cytokines, imbalance between oxygen demand and supply, and prothrombotic state [56].

The effect of immunosuppression on the course of this disease remains unclear. It is not yet known whether immunosuppression can attenuate the immune dysregulation seen in severe disease [55]. Genuardi et al. studied 99 heart transplant recipients with COVID-19 and followed them until resolution. They observed that age over 60 years old was associated with a higher risk of death (OR = 7.6.95% confidence interval [CI] 1.9-51) and the combined use of calcineurin inhibitors, antimetabolites and prednisone was associated with severe disease compared to calcineurin inhibitors and antimetabolites alone (OR = 7.3.95% CI 1.8-36.2). Perhaps this is related to the fact that severe immunosuppression regimens predispose to a higher risk of secondary infections [57]. Currently, the Clinical Practice Guideline for Solid Organ Donation and Transplantation During the COVID-19 Pandemic recommends that induction immunosuppression should not be modified to prevent the acquisition or severity of COVID-19. This recommendation is based on 9 publications of individual case reports and small case series. Furthermore, they suggest that temporary adjustment of maintenance immunosuppression may be considered for these patients. This recommendation is based on 31 publications (case report and case series), of which 6 included heart transplant recipients [58].

Complete vaccination of transplant candidates and family members is recommended. In addition, despite the vaccination status, they must continue with preventive measures (distancing, hand washing, and face mask).

Currently, donors with active COVID-19 are rejected. Although donors with epidemiological exposure, or with a history of COVID-19 can be accepted. Therefore, it is recommended to test the donors with SARS CoV-2 PCR prior to ablation.

Bacterial Infections

Bacterial Infections by Common Microorganisms in the Recipient

Bacterial infection is the most common infection and accounts for 40-50% of all infections. Within the first 30 days after transplantation, the most frequent are nosocomial infections, especially surgical site infections. The spectrum of pathogens is similar to that of major thoracic surgical procedures and other critically ill patients. Less frequent are donor-derived infections, which generally cause clinical symptoms shortly after transplantation.

Infections common to other surgical patients such as pneumonia, catheter-associated bacteremia, and urinary tract infections also occur during this period. From the third to the twelfth month after transplantation, patients with satisfactory graft function, in whom immunosuppression begins to decrease, a greater risk of infections compared to immunocompetent patients still persists. The spectrum and severity of infections generally depends on the epidemiological context of the patient [7].

Bacteremic Donors

Unexpected transmission of donor-derived diseases is rare and complicates less than 1% of transplants. In general, most donor-derived infections cause symptoms shortly after transplantation. Bacterial infections are almost always recognized within 30 days and rarely manifest after 45 days. Outcomes can be poor, with high morbidity, graft loss, and mortality rates of up to 25% in affected recipients [7].

Approximately 5% of organ donors have bacteremia at the time of organ procurement [59-61]. The risk of donor-transmitted infection varies depending on the type of bacteria causing the infection [62]. However, bacteremic donors can be used in certain circumstances [60, 61]. It is recommended that the infected donor receives specific antimicrobial treatment for at least 24-48 hours, optimally with some degree of clinical response (improved white blood cell count and hemodynamics). In this case, the recipient should be treated with a 7-to-14-day course of antibiotics directed at the organism isolated from the donor [4]. On the contrary, donation is contraindicated when donors present bacterial sepsis with septic shock or multiple organ failure, bacteremia due to highly virulence germs capable of producing distant metastases or invasion of the vascular endothelium (*Streptococcus* group A, Vancomycin-resistant *Enterococcus, Streptococcus millieri, Salmonella sp.*, fungi, mycobacteria or *Nocardia*) without adequate treatment or persistence of positive blood cultures despite treatment.

Colonization by Multi-resistant Bacteria

One of the main challenges is the global emergence of multi-resistant microorganisms. Donors have been routinely screened for the presence of multi-resistant organisms and perioperative prophylaxis has been tailored accordingly.

Major complications can occur when donors are infected or colonized with oxacillin-resistant *Staphylococcus aureus*, vancomycin-resistant *Enterococcus*, carbapenemase-producing bacteria, pan-resistant *P. aeruginosa*, and other pan-resistant gram-negative bacteria. Reports describe poor outcomes in these cases [63]. In general, these donors should be used with great caution.

The presence of multi-resistant bacteria in donors must be reported to the potential receiving center, clarifying the site of colonization, the type of microorganism and its antibiotic sensitivity. Regarding recipients, longer hospital stays, especially in intensive care units, are risk factors for colonization with multi-resistant organisms, because they have more requirements for invasive diagnostic and therapeutic procedures, and are more exposed to broad-spectrum antibiotics than other groups of patients.

Contamination of Preservation Fluid

Preservation fluid can become contaminated during handling when used on the donor, in the ablation process or when transporting the organ. The infection transmission rate from the preservation fluid reported by the different series ranges from 0% to 42.9% [64, 65]. The risk of transmission can be mitigated when the recipient receives effective prophylaxis for a minimum period of 48 hours, continuing treatment based on the cultures obtained.

Preservation fluids with the development of *Staphylococcus aureus, Enterococcus spp,* Enterobacteria, *Pseudomonas aeruginosa* and *Candida spp* represent a higher risk of recipient infection, especially at the level of the vascular sutures (mycotic aneurysms). In contrast, skin-contaminating microorganisms have rarely been implicated in infectious processes in the recipient.

Antimicrobial prophylaxis should be adjusted according to the results of the preservation fluid cultures, with a duration from 5 to 14 days depending on the virulence of the microorganism found. In the case of fungi isolation, it could last up to 4 weeks in the presence of infection and 6 weeks in the case of vascular compromise [66, 67].

Pneumonia

Pneumonia is one of the most common infections in heart transplant recipients. Opportunistic infections may occur due to the effect of immunosuppressants that predominantly inhibit the T-lymphocyte response. Humoral immunity may also be impaired, particularly with the current use of drugs such as rituximab, increasing the risk of bacterial pneumonia. In fact, neutropenia is a common complication of both immunosuppressive drugs and anti-infective agents (e.g., mycophenolate mofetil and valganciclovir) and can lead to bacterial or, less commonly, fungal infections.

Chest tomography is superior to plain radiography in detecting less dense infiltrates, such as ground glass opacities, locating lesions, and detecting complications (pleural effusion, abscesses, and cavitations). Ventilation-associated pneumonia and hospital-acquired pneumonia in non-ventilated patients are important perioperative complications of transplant recipients.

The choice of treatment of these entities should be based on the local epidemiology of the pathogens and their antimicrobial susceptibilities. It is recommended to include empirical coverage for *Staphylococcus aureus, Pseudomonas aeruginosa*, and other gram-negative bacilli [68]. In patients with risk factors for *Pseudomonas spp* or those who present septic shock, they require a broader empirical coverage [69]. Finally, one of the leading agents of community-acquired pneumonia in recipients is *Streptococcus pneumoniae*, and it is associated with significant morbidity and mortality.

Mediastinitis

In heart transplant recipients, surgical wound complications are seen in 8% to 15% of patients, but much higher incidences of up to 40% have also been reported. Superficial wound infections range from 3.9% to 16% in heart transplant recipients. Mediastinitis after heart transplantation was at least twice as likely to occur when compared with non-transplant cardiac operations [70]. Deep wound infections, including mediastinitis, are reported with incidences of 2.4% to 35%. Sternal dehiscence occurs in 12.5% to 25%. In most reports of general cardiac surgery and heart transplantation, gram-positive microorganisms, especially *Staphylococcus aureus*, often methicillin-resistant and *Enterococcus faecalis*, have been isolated from infected sternal wounds. Furthermore, cases of gram-negative organisms, such as *Escherichia coli* and *Acinetobacter spp*, have also been reported. In particular, a higher incidence of fungal wound infections was described after heart transplantation compared with other cardiac surgeries [71].

Commonly described risk factors for surgical wound complications in general cardiac surgery, such as diabetes, reoperation, and increased body mass index, are also of relevance in heart transplantation. In addition, other risk factor specific to heart transplantation are [71]:

- Immunosuppression
- Poorer health status of patients who usually remain hospitalized for a long time before transplantation
- Renal kidney failure
- Mechanical circulatory support as a bridge to transplantation.

After the initial diagnosis of mediastinitis, prompt aggressive surgical treatment with surgical debridement, including radical excision of necrotic tissue, is essential. Additionally, at least 4 to 6 weeks of antibiotic treatment should be implemented [71].

Central Nervous System Infections

Central nervous system infections occur in 5 to 10% of transplant recipients. After transplantation, the risk intervals for infection are classified into three time periods, although this timeline is influenced and altered by anti-infective prophylaxis, intensity of immunosuppression, and the development of allograft rejection [72].

In the first month after transplantation, these infections are rare and are most often attributed to herpes simplex virus, *Aspergillus* or donor-transmitted infections.

The classic opportunistic infections occur between 2 to 6 months after transplantation and coincide with the peak effects of immunosuppression, resulting in the reactivation of latent infections hosted by the recipient, transmitted by the donor, or acquired in the community. Typical pathogens during this period include CMV, *Toxoplasma gondii*, and *Mycobacterium tuberculosis*. After 6 months, *Cryptococcus spp* is the third most common invasive fungal infection in transplant recipients [73].

In the late post-transplant period, the risk of opportunistic infections decreases, but they can still occur. The most common pathogens causing bacterial meningitis in recipients are *Streptococcus pneumoniae* and *Listeria monocytogenes*.

Infections Associated with Devices

Devices used in heart transplant candidates such as ventricular assist devices, extracorporeal membrane oxygenation, central venous catheters, pacemakers or implantable cardioverter defibrillators can be the source of infections.

Infections related to ventricular assist devices can occur in the postoperative period, after the device has been removed. This is due to partial treatment of infection in the recipient or due to material retained from the infected device or from other retained foreign bodies.

The rates of bloodstream infections in patients with ventricular assist devices are around 20-27% [74]. The risk of infection is highest in the first month after implantation, and when bacteremia occurs, mortality increases. The most frequent microorganisms are *Staphylococcus sp* (> 50%) with a predominance of *Staphylococcus aureus* and *S.epidermidis*, followed by gram-negative bacteria with a predominance of *Pseudomonas sp.* (up to 28%), *Serratia sp.* (9%), *Enterobacter sp.* (2%), and *Klebsiella sp.* (2%). Fungal infections account for less than 10%, predominantly *Candida sp* [75]. Atypical mycobacterial have been reported rarely [76].

The factors that contribute to the development of endovascular infections in these patients are similar to those observed in infections due to extracorporeal membrane oxygenation or central venous catheters. Some of these factors are the presence of thrombi, device surface characteristics, blood flow dynamics, device internal surface area, and coagulopathy

The primary approach is to remove the entire device at the time of heart transplantation and also consider removal or replacement of other devices that were present with the infected ventricular assist device (e.g., implantable cardioverter defibrillator, pacemaker). In the post-transplant period, antibiotics directed to the specific pathogen and the type of infection should be used, and embolic phenomena should be ruled out in addition to endocarditis [75].

Tuberculosis

Tuberculosis (TBC) is caused by *Mycobacterium tuberculosis*. There are three possible different clinical courses of this disease: cure, with the elimination of the microorganism; primary disease; or latent disease, with the possibility of reactivation [77]. The incidence of TBC in cardiac recipients is estimated at 1.46% with variations between endemic and non-endemic countries [78].

The clinical presentation can be insidious and atypical in transplant recipients with a higher incidence of extrapulmonary (30%) and disseminated TBC (16%). However, pulmonary disease continues to be the most frequent presentation (54%) (Figure 2). Mortality in cardiac recipients is approximately 24% [78].

Documented cases of primary infection are rare in transplantation. Instead, active TBC is generally caused by reactivation of an untreated, latent or cured primary infection. Therefore, TBC screening should be performed in all transplant candidates, including an epidemiological history, purified protein derivative (PPD) or Interferon-Gamma Release Assay (IGRA) test, and chest x-ray or computed tomography scan. Those with positive PPD or IGRA should undergo chemoprophylaxis once active tuberculosis has been ruled out. In cases where a high epidemiological risk is considered and/or lesions compatible with tuberculosis are observed without a history of having received adequate treatment, chemoprophylaxis should be performed regardless of the result of the PPD or IGRA test [77, 78]. Transplant candidates diagnosed with active TBC must complete treatment before heart transplantation.

On the other hand, TBC can also be transmitted by the donor through organs and tissues [79]. It is estimated that this route represents less than 5% of active TBC cases; however, it can have great impact on morbidity and mortality. The diagnosis of active TBC in the donor is a contraindication to organ donation [77].

Treatment of TBC in transplant patients is often difficult due to toxicity and interactions between anti-TBC drugs and immunosuppressants. In this population, the use of regimens without rifampicin, an induction phase with 4 drugs, a reduction to 2 or 3 drugs in the consolidation phase, and longer treatments are usually recommended [77].

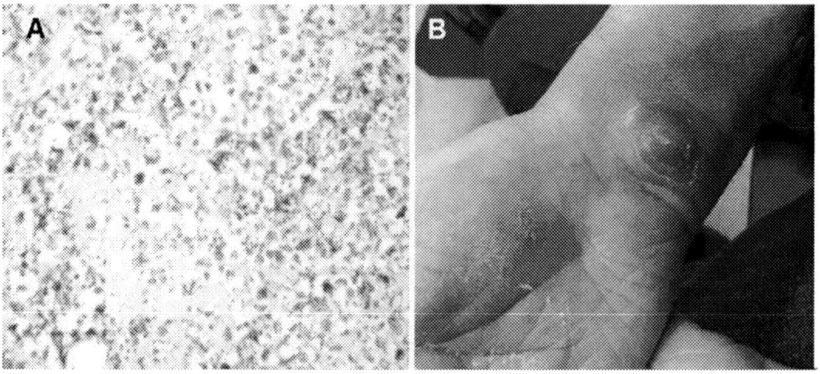

Figure 2. Manifestations of Mycobacterium tuberculosis.
A. Necrotizing pneumonia, Ziehl-Neelsen stain with numerous acid-fast bacilli. B. Metastatic tuberculous abscess.

Parasitic Infections

Toxoplasmosis

Toxoplasmosis is a parasitic disease caused by the protozoan *Toxoplasma gondii*. It has a worldwide distribution with higher incidence in endemic regions. In transplant recipients, infection can occur through ingestion of contaminated food or water, after receiving an infected allograft, or by reactivation of latent infection.

This parasite is relevant in heart transplantation due to its high affinity for muscle tissue. Heart transplant recipients who are seronegative for toxoplasmosis and receive an organ from a seropositive donor have a 57–75% risk of developing a symptomatic infection without prophylaxis, usually within 3 months after transplantation [80].

Patients may present with fever, myocarditis, lymphadenopathy, hepatosplenomegaly, meningitis, brain abscess, chorioretinitis, pneumonitis, hepatitis, pancytopenia or disseminated disease. Symptoms usually appear within 3 months after transplantation; however, late presentations can be seen, particularly after discontinuation of Trimethoprim/sulfamethoxazol (TMP/SMX) chemoprophylaxis [81]. Toxoplasmosis can cause myocarditis, heart failure, or arrhythmias, which may be clinically indistinguishable from graft rejection.

Definitive diagnosis requires identification of tachyzoites on tissue, seroconversion or PCR amplification of toxoplasma DNA from infected tissues, blood or body fluids [81, 82]. Both heart transplant donors and candidates must be screened for Toxoplasma IgG prior to transplantation [82].

After heart transplantation, routine use of TMP/SMX prophylaxis decreases the risk of toxoplasmosis reactivation. Many studies showed successful prophylaxis using TMP/SMX for different durations (ranging from 3 months to life-long schemes) [83].

Treatment of infection is based on an induction phase with pyrimethamine, sulfadiazine, and leucovorin for at least 6 weeks, followed by chronic suppressive therapy with these drugs [81].

Chagas Disease

Chagas disease (ChD) affects about 18 million people in the American continent. In endemic areas, screening for *T. cruzi* infection should be routinely performed on all candidates and potential donors. The diagnosis of ChD is based on serological tests in the pre-transplant period.

Heart grafting from donors with positive antibodies to *Trypanosoma cruzi* is contraindicated for transplantation. However, people with ChD can donate organs other than the heart.

The frequency of chagasic cardiomyopathy as cause of heart transplantation varies by countries in endemic areas (e.g., in Argentina is approximately 9% and in Brazil 13%) [84, 85]. Post-transplant evolution does not differ significantly from heart transplants of other etiologies but ChD reactivation rate is high (up to 70%) (See Chapter 16) [86]. Reactivation can be symptomatic or asymptomatic. Common clinical manifestations are panniculitis followed by myocarditis and encephalitis. Early diagnosis of reactivation and early antiparasitic treatment are important to avoid increased mortality [86].

Systematized follow-up with direct methods is recommended after transplant and after intensification of immunosuppression [87]. The Strout method detects parasites in the bloodstream but it can take days or weeks to become positive and its sensitivity is low [88]. The PCR technique is a sensitive diagnostic tool that can show positive findings days or weeks earlier than conventional parasitological methods [89, 90]. This strategy allows preemptive therapy in case of reactivation. When ChD reactivation occurs, treatment with Benznidazole or Nifurtimox is indicated for 30-60 days. The toxicity of these drugs should be monitored, as they can cause leukopenia or elevated liver enzymes. There is no evidence on the efficacy of primary or secondary prophylaxis with benznidazole for transplant recipients.

Finally, to avoid *T. cruzi* reactivation in heart transplantation, the suggested immunosuppression is with lower doses of corticosteroids, adjusted levels of cyclosporine (100–150 ng/ml) or tacrolimus, and mycophenolate-sparing regimens. There is no consensus on management of immunosuppression during reactivation episodes, but it should be reduced whenever possible [91].

Intestinal Parasitosis: Strongyloides

Strongyloides stercoralis, a globally distributed intestinal nematode, is endemic to tropical and subtropical areas. It can complete its life cycle both in the environment and in the human host. As a consequence, the parasite has a "self-infectious" cycle that produces long-term persistent infections.

Strongyloides stercoralis can affect transplant recipients by primary infection in the post-transplant period, by transmission through the graft, or by reactivation of a latent infection [92].

The effects of cell-mediated immunity, and the use of corticosteroids, are the main risk factors for the development of severe cases. Strongyloidiasis can be a devastating disease in transplant recipients; the mortality rate is close to 50% in hyperinfection syndrome and 70% in disseminated infection [93].

Clinical syndromes include acute infection, chronic infection, hyperinfection syndrome and disseminated disease. Diagnosis is usually made by serological methods, parasitological test that detect rhabditiform larvae, or molecular tests from clinical samples [94]. Pre-transplant screening of the recipient is suggested, mainly in endemic areas. Ivermectin is the treatment of choice for *Strongyloides stercoralis* infection.

Fungal Infections

Candida

Candida infection is almost always endogenous in origin and usually begins with colonization of damaged skin or mucosa, the gastrointestinal tract, or the urinary tract. *Candida Albicans* is the most common species, although other species such as *C. tropicalis, C. krusei, C. parapsilosis and C. glabrata* are increasing in frequency. During the heart procurement, the contamination of the preservation fluid is unusual. When *Candida spp.* grows, antifungal prophylaxis should be initiated [95].

Candida infections are rare after heart transplantation, and antifungal prophylaxis is not routinely recommended for these patients [95]. In heart and lung transplantation, the risk factors for *Candida spp* infection are the use of broad-spectrum and prolonged antibiotics, the presence of a central venous catheter, and dialysis. Prophylaxis for *Aspergillus spp.* in these cases also provides coverage for *Candida spp* [95].

After heart transplant, the most common clinical presentation is mucocutaneous candidiasis, such as oral thrush, esophageal candidiasis and vulvovaginitis. Invasive candidiasis, pneumonia, pericarditis, or mediastinitis are rare and have been described more frequently in heart or lung transplant patients.

Aspergillus

The incidence of Invasive Aspergillosis (IA) in heart transplant recipients ranges from 1% to 14% [96, 97]. Risk factors for the development of IA include [98, 99]:

- *Aspergillus* spores in the air in the intensive care unit
- *Aspergillus fumigatus* in bronchoalveolar lavage,
- Reoperation, thoracic surgery
- CMV disease
- Post-transplant hemodialysis
- AI episode in any patient in the heart transplant program 2 months before or after heart transplantation in the context of an outbreak.
- Allograft rejection
- Increased number of hospitalizations prior to transplantation.

AI prophylaxis is suggested if the patient meets one or more of the risk factors. Overall, 1-year mortality in heart transplant recipients with IA was approximately 67% [96]. However, in recent years mortality has decreased to 38% [100].

In case of clinical suspicion of IA, imaging studies of the suspected site of infection should be performed according to the clinical symptoms, such as computed tomography of the chest, brain and paranasal sinuses. If pulmonary infiltrates are identified, bronchoscopy with bronchoalveolar lavage is indicated to perform fungal cultures and galactomannan testing (Figure 3).

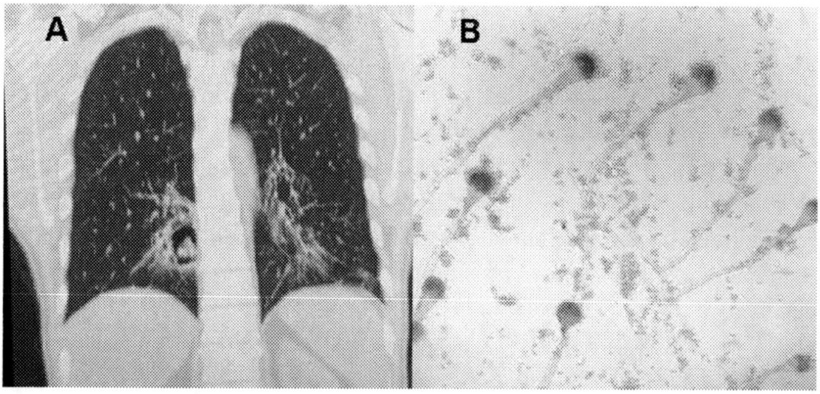

Figure 3. Pulmonary Aspergillosis.
A. Chest computed tomography, Aspergilloma within a cavern. B. *Aspergillus fumigatus* hyphae.

If a lesion is readily accessible for biopsy (i.e., skin lesion, sinusitis), the tissue should be submitted for histopathology as well as fungal culture and molecular testing.

The mainstays of IA treatment are based on antifungal therapy, assessment of the need for surgical debridement (which is not usually necessary in IA), and reduction of immunosuppression if possible. Voriconazole is the first-line treatment for IA. It is recommended to monitor plasma azole levels in all patients to ensure efficacy and avoid toxicity. When blood azole concentrations cannot be adequately documented in patients on extracorporeal membrane oxygenation, liposomal Amphotericin B may be indicated [101].

Pneumocystis Jiroveccii

Solid organ transplant patients are at risk for *Pneumocystis jirovecii* (PJP) infection. Historically, an incidence of at least 3% to 5% of PJP among transplant recipients was considered a threshold for the use of prophylaxis [102]. Major risk factors include [103]:

- Immunosuppression treatment for graft rejection
- CMV infection
- High corticosteroid dose (e.g., >20 mg daily of prednisone for at least 2 weeks)
- Flares of autoimmune disease
- Type of transplant (lung transplant).

Universal prophylaxis is generally recommended at most transplant centers, for at least 6-12 months after transplantation. For heart or lung transplants and for transplant patients with a history of prior PJP infection, lifelong prophylaxis is often indicated [103]. TMP/SMX is the drug of choice for PJP prophylaxis, although side effects require monitoring. Bone marrow suppression may occur and be potentiated by concomitant administration of other myelosuppressive agents. Rash can occur from benign reactions to Stevens-Johnson syndrome. Other potential side effects include hepatitis, interstitial nephritis, aseptic meningitis, and pancreatitis. This prophylaxis is also useful in preventing infections such as *Nocardia spp.*, *Toxoplasma gondii*, *Isospora belli*, and some community-acquired bacteria [103]. Dapsone is often used as a second-line agent for PJP prophylaxis. Its use is not recommended in patients who have experienced severe adverse effects with TMP/SMX, such as desquamation toxidermy, severe neutropenia, nephritis or hepatitis, or in patients with glucose-6-phosphate-dehydrogenase deficiency. Atovaquone, and aerosolized pentamidine are often used as alternative drugs [103].

Conclusion

Although great advances have been made in the field, infectious diseases remain a major cause of morbidity and mortality in heart transplant patients. To achieve the best possible outcomes, it is important to identify patients at highest risk, implement personalized prophylaxis when appropriate, use advanced diagnostic techniques, and choose the adequate treatment. Monitoring of side effects and interactions is also essential in this special population of immunosuppressed patients. Therefore, any healthcare provider treating heart transplant patients should be familiar with the basic concepts related to their infectious diseases.

References

[1] Multani A, Moayedi Y, Puing A, Henricksen E, Garvert DW, Gomez CA, Tremblay-Gravel M, Bunce PE, Luikart H, Ross HJ, Khush KK, Montoya JG, Teuteberg JJ. Recent Trends of Infectious Complications Following Heart Transplantation. *Transplantation.* 2020 Oct;104(10):e284-e294.

[2] Malinis M, Boucher HW; AST Infectious Diseases Community of Practice. Screening of donor and candidate prior to solid organ transplantation-Guidelines from the American Society of Transplantation Infectious Diseases Community of Practice. *Clin Transplant.* 2019 Sep;33(9):e13548.

[3] Fischer SA, Lu K; AST Infectious Diseases Community of Practice. Screening of donor and recipient in solid organ transplantation. *Am J Transplant.* 2013 Mar;13 Suppl 4(Suppl 4):9-21.

[4] Fishman JA, Greenwald MA, Grossi PA. Transmission of infection with human allografts: essential considerations in donor screening. *Clin Infect Dis.* 2012 Sep;55(5):720-7.

[5] OPTN Ad Hoc Disease Transmission Advisory Committee. Briefing to the OPTN Board of Directors on Align OPTN Policy with U.S. Public Health Service Guideline [online]. 2020 [cited 2022-Jan-20]. Available from: https://optn.transplant.hrsa.gov/media/4225/bp_202012_align_2020_phs_guideline.pdf.

[6] Seem DL, Lee I, Umscheid CA, Kuehnert MJ; United States Public Health Service. PHS guideline for reducing human immunodeficiency virus, hepatitis B virus, and hepatitis C virus transmission through organ transplantation. *Public Health Rep.* 2013 Jul;128(4):247-343.

[7] Wolfe CR, Ison MG; AST Infectious Diseases Community of Practice. Donor-derived infections: Guidelines from the American Society of Transplantation Infectious Diseases Community of Practice. *Clin Transplant.* 2019 Sep;33 (9):e13547.

[8] Jones JM, Kracalik I, Levi ME, Bowman JS 3rd, Berger JJ, Bixler D, Buchacz K, Moorman A, Brooks JT, Basavaraju SV. Assessing Solid Organ Donors and Monitoring Transplant Recipients for Human Immunodeficiency Virus, Hepatitis B Virus, and Hepatitis C Virus Infection - U.S. Public Health Service Guideline, 2020. *MMWR Recomm Rep.* 2020 Jun 26;69(4):1-16.

[9] Razonable RR, Humar A. Cytomegalovirus in solid organ transplant recipients-Guidelines of the American Society of Transplantation Infectious Diseases Community of Practice. *Clin Transplant.* 2019 Sep;33(9):e13512.

[10] Meesing A, Razonable RR. New Developments in the Management of Cytomegalovirus Infection After Transplantation. *Drugs.* 2018 Jul;78(11):1085-1103.

[11] Ljungman P, Boeckh M, Hirsch HH, Josephson F, Lundgren J, Nichols G, Pikis A, Razonable RR, Miller V, Griffiths PD; Disease Definitions Working Group of the Cytomegalovirus Drug Development Forum. Definitions of Cytomegalovirus Infection and Disease in Transplant Patients for Use in Clinical Trials. *Clin Infect Dis.* 2017 Jan 1;64(1):87-91.

[12] Razonable RR, Hayden RT. Clinical utility of viral load in management of cytomegalovirus infection after solid organ transplantation. *Clin Microbiol Rev.* 2013 Oct;26(4):703-27.

[13] Gliga S, Korth J, Krawczyk A, Wilde B, Horn PA, Witzke O, Lindemann M, Fiedler M. T-Track-CMV and QuantiFERON-CMV assays for prediction of protection from CMV reactivation in kidney transplant recipients. *J Clin Virol.* 2018 Aug;105:91-96.

[14] Kotton CN, Kumar D, Caliendo AM, Huprikar S, Chou S, Danziger-Isakov L, Humar A; The Transplantation Society International CMV Consensus Group. The Third International Consensus Guidelines on the Management of Cytomegalovirus in Solid-organ Transplantation. *Transplantation.* 2018 Jun;102(6):900-931.

[15] Cherrier L, Nasar A, Goodlet KJ, Nailor MD, Tokman S, Chou S. Emergence of letermovir resistance in a lung transplant recipient with ganciclovir-resistant cytomegalovirus infection. *Am J Transplant.* 2018 Dec;18(12):3060-3064.

[16] Lee DH, Zuckerman RA; AST Infectious Diseases Community of Practice. Herpes simplex virus infections in solid organ transplantation: Guidelines from the American Society of Transplantation Infectious Diseases Community of Practice. *Clin Transplant.* 2019 Sep;33(9):e13526.

[17] Pergam SA, Limaye AP; AST Infectious Diseases Community of Practice. Varicella zoster virus in solid organ transplantation: Guidelines from the American Society of Transplantation Infectious Diseases Community of Practice. *Clin Transplant.* 2019 Sep;33(9):e13622.

[18] Taylor AL, Marcus R, Bradley JA. Post-transplant lymphoproliferative disorders (PTLD) after solid organ transplantation. *Crit Rev Oncol Hematol.* 2005 Oct;56(1):155-67.

[19] Gulley ML, Swinnen LJ, Plaisance KT Jr, Schnell C, Grogan TM, Schneider BG; Southwest Oncology Group. Tumor origin and CD20 expression in posttransplant lymphoproliferative disorder occurring in solid organ transplant recipients: implications for immune-based therapy. *Transplantation.* 2003 Sep 27;76(6):959-64.

[20] Olagne J, Caillard S, Gaub MP, Chenard MP, Moulin B. Post-transplant lymphoproliferative disorders: determination of donor/recipient origin in a large cohort of kidney recipients. *Am J Transplant.* 2011 Jun;11(6):1260-9.

[21] Sampaio MS, Cho YW, Qazi Y, Bunnapradist S, Hutchinson IV, Shah T. Posttransplant malignancies in solid organ adult recipients: an analysis of the U.S. National Transplant Database. *Transplantation.* 2012 Nov 27;94(10):990-8.

[22] Allen UD, Preiksaitis JK; AST Infectious Diseases Community of Practice. Post-transplant lymphoproliferative disorders, Epstein-Barr virus infection, and disease in solid organ transplantation: Guidelines from the American Society of Transplantation Infectious Diseases Community of Practice. *Clin Transplant.* 2019 Sep;33(9):e13652.

[23] AlDabbagh MA, Gitman MR, Kumar D, Humar A, Rotstein C, Husain S. The Role of Antiviral Prophylaxis for the Prevention of Epstein-Barr Virus-Associated Posttransplant Lymphoproliferative Disease in Solid Organ Transplant Recipients: A Systematic Review. *Am J Transplant.* 2017 Mar;17(3):770-781.

[24] Lautenschlager I, Razonable RR. Human herpesvirus-6 infections in kidney, liver, lung, and heart transplantation: review. *Transpl Int.* 2012 May;25(5):493-502.

[25] Manuel O, Ison MG. *Infectious Diseases in Solid-organ Transplant Recipients: A Practical Approach.* 1st Edition. Germany: Springer; 2019.

[26] Pellett Madan R, Hand J; AST Infectious Diseases Community of Practice. Human herpesvirus 6, 7, and 8 in solid organ transplantation: Guidelines from the

American Society of Transplantation Infectious Diseases Community of Practice. *Clin Transplant.* 2019 Sep;33(9):e13518.
[27] Horan JL, Stout JE, Alexander BD. Hepatitis B core antibody-positive donors in cardiac transplantation: a single-center experience. *Transpl Infect Dis.* 2014 Oct;16(5):859-63.
[28] Te H, Doucette K. Viral hepatitis: Guidelines by the American Society of Transplantation Infectious Disease Community of Practice. *Clin Transplant.* 2019 Sep;33(9):e13514.
[29] Vitrone M, Iossa D, Rinaldi L, Pafundi PC, Molaro R, Parrella A, Andini R, Ragone E, Maiello C, Zampino R, Durante-Mangoni E. Hepatitis B virus reactivation after heart transplant: Incidence and clinical impact. *J Clin Virol.* 2017 Nov;96:54-59.
[30] Theodoropoulos NM, La Hoz RM, Wolfe C, Vece G, Bag R, Berry GJ, Bucio J, Danziger-Isakov L, Florescu DF, Goldberg D, Ho CS, Lilly K, Malinis M, Mehta AK, Nalesnik MA, Sawyer R, Strasfeld L, Wood RP, Michaels MG. Donor derived hepatitis B virus infection: Analysis of the Organ Procurement & Transplantation Network/United Network for Organ Sharing Ad Hoc Disease Transmission Advisory Committee. *Transpl Infect Dis.* 2021 Feb;23(1):e13458.
[31] Shin HS, Cho HJ, Jeon ES, Hwang HY, Kim JJ, Kim KB, Oh BH, Lee HY. The impact of hepatitis B on heart transplantation: 19 years of national experience in Korea. *Ann Transplant.* 2014 Apr 23;19:182-7.
[32] Rochlani Y, Diab K, Jorde UP. Hepatitis C-Positive Donors in Cardiac Transplantation: Problems and Opportunities. *Curr Heart Fail Rep.* 2020 Aug;17(4):106-115.
[33] Levitsky J, Formica RN, Bloom RD, Charlton M, Curry M, Friedewald J, Friedman J, Goldberg D, Hall S, Ison M, Kaiser T, Klassen D, Klintmalm G, Kobashigawa J, Liapakis A, O'Conner K, Reese P, Stewart D, Terrault N, Theodoropoulos N, Trotter J, Verna E, Volk M. The American Society of Transplantation Consensus Conference on the Use of Hepatitis C Viremic Donors in Solid Organ Transplantation. *Am J Transplant.* 2017 Nov;17(11):2790-2802.
[34] Raasikh T, Jamali T, Flores A, Cotton RT, Ramanathan V, Tan HP, Hernaez R. Systematic review: hepatitis C viraemic allografts to hepatitis C-negative recipients in solid organ transplantation. *Aliment Pharmacol Ther.* 2021 Sep;54(5):571-582.
[35] Kaul DR, Sharma TS; AST ID Community of Practice. Human T-cell lymphotrophic virus in solid-organ transplant recipients: Guidelines from the American society of transplantation infectious diseases community of practice. *Clin Transplant.* 2019 Sep;33(9):e13575.
[36] Castel MA, Pérez-Villa F, Miró JM. Heart transplantation in HIV-infected patients: more cases in Europe. *J Heart Lung Transplant.* 2011 Dec;30(12):1418.
[37] Agüero F, Castel MA, Cocchi S, Moreno A, Mestres CA, Cervera C, Pérez-Villa F, Tuset M, Cartañà R, Manzardo C, Guaraldi G, Gatell JM, Miró JM. An Update on Heart Transplantation in Human Immunodeficiency Virus-Infected Patients. *Am J Transplant.* 2016 Jan;16(1):21-8.
[38] Boignard A, Blanc M, Chavanon O. High-urgency priority heart transplantation in HIV-positive patients on life support: breaking barriers? *J Heart Lung Transplant.* 2011 Aug;30(8):968-9.

[39] Sims DB, Uriel N, González-Costello J, Deng MC, Restaino SW, Farr MA, Takayama H, Mancini DM, Naka Y, Jorde UP. Human immunodeficiency virus infection and left ventricular assist devices: a case series. *J Heart Lung Transplant.* 2011 Sep;30(9):1060-4.

[40] Gupta S, Markham DW, Mammen PP, Kaiser P, Patel P, Ring WS, Drazner MH. Long-term follow-up of a heart transplant recipient with documented seroconversion to HIV-positive status 1 year after transplant. *Am J Transplant.* 2008 Apr;8(4):893-6.

[41] Koval CE, Farr M, Krisl J, Haidar G, Pereira MR, Shrestha N, Malinis MF, Mueller NJ, Hannan MM, Grossi P, Huprikar S. Heart or lung transplant outcomes in HIV-infected recipients. *J Heart Lung Transplant.* 2019 Dec;38(12):1296-1305.

[42] Chen C, Wen X, Yadav A, Belviso N, Kogut S, McCauley J. Outcomes in human immunodeficiency virus-infected recipients of heart transplants. *Clin Transplant.* 2019 Jan;33(1):e13440.

[43] Lee I, Blumberg E. HIV and organ transplantation. *Curr Opin Organ Transplant.* 2020 Aug;25(4):371-376.

[44] Sénéchal I, Châteauvert N, Gervais P, Voisine P, Dubois M, Sénéchal M. Complex drug interactions in an HIV-seropositive heart transplant recipient. *Turk Kardiyol Dern Ars.* 2020 Mar;48(2):180-184.

[45] Durand CM, Segev D, Sugarman J. Realizing HOPE: The Ethics of Organ Transplantation From HIV-Positive Donors. *Ann Intern Med.* 2016 Jul 19;165(2):138-42.

[46] Vigil D, Konstantinov NK, Barry M, Harford AM, Servilla KS, Kim YH, Sun Y, Ganta K, Tzamaloukas AH. BK nephropathy in the native kidneys of patients with organ transplants: Clinical spectrum of BK infection. *World J Transplant.* 2016 Sep 24;6(3):472-504.

[47] Lavien G, Alger J, Preece J, Alexiev BA, Alexander RB. BK Virus-Associated Invasive Urothelial Carcinoma With Prominent Micropapillary Carcinoma Component in a Cardiac Transplant Patient: Case Report and Review of Literature. *Clin Genitourin Cancer.* 2015 Dec;13(6):e397-9.

[48] Nieto-Ríos JF, Benavides-Henao DA, Aristizabal-Alzate A, Morales-Contreras C, Chacón-Jaimes DC, Zuluaga-Valencia G, Serna-Higuita LM. BK virus nephropathy in a heart transplant recipient. *J Bras Nefrol.* 2021 Jul-Sep;43(3):434-439.

[49] Joseph A, Pilichowska M, Boucher H, Kiernan M, DeNofrio D, Inker LA. BK Virus Nephropathy in Heart Transplant Recipients. *Am J Kidney Dis.* 2015 Jun;65(6):949-55.

[50] Johns Hopkins University of Medicine. Coronavirus Resource Center, COVID19 Dashboard. [online]. 2020 [cited 2022-Jan-20]. Available from: https://corona virus.jhu.edu/map.html.

[51] Marcondes-Braga FG, Murad CM, Belfort DSP, Dantas RCT, Lira MTSS, Aragão CAS, Siciliano RF, Mangini S, Seguro LFBC, Campos IW, Avila MS, Bello MVO, Dos Santos FBA, Strabelli TMV, Gaiotto FA, Bacal F. Characteristics and

Outcomes of Heart Transplant Recipients with Coronavirus-19 Disease in A High-Volume Transplant Center. *Transplantation.* 2021 Mar 22.

[52] Lima B, Gibson GT, Vullaganti S, Malhame K, Maybaum S, Hussain ST, Shah S, Majure DT, Wallach F, Jang K, Bijol V, Esposito MJ, Williamson AK, Thomas RM, Bhuiya TA, Fernandez HA, Stevens GR. COVID-19 in recent heart transplant recipients: Clinicopathologic features and early outcomes. *Transpl Infect Dis.* 2020 Oct;22(5):e13382.

[53] Rivinius R, Kaya Z, Schramm R, Boeken U, Provaznik Z, Heim C, Knosalla C, Schoenrath F, Rieth A, Berchtold-Herz M, Barten MJ, Rauschning D, Mücke VT, Heyl S, Pistulli R, Grinninger C, Hagl C, Gummert JF, Warnecke G, Schulze PC, Katus HA, Kreusser MM, Raake PW. COVID-19 among heart transplant recipients in Germany: a multicenter survey. *Clin Res Cardiol.* 2020 Dec;109(12):1531-1539.

[54] Kittleson MM, Chambers DC, Cypel M, Potena L. Covid-19 in recipients of heart and lung transplantation: Learning from experience. *J Heart Lung Transplant.* 2021 Sep;40(9):948-950.

[55] Latif F, Farr MA, Clerkin KJ, Habal MV, Takeda K, Naka Y, Restaino S, Sayer G, Uriel N. Characteristics and Outcomes of Recipients of Heart Transplant With Coronavirus Disease 2019. *JAMA Cardiol.* 2020 Oct 1;5(10):1165-1169.

[56] Wang D, Hu B, Hu C, Zhu F, Liu X, Zhang J, Wang B, Xiang H, Cheng Z, Xiong Y, Zhao Y, Li Y, Wang X, Peng Z. Clinical Characteristics of 138 Hospitalized Patients With 2019 Novel Coronavirus-Infected Pneumonia in Wuhan, China. *JAMA.* 2020 Mar 17;323(11):1061-1069.

[57] Genuardi MV, Moss N, Najjar SS, Houston BA, Shore S, Vorovich E, Atluri P, Molina M, Chambers S, Sharkoski T, Hsich E, Estep JD, Owens AT, Alexander KM, Chaudhry SP, Garcia-Cortes R, Molina E, Rodrigo M, Wald MJ, Margulies KB, Hanff TC, Zimmer R, Kilic A, Mclean R, Vidula H, Dodd K, Blumberg EA, Mazurek JA, Goldberg LR, Alvarez-Garcia J, Mancini D, Teuteberg JJ, Tedford RJ, Birati EY. Coronavirus disease 2019 in heart transplant recipients: Risk factors, immunosuppression, and outcomes. *J Heart Lung Transplant.* 2021 Sep;40(9):926-935.

[58] Weiss MJ, Hornby L, Foroutan F, Belga S, Bernier S, Bhat M, Buchan CA, Gagnon M, Hardman G, Ibrahim M, Luo C, Luong ML, Mainra R, Manara AR, Sapir-Pichhadze R, Shalhoub S, Shaver T, Singh JM, Srinathan S, Thomas I, Wilson LC, Wilson TM, Wright A, Mah A. Clinical Practice Guideline for Solid Organ Donation and Transplantation During the COVID-19 Pandemic. *Transplant Direct.* 2021 Sep 7;7(10):e755.

[59] Ison MG, Nalesnik MA. An update on donor-derived disease transmission in organ transplantation. *Am J Transplant.* 2011 Jun;11(6):1123-30.

[60] Lumbreras C, Sanz F, González A, Pérez G, Ramos MJ, Aguado JM, Lizasoain M, Andrés A, Moreno E, Gómez MA, Noriega AR. Clinical significance of donor-unrecognized bacteremia in the outcome of solid-organ transplant recipients. *Clin Infect Dis.* 2001 Sep 1;33(5):722-6.

[61] Singh N. Impact of donor bacteremia on outcome in organ transplant recipients. *Liver Transpl.* 2002 Oct;8(10):975-6.

[62] Nguyen M, Eschenauer GA, Bryan M, O'Neil K, Furuya EY, Della-Latta P, Kubin CJ. Carbapenem-resistant Klebsiella pneumoniae bacteremia: factors correlated with clinical and microbiologic outcomes. *Diagn Microbiol Infect Dis.* 2010 Jun;67(2):180-4.

[63] Sifri CD, Ison MG. Highly resistant bacteria and donor-derived infections: treading in uncharted territory. *Transpl Infect Dis*. 2012 Jun;14(3):223-8.

[64] Mattner F, Kola A, Fischer S, Becker T, Haverich A, Simon A, Suerbaum S, Gastmeier P, Weissbrodt H, Strüber M. Impact of bacterial and fungal donor organ contamination in lung, heart-lung, heart and liver transplantation. *Infection.* 2008 Jun;36(3):207-12.

[65] Yansouni CP, Dendukuri N, Liu G, Fernandez M, Frenette C, Paraskevas S, Sheppard DC. Positive cultures of organ preservation fluid predict postoperative infections in solid organ transplantation recipients. *Infect Control Hosp Epidemiol.* 2012 Jul;33(7):672-80.

[66] Chong PP, Razonable RR. Diagnostic and management strategies for donor-derived infections. *Infect Dis Clin North Am.* 2013 Jun;27(2):253-70.

[67] El-Bandar N, Kroy DC, Fuller TF, Kramer J, Liefeldt L, Budde K, Blobel C, Miller K, Friedersdorff F. Development of Graft-Site Candidiasis in 3 Solid Organ Transplant Recipients from the Same Donor. *Am J Case Rep.* 2017 Jul 11;18:777-781.

[68] Kalil AC, Metersky ML, Klompas M, Muscedere J, Sweeney DA, Palmer LB, Napolitano LM, O'Grady NP, Bartlett JG, Carratalà J, El Solh AA, Ewig S, Fey PD, File TM Jr, Restrepo MI, Roberts JA, Waterer GW, Cruse P, Knight SL, Brozek JL. Management of Adults With Hospital-acquired and Ventilator-associated Pneumonia: 2016 Clinical Practice Guidelines by the Infectious Diseases Society of America and the American Thoracic Society. *Clin Infect Dis.* 2016 Sep 1;63(5):e61-e111.

[69] Dulek DE, Mueller NJ; AST Infectious Diseases Community of Practice. Pneumonia in solid organ transplantation: Guidelines from the American Society of Transplantation Infectious Diseases Community of Practice. *Clin Transplant.* 2019 Sep;33(9):e13545.

[70] Sénéchal M, LePrince P, Tezenas du Montcel S, Bonnet N, Dubois M, El-Serafi M, Ghossoub JJ, Pavie A, Gandjbakhch I, Dorent R. Bacterial mediastinitis after heart transplantation: clinical presentation, risk factors and treatment. *J Heart Lung Transplant.* 2004 Feb;23(2):165-70.

[71] Zuckermann A, Barten MJ. Surgical wound complications after heart transplantation. *Transpl Int.* 2011 Jul;24(7):627-36.

[72] Cohen BA, Stosor V. Opportunistic infections of the central nervous system in the transplant patient. *Curr Neurol Neurosci Rep.* 2013 Sep;13(9):376.

[73] Pappas PG, Alexander BD, Andes DR, Hadley S, Kauffman CA, Freifeld A, Anaissie EJ, Brumble LM, Herwaldt L, Ito J, Kontoyiannis DP, Lyon GM, Marr KA, Morrison VA, Park BJ, Patterson TF, Perl TM, Oster RA, Schuster MG, Walker R, Walsh TJ, Wannemuehler KA, Chiller TM. Invasive fungal infections

among organ transplant recipients: results of the Transplant-Associated Infection Surveillance Network (TRANSNET). *Clin Infect Dis.* 2010 Apr 15;50(8):1101-11.

[74] Nienaber J, Wilhelm MP, Sohail MR. Current concepts in the diagnosis and management of left ventricular assist device infections. *Expert Rev Anti Infect Ther.* 2013 Feb;11(2):201-10.

[75] Kusne S, Mooney M, Danziger-Isakov L, Kaan A, Lund LH, Lyster H, Wieselthaler G, Aslam S, Cagliostro B, Chen J, Combs P, Cochrane A, Conway J, Cowger J, Frigerio M, Gellatly R, Grossi P, Gustafsson F, Hannan M, Lorts A, Martin S, Pinney S, Silveira FP, Schubert S, Schueler S, Strueber M, Uriel N, Wrightson N, Zabner R, Huprikar S. An ISHLT consensus document for prevention and management strategies for mechanical circulatory support infection. *J Heart Lung Transplant.* 2017 Oct;36(10):1137-1153.

[76] Balsam LB, Louie E, Hill F, Levine J, Phillips MS. Mycobacterium chimaera left ventricular assist device infections. *J Card Surg.* 2017 Jun;32(6):402-404.

[77] Subramanian AK, Theodoropoulos NM; Infectious Diseases Community of Practice of the American Society of Transplantation. Mycobacterium tuberculosis infections in solid organ transplantation: Guidelines from the infectious diseases community of practice of the American Society of Transplantation. *Clin Transplant.* 2019 Sep;33(9):e13513.

[78] Abad CLR, Razonable RR. Mycobacterium tuberculosis after solid organ transplantation: A review of more than 2000 cases. *Clin Transplant.* 2018 Jun;32(6):e13259.

[79] Weile J, Eickmeyer H, Dreier J, Liebke M, Fuchs U, Wittke JW, Richter E, Gummert J, Knabbe C, Schulz U. First case of Mycobacterium tuberculosis transmission by heart transplantation from donor to recipient. *Int J Med Microbiol.* 2013 Dec;303(8):449-51.

[80] Wreghitt TG, Hakim M, Gray JJ, Balfour AH, Stovin PG, Stewart S, Scott J, English TA, Wallwork J. Toxoplasmosis in heart and heart and lung transplant recipients. *J Clin Pathol.* 1989 Feb;42(2):194-9.

[81] La Hoz RM, Morris MI; Infectious Diseases Community of Practice of the American Society of Transplantation. Tissue and blood protozoa including toxoplasmosis, Chagas disease, leishmaniasis, Babesia, Acanthamoeba, Balamuthia, and Naegleria in solid organ transplant recipients- Guidelines from the American Society of Transplantation Infectious Diseases Community of Practice. *Clin Transplant.* 2019 Sep;33(9):e13546.

[82] Montoya JG. Laboratory diagnosis of Toxoplasma gondii infection and toxoplasmosis. *J Infect Dis.* 2002 Feb 15;185 Suppl 1:S73-82.

[83] Muñoz P, Arencibia J, Rodríguez C, Rivera M, Palomo J, Yañez J, Bouza E. Trimethoprim-sulfamethoxazole as toxoplasmosis prophylaxis for heart transplant recipients. *Clin Infect Dis.* 2003 Apr 1;36(7):932-3; author reply 933.

[84] Peradejordi Lastras MA, Favaloro LE, Vigliano C, Renedo MF, Martínez L, Moscoloni SE, Abud J, Absi DO, Favaloro RR, Bertolotti AM. Outcomes of Heart Transplantation Based on Recipient's Clinical Profile: 21-Year Experience. *Rev Argent Cardiol* 2016 Jun;84(3):235-241

[85] de Carvalho VB, Sousa EF, Vila JH, da Silva JP, Caiado MR, Araujo SR, Macruz R, Zerbini EJ. Heart transplantation in Chagas' disease. 10 years after the initial experience. *Circulation.* 1996 Oct 15;94(8):1815-7.

[86] Bocchi EA, Bellotti G, Mocelin AO, Uip D, Bacal F, Higuchi ML, Amato-Neto V, Fiorelli A, Stolf NA, Jatene AD, Pileggi F. Heart transplantation for chronic Chagas' heart disease. *Ann Thorac Surg.* 1996 Jun;61(6):1727-33.

[87] Altclas JD, Barcan L, Nagel C, Lattes R, Riarte A. Organ transplantation and Chagas disease. *JAMA.* 2008 Mar 12;299(10):1134; author reply 1134-5.

[88] Barcán L, Luna C, Clara L, Sinagra A, Valledor A, De Rissio AM, Gadano A, García MM, de Santibañes E, Riarte A. Transmission of T. cruzi infection via liver transplantation to a nonreactive recipient for Chagas' disease. *Liver Transpl.* 2005 Sep;11(9):1112-6.

[89] Diez M, Favaloro L, Bertolotti A, Burgos JM, Vigliano C, Lastra MP, Levin MJ, Arnedo A, Nagel C, Schijman AG, Favaloro RR. Usefulness of PCR strategies for early diagnosis of Chagas' disease reactivation and treatment follow-up in heart transplantation. *Am J Transplant.* 2007 Jun;7(6):1633-40.

[90] Schijman AG, Bisio M, Orellana L, Sued M, Duffy T, Mejia Jaramillo AM, Cura C, Auter F, Veron V, Qvarnstrom Y, Deborggraeve S, Hijar G, Zulantay I, Lucero RH, Velazquez E, Tellez T, Sanchez Leon Z, Galvão L, Nolder D, Monje Rumi M, Levi JE, Ramirez JD, Zorrilla P, Flores M, Jercic MI, Crisante G, Añez N, De Castro AM, Gonzalez CI, Acosta Viana K, Yachelini P, Torrico F, Robello C, Diosque P, Triana Chavez O, Aznar C, Russomando G, Büscher P, Assal A, Guhl F, Sosa Estani S, DaSilva A, Britto C, Luquetti A, Ladzins J. International study to evaluate PCR methods for detection of Trypanosoma cruzi DNA in blood samples from Chagas disease patients. *PLoS Negl Trop Dis.* 2011 Jan 11;5(1):e931.

[91] Nogueira SS, Felizardo AA, Caldas IS, Gonçalves RV, Novaes RD. Challenges of immunosuppressive and antitrypanosomal drug therapy after heart transplantation in patients with chronic Chagas disease: A systematic review of clinical recommendations. *Transplant Rev* (Orlando). 2018 Jul;32(3):157-167.

[92] Abanyie FA, Gray EB, Delli Carpini KW, Yanofsky A, McAuliffe I, Rana M, Chin-Hong PV, Barone CN, Davis JL, Montgomery SP, Huprikar S. Donor-derived Strongyloides stercoralis infection in solid organ transplant recipients in the United States, 2009-2013. *Am J Transplant.* 2015 May;15(5):1369-75.

[93] Geri G, Rabbat A, Mayaux J, Zafrani L, Chalumeau-Lemoine L, Guidet B, Azoulay E, Pène F. Strongyloides stercoralis hyperinfection syndrome: a case series and a review of the literature. *Infection.* 2015 Dec;43(6):691-8.

[94] Buonfrate D, Formenti F, Perandin F, Bisoffi Z. Novel approaches to the diagnosis of Strongyloides stercoralis infection. *Clin Microbiol Infect.* 2015 Jun;21(6):543-52.

[95] Aslam S, Rotstein C; AST Infectious Disease Community of Practice. Candida infections in solid organ transplantation: Guidelines from the American Society of Transplantation Infectious Diseases Community of Practice. *Clin Transplant.* 2019 Sep;33(9):e13623.

[96] Muñoz P, Singh N, Bouza E. Treatment of solid organ transplant patients with invasive fungal infections: should a combination of antifungal drugs be used? *Curr Opin Infect Dis.* 2006 Aug;19(4):365-70.

[97] Neofytos D, Chatzis O, Nasioudis D, Boely Janke E, Doco Lecompte T, Garzoni C, Berger C, Cussini A, Boggian K, Khanna N, Manuel O, Mueller NJ, van Delden C; Swiss Transplant Cohort Study. Epidemiology, risk factors and outcomes of invasive aspergillosis in solid organ transplant recipients in the Swiss Transplant Cohort Study. *Transpl Infect Dis.* 2018 Aug;20(4):e12898.

[98] Muñoz P, Alcalá L, Sánchez Conde M, Palomo J, Yáñez J, Pelaez T, Bouza E. The isolation of Aspergillus fumigatus from respiratory tract specimens in heart transplant recipients is highly predictive of invasive aspergillosis. *Transplantation.* 2003 Feb 15;75(3):326-9.

[99] Peláez T, Muñoz P, Guinea J, Valerio M, Giannella M, Klaassen CH, Bouza E. Outbreak of invasive aspergillosis after major heart surgery caused by spores in the air of the intensive care unit. *Clin Infect Dis.* 2012 Feb 1;54(3):e24-31.

[100] Muñoz P, Cerón I, Valerio M, Palomo J, Villa A, Eworo A, Fernández-Yáñez J, Guinea J, Bouza E. Invasive aspergillosis among heart transplant recipients: a 24-year perspective. *J Heart Lung Transplant.* 2014 Mar;33(3):278-88.

[101] Husain S, Camargo JF. Invasive Aspergillosis in solid-organ transplant recipients: Guidelines from the American Society of Transplantation Infectious Diseases Community of Practice. *Clin Transplant.* 2019 Sep;33(9):e13544.

[102] Fishman JA. Prevention of infection caused by Pneumocystis carinii in transplant recipients. *Clin Infect Dis.* 2001 Oct 15;33(8):1397-405.

[103] Fishman JA, Gans H; AST Infectious Diseases Community of Practice. Pneumocystis jiroveci in solid organ transplantation: Guidelines from the American Society of Transplantation Infectious Diseases Community of Practice. *Clin Transplant.* 2019 Sep;33(9):e13587.

Chapter 14

Nursing Care and Follow-Up of the Heart Transplant Patient

Teresa Patricia Ibañez, Norma Graciela Yakobas and Orlando Omar Zacarias*
Heart Failure and Heart Transplantation, Favaloro Foundation University Hospital, Buenos Aires, Argentina

Abstract

Heart transplantation is a highly complex surgery that impacts on the physical, mental and social dimension of patients and their environment. In this sense, heart transplant coordinator nurses have a fundamental role, providing education for health promotion and the tools and knowledge necessary for self-care, as well as for adequate adherence to treatment. Their multiple roles, tasks, and responsibilities are focused on promoting the well-being of the patient. Furthermore, nurses play an active role in the development and execution of the post-transplant follow-up protocol that is essential to detect the different types of rejection and act in the event of possible complications.

Keywords: nursing care, education, follow-up studies

Introduction

Organ transplantation has been one of the most spectacular milestones in 20th century medicine, and its advances and good results highlight the importance

* Corresponding Author's E-mail: coordinadoresenfermeriatx@ffavaloro.org.

In: Heart Transplantation
Editor: Elian Facundo Giordanino
ISBN: 978-1-68507-759-4

of the cooperation of a multidisciplinary team to carry out an organ transplantation program.

Heart transplantation is the treatment of choice for end-stage heart failure when survival and quality of life cannot be improved with conventional treatments.

The first human-to-human heart transplant (HTx) was performed by the team of South African surgeon Christian Barnard at the Groote Schuur Hospital in Cape Town, South Africa on December 3, 1967.

In 1968, Dr. Miguel Bellizi carried out the first HTx in Argentina, number nineteen worldwide, at the Lanus Model Clinic. The patient survived 94 hours after surgery. In the eighties, Dr. René G. Favaloro developed the first national heart transplant program at the Güemes Hospital, where the first HTx with long-term survival was performed [1].

The success of heart transplantation is due to the important development in recent years of immunosuppressive treatment with the appearance of cyclosporine in 1972 as well as advances in the treatment of infections, improvement in rejection detection methods, proper preservation of the organ, the correct selection of the recipient and enhancement in the postoperative care.

Heart Transplant Nurse Qualifications

The American Nurses Association and International Transplant Nurses Society defined transplant nursing practice as: "Specialized nursing care focused on the protection, promotion, and optimization of the health and abilities of both the transplant recipient and the living donor across the lifespan. The depth and breadth in which individual registered nurses engage in the total scope of nursing practice is dependent upon education, experience, role, and the population served" [2].

The care of the HTx patient requires the proper organization and multidisciplinary approach of the health team, especially the nursing professional, who must have specific expertise. This includes an adequate set of knowledge, skills and abilities in the approach to the HTx patient. The experience of the HTx nurses helps to optimize logistical issues from the moment the patient is admitted to hospital to the moment the HTx is performed, as well as to improve immediate, mediate and distant follow-up. It is important to highlight the application of the nursing care process for the comprehensive care of the person and to obtain good results in the quality of life of the patients.

The achievements obtained in heart transplantation and the better survival of these patients has increased the demand for care. Due to this reality, the figure of the heart transplant coordinator nurses emerges. They become the reference for patients and their families throughout the healthcare process and they promote family involvement in heart transplantation through education and therapeutic co-responsibility.

To be able to modify the behavior of patients, education implies an interactive process, so the nurse manager must have skills such as clinical experience, specific knowledge of the pathology and the treatments used, be a good communicator and educator as well as possess the ability to work as a team, with the aim of ensuring the continuity of care.

Education for the Heart Transplant Patient

Since the beginning of heart transplantation, there have been advances aimed to improve survival such as:

- Detection and maintenance of the potential donor
- Development of surgical techniques
- Preservation and maintenance of implanted organs
- Pre, intra- and post-transplant care
- Immunosuppressive therapy
- Control, prevention and treatment of complications
- Cardiac rehabilitation

However, education also plays a fundamental role for survival and to improve the quality of life of the HTx patient in aspects such as:

- Nutritional education
- Obesity prevention
- Early identification of signs and symptoms
- Return to activities of daily living
- Return to sexual life
- Psychological and social stability

Table 1. Barriers to learning. Heart transplant coordinator nurses must take these barriers into account when educating the patient

Physical factors (pain, fatigue)
Psychological factors (Anxiety, resilience, past experiences, personal values and motivation)
Social factors (social support network)
Cognitive factors (memory impairment)
Educational factors (level of education)
Others (environment, time)

Data from Solis Muñoz M. Enfermeria en trasplante [Transplant Nursing] Madrid: *Difusion Avances de Enfermeria*, 2005, 586-894.

Proper planning of nursing care in HTx patients and adequate health education before discharge are essential. More and more individuals receive a HTx and more and more professionals are involved in the task to provide knowledge and skills to promote the independence of these patients [2, 3]. There are different barriers to learning that the nurse must help the patient overcome (Table 1).

Some of the elements that may facilitate learning are:

- Dedicate time to establish a positive nurse-patient and nurse-family relationship
- Set the expected objectives during the session and promote collaboration and maximum participation
- Adapt communications to the patient's level of understanding
- Let the patient and family express their enthusiasm or concern
- Make sessions as enjoyable as possible
- Give time to assimilate the information
- Highlight the positive aspects and acknowledge what the patient has learned

Nurse-Patient Encounters

There are different nurse-patient encounters that aim to provide knowledge and tools for the post-transplant setting.

These encounters can be organized as follows:

Encounter nº 1: Singularities of heart transplantation, cardiac denervation and graft rejection.

- Increase the level of knowledge about heart transplantation of the patients and their relatives
- Special considerations of the denervated heart
- Definition, diagnosis and treatment of graft rejection

Encounter nº 2: immunosuppressive therapy and its complications

- Explain the immunosuppressive therapy (Figure 1)
- Secondary effects, how to prevent them
- Early detection of secondary effects

Encounter nº 3: Infections, prevention and early detection

- Explain the increased risk of infections
- How to prevent them
- Early detection of infections

Encounter nº 4: Nutritional advice.

- Importance of a healthy diet
- Food not allowed during the different stages of the post-transplant life
- Food handling

Encounter nº 5: Potential psychological disorders of the patients and their relatives, return to activities of daily living

- Explain possible psychological disorders after heart transplantation and their potential treatment
- Promote increased level of independence
- How to recognize and take advantage of their available resources to improve their health

Encounter nº 6: Sexuality. Special considerations in female patients

- Increase the level of knowledge about aspects related to sexuality

- Female HTx recipients, aspects related to menstrual cycle, contraception, pregnancy and lactation.

FUNDACIÓN FAVALORO

FAVALORO FOUNDATION UNIVERSITY HOSPITAL

Name:

Transplant date: Discharge date:

IMMUNOSUPPRESSION

Drug	Dose	Posology
Tacrolimus 5mg	5mg	8hs 20hs
Mycophenolate Mofetil 500mg	1500 mg	8 hs 20 hs
Prednisone 40mg	20mg	8 hs

PROPHYLAXIS

Drug	Dose	Posology
Sulfamethoxazole / trimethoprim 160+800mg	1 tablet (3 times a week)	Mon Wed Fri
Nystatin	4ml	After meals

OTHERS

Drug	Dose	Posology
Omeprazole 20mg	20mg	Before breakfast
Folic acid 10mg	10mg	8hs
Theophylline 300mg	100mg	08hs 16hs 24hs
Vitamin B Complex	1 tablet	16hs
Acetylsalicylic acid 100mg	100 mg	12hs
Atorvastatin 20 mg	20 mg	20hs
Alendronate	70 mg	weekly
Calcium carbonate	1250 mg	10 hs
Magnesium citrate	2 tablets	With meals
Potassium chloride 600mg	2 tablets	With meals

Emergency mobile number: (12) 1234-5678

Figure 1. Example of indication sheet for patients.

Post-Transplant Follow-Up Protocol

Heart transplant patients are put through very complex procedures and are exposed to a series of complications derived from the heart transplant itself, such as graft rejection, among others.

Strict controls allow healthcare professionals to detect complications early and, therefore, treat them as quickly and efficiently as possible.

The post-transplant follow-up protocol aims to detect rejection early, evaluate graft function, carry out a general assessment of the recipient's health status, and rule out possible complications related to transplantation. This protocol may vary depending on each institution, but in general terms it implies the performance of periodic supplementary tests that decrease in frequency over time.

It is important to highlight the role of telemedicine, mainly through telephone calls, as an important follow-up tool that allows early detection of signs and symptoms, as well as provides confidence to patients at home [4].

Endomyocardial Biopsies

Endomyocardial biopsy (EMB) remains as the gold standard for the diagnosis of graft rejection in heart transplantation [5]. Although there is no universal schedule for surveillance EMB, the main principle is to perform this procedure more frequently during the first period of follow-up. In our experience at the Favaloro Foundation University Hospital the EMB schedule is as follows:

- From day 1 to 30: weekly EMB.
- From day 30 to 60: fortnightly EMB
- From day 60 to 180: monthly EMB
- From day 180 to 360: EMB every 3 months
- After one year: EMB every 6 months or every year according to each patient, with physician evaluation every 3 months. Annually, patients are also screened for the presence of donor specific antibodies.

Along with the EMB, a complete laboratory test is performed, including thyroid hormones, cytomegalovirus detection and monitoring of immunosuppressant levels, among others. Additionally, an electrocardiogram, chest radiography and echocardiogram are performed. All these supplementary tests are assessed by the physician together with the anamnesis and physical examination.

EMB are performed as an outpatient procedure and additional laboratory and imaging tests are carried out within the previous 48 hours. After the patient is examined by the physicians and upon their approval for the procedure, the EMB is performed in the catheterization laboratory with local anesthesia. Afterwards, a chest radiography and physical examination are carried out to detect any complications related to the procedure and the patient is discharged home. Once the result of the EMB has been reported by the pathologist, the patients are called in order to make the necessary adjustments in their treatment.

Other Tests

Apart from EMB, there are several other supplementary tests that are necessary for an adequate follow-up of the HTx recipient. Coronary angiography, ideally with intravascular ultrasound, is mandatory for detecting cardiac allograft vasculopathy (see Chapter 12) [6]. In case there are contraindications for this test, an alternative procedure is a Dipyridamole Single-photon emission computed tomography (SPECT). These tests are performed annually, generally in conjunction with the EMB.

Every 3 months, the patient should assist to a medical visit with the heart transplant physician, either during the frequent EMB appointments at the early stages of the follow-up or during a scheduled appointment that includes complete laboratory tests with monitoring of immunosuppressant levels and an echocardiogram. Furthermore, there are some tests that should be performed in an annual basis in all patients:

- Renal ultrasound with renal artery doppler ultrasound
- 24-hour Holter monitoring
- Bone densitometry
- Psychological consultation
- Dental consultation
- Nutritional consultation
- Infectious diseases specialist consultation
- Cardiac rehabilitation

These should be accompanied by frequent consultations with dermatology, urology and gynecology. Figure 2 shows the follow-up schedule for HTx patients at Favaloro Foundation University Hospital.

Detection of Complications after Heart Transplantation

The extensive clinical experience acquired by the heart transplant groups has been a determining factor in reducing the main postoperative complications, infections and rejections. The role of the transplant nurse is essential for the early detection of complications that may arise in the follow-up of the heart transplant patient. In order to do this, it is important to understand the basic principles behind these complications [7].

Infections

Infections represent one of the main complications after heart transplantation and occur more frequently during the first semester as a consequence of the requirement of high doses of immunosuppressants. During this period, there are various viruses such as cytomegalovirus, herpes simplex virus, Epstein-Barr virus, Varicella zoster virus, as well as other microorganisms such as pneumocystis carinii, legionella, mycobacteria, nocardia, toxoplasmosis, candida, aspergillosis or cryptococcus. (See Chapter 13) [8].

Heart transplant coordinator nurses need to appropriately question patients for signs or symptoms that may be manifestations of such infections. Among them, there are easily detectable symptoms such as fever, diarrhea or cough but others are more subtle such as skin lesions, fatigue or weight loss, which are generally not reported by patients and therefore should be questioned by heart transplant nurses.

Cardiac Allograft Rejection

Cardiac allograft rejection is the process by which the body recognizes the transplanted heart as a foreign agent, rejecting it by activating the immune system. To reduce the likelihood of rejection, HTx patients must be treated with immunosuppressants throughout their entire lives (See Chapter 11).

		EMB	EMB +IHC	Medical visit	Echo	CA +IVUS	DSA
1° M	1° W	X			X		
	2° W	X	X				X
	3° W	X					
	4° W	X	X				X
2° M	5° W				X		
	6° W	X					
	7° W						
	8° W	X	X				X
3° M		X			X		
4° M							
5° M				X	X		
6° M		X	X				X
7° M				X	X		
8° M							
9° M		X					
10° M				X	X		
11° M							
12° M		X	X			X	X

Figure 2. Follow-up Schedule for Heart Transplant Patients at Favaloro Foundation University Hospital. After 1 year, EMB is performed every 6 to 12 months and CA+IVUS every 12 months. CA, coronary angiography; DSA, donor specific antibodies screening; Echo, echocardiography; EMB, endomyocardial biopsy; IHC, immunohistochemistry, IVUS, intravascular ultrasound; M, month; W, week.

There are different types of cardiac allograft rejection [9]:

- Acute cellular rejection: it is the most common and it appears when the T cells of the immune system attack the cells of the donor heart. It usually occurs most often during the first three to six months after transplant.
- Antibody mediated rejection: it is less frequent than cellular rejection. It can occur at any time during the follow-up of the heart transplant patient and can sometimes present with severe hemodynamic compromise. It is produced by the formation of antibodies against the donor's heart.

- Cardiac allograft vasculopathy: This is a form of chronic rejection that affects coronary arteries and can lead to a reduction in coronary blood flow to the graft.

Rejection after heart transplantation is common and most patients suffer from it at some point in their clinical course. Transplant recipients should be informed that there is a possibility of rejection at any point in their post-transplant life, although it is more frequent during the first year. Even though cardiac allograft rejection may sometimes be asymptomatic, the heart transplant coordinator nurse should be aware of the main signs and symptoms that may raise suspicion of allograft rejection in order to promptly alert the medical team and arrange an urgent EMB. These symptoms can be palpitations, exercise intolerance, dizziness, lower limb edema, asthenia, shortness of breath, syncope, among others. In case allograft rejection is diagnosed by EMB, hospitalization for intravenous treatment may be necessary [10].

Other Complications

Malignancy

It has a higher incidence than in the general population, the most frequent being skin tumors. Excessive immunosuppression and monoclonal antibody treatment have contributed to the increase in lymphomas [8]. Treatment can be effective in one third of patients and consists mainly of reduction of immunosuppression, resection of lesions, and radiation therapy or chemotherapy as appropriate. These patients should be monitored more frequently with laboratory test, echocardiograms and periodic clinical visits to the transplant team during the treatment period.

Arterial Hypertension, Dyslipidemia and Post-Transplant Diabetes Mellitus

These conditions might be exacerbated by immunosuppressant agents and can accelerate the development of cardiac allograft vasculopathy. Almost 50% of patients may develop arterial hypertension alter one year of HTx and 77% after 4 years [11]. The prevalence of dyslipidemia might be up to 50% after 5 years of HTx whereas diabetes mellitus can occur in approximately 30% of patients in the same period [12, 13].

Osteoporosis

It is another complication of heart transplantation, mainly due to the use of corticosteroids. It can lead to bone fractures, which is why it is necessary to prevent it with different therapies and to diagnose it early by means of a bone densitometry.

Renal Failure

Although the development of new immunosuppressive schemes has considerably reduced the incidence of kidney failure in transplant patients, this condition continues to be observed frequently; therefore the *'personified and artisanal'* administration of immunosuppressive drugs is decisive to avoid many of these episodes [6].

In this sense, the role of heart transplant coordinator nurses is key in making the patient aware of the need for and importance of periodic medical visits in order to prevent or treat the complications that arise throughout the life of the transplanted patient.

Conclusion

The heart transplant coordinator nurse plays a fundamental role in the interdisciplinary HTx team, providing the education, tools and knowledge necessary to stimulate healthy lifestyle habits, self-care and adherence to treatment. Additionally, it is the health professional that is present in the short-, medium- and long-term follow-up, being the link between the patient, the environment and the medical team. The heart transplant coordinator nurse is essential for the correct organization of the follow-up tests and clinical visits of the HTx patients and also serves as the first contact with them, detecting the possible complications that may arise. Nursing carries out multiple functions, tasks and responsibilities and its goal is always the well-being of the patient.

References

[1] Peradejordi M, Favaloro R, Bertolotti A, Abud J, Gomez C, Absi D, Favaloro L, Diez, M, Martinez L, Moscoloni, S. Orthotopic Heart Transplantation: Results from the Hospital Universitario Fundación Favaloro. *Rev. Argent Cardiol.* 2011 Nov-Dec;79(6):508-513.

[2] Coleman B, Blumenthal N, Currey J, Dobbels F, Velleca A, Grady KL, Kugler C, Murks C, Ohler L, Sumbi C, Luu M, Dark J, Kobashigawa J, White-Williams C. Adult cardiothoracic transplant nursing: an ISHLT consensus document on the current adult nursing practice in heart and lung transplantation. *J. Heart Lung Transplant*. 2015 Feb;34(2):139-48.

[3] Solis Muñoz M. Educación para la salud al trasplantado cardiopulmonar, In: Solis Muñoz M. Enfermeria en trasplante [*Health education for cardiopulmonary transplant patients, In Transplant Nursing*]. Madrid: Difusion Avances de Enfermeria, 2005, 586-894.

[4] Freeman R, Koerner E, Clark C, Halabicky K. Cardiac Transplant Postoperative Management and Care. *Crit. Care Nurs. Q*. 2016 Jul-Sep;39(3):214-26.

[5] Kiamanesh O, Toma M. The State of the Heart Biopsy: A Clinical Review. *CJC Open*. 2020 Dec 1;3(4):524-531.

[6] Costanzo MR, Dipchand A, Starling R, Anderson A, Chan M, Desai S, Fedson S, Fisher P, Gonzales-Stawinski G, Martinelli L, McGiffin D, Smith J, Taylor D, Meiser B, Webber S, Baran D, Carboni M, Dengler T, Feldman D, Frigerio M, Kfoury A, Kim D, Kobashigawa J, Shullo M, Stehlik J, Teuteberg J, Uber P, Zuckermann A, Hunt S, Burch M, Bhat G, Canter C, Chinnock R, Crespo-Leiro M, Delgado R, Dobbels F, Grady K, Kao W, Lamour J, Parry G, Patel J, Pini D, Towbin J, Wolfel G, Delgado D, Eisen H, Goldberg L, Hosenpud J, Johnson M, Keogh A, Lewis C, O'Connell J, Rogers J, Ross H, Russell S, Vanhaecke J; International Society of Heart and Lung Transplantation Guidelines. The International Society of Heart and Lung Transplantation Guidelines for the care of heart transplant recipients. *J. Heart Lung Transplant*. 2010 Aug;29(8):914-56.

[7] Bahruth AJ. What every patient should know... pretransplantation and posttransplantation. *Crit. Care Nurs. Q*. 2004 Jan-Mar;27(1):31-60.

[8] Revuelta JM, Sarralde A. Complicaciones del trasplante cardíaco, In: Parrilla P, Ramírez P, Ríos A. Manual sobre donación y trasplante de órganos [*Complications in heart transplatation, In Handbook on Organ Donation and Transplantation*] Madrid: Aran Editions, 2008, 389-391.

[9] Colvin MM, Cook JL, Chang P, Francis G, Hsu DT, Kiernan MS, Kobashigawa JA, Lindenfeld J, Masri SC, Miller D, O'Connell J, Rodriguez ER, Rosengard B, Self S, White-Williams C, Zeevi A; American Heart Association Heart Failure and Transplantation Committee of the Council on Clinical Cardiology; American Heart Association Heart Failure and Transplantation Committee of the Council on Cardiopulmonary Critical Care, Perioperative and Resuscitation; American Heart Association Heart Failure and Transplantation Committee of the Council on Cardiovascular Disease in the Young; American Heart Association Heart Failure

and Transplantation Committee of the Council on Clinical Cardiology, Council on Cardiovascular and Stroke Nursing; American Heart Association Heart Failure and Transplantation Committee of the Council on Cardiovascular Radiology and Intervention; American Heart Association Heart Failure and Transplantation Committee of the Council on Cardiovascular Surgery and Anesthesia. Antibody-mediated rejection in cardiac transplantation: emerging knowledge in diagnosis and management: a scientific statement from the American Heart Association. *Circulation*. 2015 May 5;131(18):1608-39.

[10] Revuelta JM, Sarralde A, Portón A. Resultados y calidad de vida en el trasplante cardiaco, In: Parrilla P, Ramírez P, Ríos A. Manual sobre donación y trasplante de órganos [*Results and quality of life in heart transplantation In Handbook on Organ Donation and Transplantation*] Madrid: Aran Editions, 2008, 401-405.

[11] Ozdogan E, Banner N, Fitzgerald M, Musumeci F, Khaghani A, Yacoub M. Factors influencing the development of hypertension after heart transplantation. *J. Heart Transplant*. 1990 Sep-Oct;9(5):548-53. PMID: 2231094.

[12] Marchetti P. New-onset diabetes after transplantation. *J. Heart Lung Transplant*. 2004 May;23(5 Suppl):S194-201.

[13] Agarwal A, Prasad GV. Post-transplant dyslipidemia: Mechanisms, diagnosis and management. *World J. Transplant*. 2016 Mar 24;6(1):125-34.

Part IV: Special Situations

Chapter 15

Pediatric Heart Transplantation

Julio Jorge Trentadue*
Department of Pediatrics, Favaloro Foundation University Hospital, Buenos Aires, Argentina

> So, when they change my heart for another, will I stop loving those I loved?
>
> María, 6 years old, hospitalized with inotropes, waiting for her new heart…

Abstract

As more and more children with congenital heart disease are operated on around the world, a group of them are faced with the limitations on their survival imposed by the type of surgery they faced. Many of those who were candidates for transplantation during the eighties and nineties due to the inoperability of their heart disease (like some variants of left heart hypoplasia) had neonatal surgery as their first option. Therefore, they underwent right ventricular bypass surgeries that limited the life expectancy of some of them. These patients began thus to expand the list of candidates for heart transplantation, changing the profile of pre-transplant diagnoses from the group of cardiomyopathies towards that of congenital heart disease.

Pediatric heart transplantation is a fascinating tool for the treatment of end-stage heart disease in a heterogeneous group of patients whose common characteristic is their advanced heart failure, but that have different etiologies and needs that are according to the varied age range that pediatrics entails. This chapter describes the current state of pediatric heart transplantation and its most relevant aspects in this regard and those that determine its results.

Keywords: heart transplantation, pediatrics, complications

---

* Corresponding Author's E-mail: jtrentadue@ffavaloro.org.

In: Heart Transplantation
Editor: Elian Facundo Giordanino
ISBN: 978-1-68507-759-4

Introduction

The first pediatric heart transplantation was performed in December 1967 a few days after the first adult heart transplantation was performed. Although it was a milestone in the history of medicine, the patient survived only a few hours. Long-term survival was not achieved in the ensuing years, primarily because of a lack of effective immunosuppressive medications. Interest in heart transplantation decreased in the 1970s and it was not until the introduction of cyclosporine-based immunosuppressive regimens in 1979 that long-term survival became feasible. Denton Cooley performed the first successful orthotopic heart transplantation in 1984 while Bailey performed the first successful neonatal orthotopic heart transplantation in 1985 [1].

In the 1980s and 1990s, a resurgence in interest and dramatic strides in adult and pediatric heart transplantation occurred. These advances included better donor and recipient selection, improvement in the preservation of donor hearts, refinements in surgical technique and in pre- and postoperative complications. Furthermore, the ability to detect and treat allograft rejection contributed to the length of patient survival and improved quality of life. However, significant limitations still exist including the need for lifelong immunosuppressive medications and the potential toxicities associated with the continued use of these drugs, the development of post-transplant lymphoproliferative disease and chronic rejection or transplant coronary vascular disease.

This chapter updates the clinician who deals with this peculiar population regarding the current status of pediatric heart transplantation, highlights advances in the field, identifies ongoing controversies and problematic areas of management, and introduces potentially new perspectives for the future management of these challenging patients.

Indications for Heart Transplantation

At our institution, heart transplantation is considered an alternative therapy when no other form of long-term palliation is possible. Dilated cardiomyopathy is the primary diagnosis for most of the patients, but is not the same for the International Society for Heart and Lung Transplantation (ISHLT) registry where congenital heart disease has been an important indication for heart transplantation (Figures 1 and 2) [2].

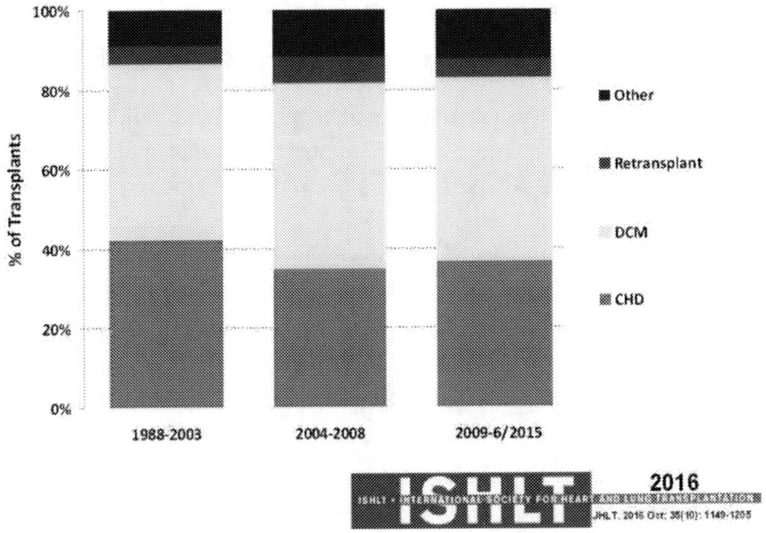

Figure 1. Diagnosis distribution by era. CHD, congenital heart disease; DCM, dilated cardiomyopathy. (Data from ISHLT. 2016. *Pediatric Heart Transplantation Statistics.* Accessed 15 Dec 2021. https://ishltregistries.org/registries/slides.asp).

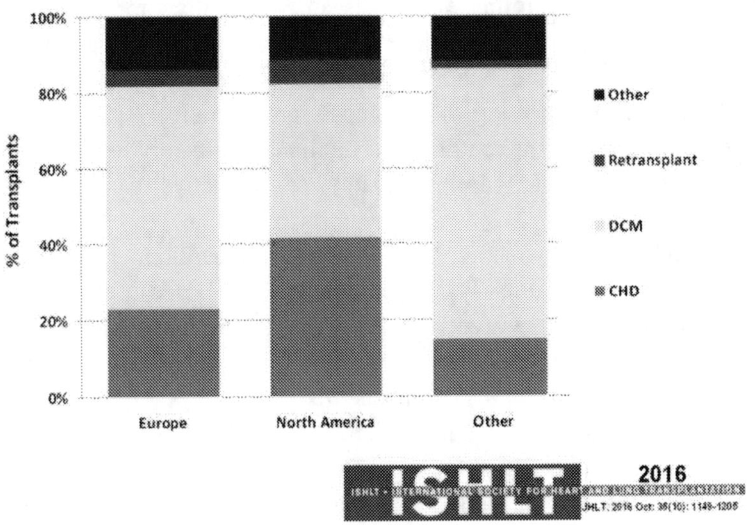

Figure 2. Diagnosis distribution by location (January 2004 to June 2015). CHD, congenital heart disease; DCM, dilated cardiomyopathy. (Data from ISHLT. 2016. *Pediatric Heart Transplantation Statistics.* Accessed 15 Dec 2021. https://ishltregistries.org/registries/slides.asp).

Heart failure refractory to appropriate medical therapy is the main indication for heart transplantation in this patient population. However, defining refractoriness to appropriate medical therapy can be challenging sometimes. Examples of this situation are patients with heart failure symptoms who cannot be weaned from intravenous support or patients under appropriate oral medical treatment with persistent New York Heart Association class III/IV.

Dilated cardiomyopathy is the most common cardiomyopathy in children, accounting for more than half of cases. It is characterized by left ventricular or biventricular dilation with impaired contraction and it can be congenital or acquired. Familiar causes were previously thought to be rare but it is now known that up to 50% of cases involve patients with an underlying genetic abnormality [3]. Among the acquired causes, viruses are a significant etiology [4]. Dilated cardiomyopathy secondary to adriamycin might be challenging given that malignancy can be a contraindication to transplantation, especially in some tumors where patients must be in remission at least 5 years before heart transplantation.

Hypertrophic cardiomyopathy is the second most common cardiomyopathy seen in children. Several gene mutation have been described. There are no acquired forms of the disease. It is often found to be the underlying pathology in young people who suffer from sudden cardiac death [5]. Hypertrophic cardiomyopathy less often leads to transplantation, with only 5% of patients carrying the diagnosis pre-operatively [6]. It is only considered when there are ventricular arrhythmias refractory to treatment or when features of dilate cardiomyopathy or restrictive cardiomyopathy develop.

Restrictive cardiomyopathy is the least common cardiomyopathy seen in children and represents only 3% of pediatric cases [7]. Because of the rapid development of pulmonary hypertension, we advocate immediate listing for transplantation. Restrictive cardiomyopathy has a mean survival of approximately 2 years from the diagnosis [8].

Patients with surgically palliated congenital heart disease no longer amenable to additional surgery who have ongoing heart failure symptoms or a degree of cyanosis that severely limits their activities constitute an important group of patients undergoing heart transplantation. Sometimes, patients have what is otherwise considered inoperable congenital heart defects (e.g., hypoplastic left heart syndrome with challenging anatomy, depressed right ventricular function or both; or certain severe cases of Ebstein anomaly), and heart transplantation should be considered as a primary therapeutic option.

More controversial is heart transplantation as primary therapy for patients with uncomplicated hypoplastic left heart syndrome. Most centers today perform staged reconstruction with some modification of the Norwood approach with excellent short-term results. Failing Fontan circulation due to either low pulmonary blood flow, recurrent ascites, protein-losing enteropathies, or plastic bronchitis are raising etiology for the procedure (See Chapter 17).

Other heart diseases with a high risk for sudden death without heart transplantation (i.e., restrictive cardiomyopathy, intractable ventricular arrhythmias, Kawasaki disease with giant coronary artery aneurysms) constitute a small but important group in which heart transplantation should be considered. Unresectable cardiac tumors that cause outflow or inflow obstruction, ventricular dysfunction, or malignant arrhythmias are also considered among the indications for heart transplantation.

Contraindications for the procedure could be absolute or relative [1, 6]. Absolute contraindications include:

- Active malignancy or a history of malignancy with a high risk of recurrence.
- Decompensated liver cirrhosis (contraindication for heart transplantation alone, combined heart and liver transplantation can be performed in some cases)
- Severe renal abnormality/dysfunction not likely to be reversible and not suitable for continuing dialysis or renal transplant at a later stage (contraindication for heart transplantation alone, combined heart and kidney transplantation can be performed in some cases).
- Progressive or refractory multisystem organ failure unlikely to be resolved by heart transplantation.
- Progressive systemic disease with early mortality (genetic, metabolic, or neurological disease).
- Anatomical concerns regarding appropriate anastomosis, particularly hypoplastic pulmonary arteries and veins and severe hypoplasia of the thoracic aorta.
- Severe, fixed elevation of pulmonary vascular (contraindication for heart transplantation alone, combined heart and lung transplantation can be performed in some cases).

- Significant organ dysfunction (including neurodevelopmental delay) likely to result in an inability to comply with post-transplant treatment regimens or leading to poor quality of life.
- History of recurrent medical non-compliance despite appropriate caregivers and multidisciplinary team involvement.
- Non-treatable psychological or psychiatric conditions that lead to non-compliance.
- Lack of adequate social support to allow adherence to treatment regimens after transplantation.

Relative contraindications include:

- Malignancy in remission. Patients should be assessed on an individual basis.
- Active sepsis from bacterial, fungal or severe viral infection. Patients need to be assessed on an individual basis after appropriate treatment is initiated.
- Sensitized patients with high levels of human leukocyte antigen (HLA) antibodies
- Diabetes mellitus with evidence of severe end-organ damage.
- Morbid obesity.
- Limited venous access.

The main Indication for retransplantation is significant cardiac allograft vasculopathy with graft dysfunction without evidence of acute graft rejection.

Evaluation of the Recipient

A team of specialists, including cardiologists, infectious disease physicians, nutritionists, social workers, psychologists, oral health specialists and other professionals according to the associated pathologies, evaluates every potential recipient.

Pretransplant evaluation includes a detailed history, physical examination, hemodynamic assessment by cardiac catheterization, and a complete anatomic evaluation of the heart and pulmonary vasculature. Estimation of indexed pulmonary vascular resistance (PVR) is a vital component in determining suitability for transplantation. Determination of ABO type, determination of the presence of HLA antibodies and screening for serologic evidence of prior exposure to several infectious agents such as Toxoplasma, Cytomegalovirus (CMV), Epstein-Barr virus (EBV), Varicella Zoster, Herpes Simplex, Hepatitis A through D, measles and human immunodeficiency virus, are performed. Evaluation of the function of other organs using biochemical techniques and imaging is essential to determine the suitability and risk of transplantation and to plan immediate postoperative care.

Management of pretransplant patients poses many challenges. A high percentage of patients require intravenous inotropic support and await heart transplantation while hospitalized. Patients managed on an outpatient basis return to the clinic at least once every four weeks. Optimizing nutrition and maintaining overall conditioning can be difficult in this end-stage population but are paramount to the overall success of the patient's perioperative course. Malnutrition and growth failure are common and secondary to anorexia and vomiting associated with high venous pressure and low cardiac output and are worsened by the malabsorptive and hypermetabolic state of heart failure. Comorbidities such as protein losing enteropathy and chronic liver and renal disease may contribute to ongoing nutritional disorders. Before transplantation immunizations should be given according to current recommendations unless the probability of transplantation within the next month is high. Waiting times for heart transplant candidates vary widely between different centers and countries and are based on factors such as the severity of the patient's illness, blood type, and anthropometric size. In general, the highest priority is given to the sickest patients.

The proper assessment of PVR is crucial in the evaluation of any candidate for heart transplantation. If PVR is excessive and fixed, the thin-walled right ventricle of the donor heart, especially after an imposed ischemic time, fails acutely and, therefore, patient cannot be weaned from cardiopulmonary bypass. The absolute upper limit of PVR index that is acceptable in the pediatric population is uncertain and institutional practice varies. In adults, PVR greater than 5 Wood units or a transpulmonary gradient greater than 15 mmHg correlate with an increase in perioperative mortality [9]. However, children may be able to undergo successful transplantation with higher PVR indices than adults [10]. At many institutions, patients with a PVR index greater than 4 Wood units at cardiac catheterization undergo additional testing for reactivity of the pulmonary vascular bed in response to 100% oxygen and, if necessary, with the subsequent administration of inhaled nitric oxide up to 80 ppm. A fixed PVR index greater than 10 Wood units is considered a contraindication to heart transplantation [11].

Surgical Considerations in Pediatric Heart Transplantation

For patients with non-complex anatomy, two basic surgical techniques have been employed. For many years, biatrial anastomoses were performed avoiding systemic and pulmonary venous connections. However, patients were left with spacious chambers comprising donor and recipient components, thus contracting asynchronously. Furthermore, this method led to complications such as tricuspid regurgitation, reduced right ventricular function and arrhythmias [12]. Since 1999, surgeons have removed the entire right atrium, leaving only a small cuff of left atrial tissue that incorporates the pulmonary veins. The donor's left atrium is sewn into place, and bicaval anastomoses are performed, with a more normal anatomical result. Theoretically, this technique is believed to improve sinus node function, produce less tricuspid regurgitation, and improve cardiac output [13, 14]. There are also advantages in using the bicaval method for patients who have already had Mustard or Senning procedures for congenital heart diseases. However, superior vena cava stenosis has been associated with complications in bicaval anastomoses, especially in infants [15].

Children with complex congenital heart disease represent about one half of all referrals for consideration for transplantation. Except from newborns with hypoplastic left heart syndrome, most of these children have undergone multiple prior surgical palliative or corrective procedures [16]. Frequently, there are multiple alterations in the anatomy of the branches of the pulmonary arteries. Anomalies of systemic and pulmonary venous return, particularly in the context of atrial isomerism or mirror-imaged atrial arrangement, pose additional challenges for the surgeon. In experienced centers, survival has been comparable with patients transplanted due to dilated cardiomyopathy, although the donor ischemic times, postoperative stays in the intensive care unit, and length of hospitalization are prolonged compared with patients with dilated cardiomyopathy [16-18]. Failure to recognize the presence of significant aortopulmonary collateral circulation in patients with cyanotic heart disease may contribute to high output failure occurring soon after transplantation [19]. This situation emphasizes the importance of comprehensive preoperative anatomic evaluation and planning in this difficult group of patients.

A patient with failed Fontan procedure poses additional challenges related to premorbid states, such as protein-losing enteropathy, chronic liver disease and pulmonary arteriovenous malformations. The latter are most common in patients with previous classic Glenn anastomosis and when hepatic venous return is excluded from the cavopulmonary repair, especially in the setting of left isomerism. Resolution of small pulmonary arteriovenous malformations may occur after transplantation, although it would seem unlikely that large lesions would regress rapidly. In this situation, patients may remain cyanotic after surgery, potentially leading to primary failure of the transplanted heart from hypoxemia. Aggressive pre-heart transplant embolization of aortopulmonary collateral vessels increases systemic flow before transplantation and may decrease bleeding after heart transplantation [20].

Early studies of outcomes after heart transplantation in Fontan patients showed lower survival after transplantation compared to other heart transplant patients [21-23]. Recent studies are more optimistic and suggest that survival for pediatric Fontan patients after heart transplantation is similar to non-Fontan congenital heart disease patients [24-26]. More details about surgical aspects in heart transplantation are discussed in Chapter 8.

Immunosuppressive Therapy for Heart Transplantation

The recipient of a transplanted heart invariably mounts an immune response to foreign antigens contained within the graft. All recipients, even neonates, require potent immunosuppressive therapy. This immune response is most vigorous in the first weeks and months after heart transplantation and is believed to persist throughout the life of the graft. In contrast to liver transplant recipients, there is no evidence that heart transplant recipients can be withdrawn from immunosuppressive therapy, even late after transplantation.

Clinical management of immunosuppression aims to prevent or minimize the host's immune response to donor antigens, while trying to avoid complications of immunodeficiency, such as infections and malignancies. It is also important to minimize non-immune toxicities, including diabetes, nephrotoxicity, neurotoxicity, hyperlipidemia, bone marrow suppression and steroids side effects.

Immunosuppressive therapy can be divided into induction therapy, maintenance therapy, and rescue therapy in cases of acute rejection.

Induction Therapy

Induction therapy has continued to be used in most pediatric heart transplant recipients, with increasing utilization over the last decade (Figure 3). It is used to rapidly produce an immunosuppressed state in the patient immediately after transplant surgery. Drugs available for this purpose include monoclonal or polyclonal antibody preparations. Monoclonal antibodies directed against the alpha chain of the interleukin-2 receptor are Basiliximab and Daclizumab.

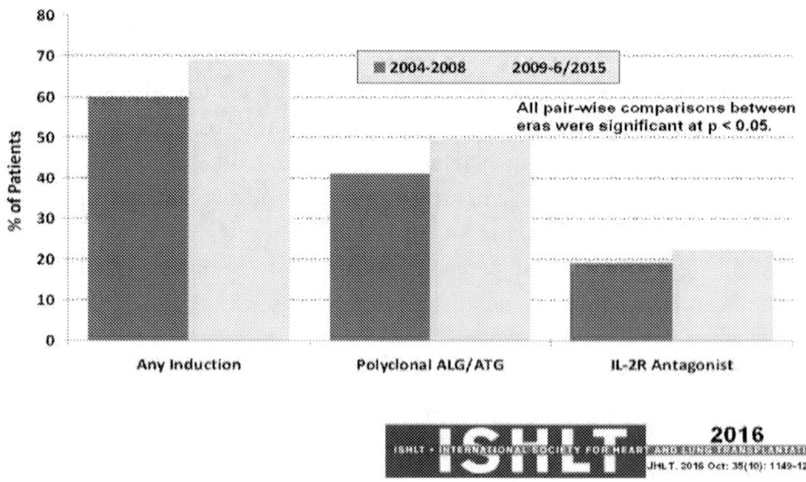

Figure 3. Induction immunosuppression by era (January 2004 to June 2015). ALG, anti-lymphocyte globulin; ATG, anti-thymocyte globulin; IL-2R, interleukin-2 receptor. (Data from ISHLT. 2016. *Pediatric Heart Transplantation Statistics.* Accessed 15 Dec 2021. https://ishltregistries.org/registries/slides.asp).

Polyclonal antibodies directed against T cells are antithymocyte globulin. No survival benefit has been shown from induction therapy, but recent registry reports have demonstrated a slight advantage in freedom from coronary allograft vasculopathy [27]. Induction therapy also allows for delayed introduction of nephrotoxic immunosuppressive agents in the early postoperative period at a time when the kidney is particularly vulnerable [28].

Maintenance Immunosuppression

Maintenance immunosuppression regimens used in pediatric heart transplant recipients tend to be individual-specific and institution-specific. The strategies take advantage of the selectivity of immunosuppressive agents for critical pathways in graft rejection. Virtually all immunosuppressive regimens in children are based on the use of calcineurin inhibitors, such as tacrolimus or cyclosporine, and an antiproliferative agent, such as mycophenolate mofetil or mycophenolic acid. Corticosteroids are typically started in the operating room and continued in the early postoperative period, with most centers now tapering or discontinuing steroids from the long-term maintenance regimen. Long term corticosteroid use in pediatric patients has been linked in some centers to several undesirable risks such as higher rate of opportunistic infections, diabetes, and bone demineralization [28]. We gradually withdraw corticosteroid therapy between 6 and 12 months after transplantation if the patient did not have graft rejection.

Over the last decade, tacrolimus use has increased from 65% to 85% and mycophenolate mofetil or mycophenolic acid increased from 78% to 92%, whereas prednisone has decreased from 75% to 70%. Cyclosporine use has decreased from 33% (2004-2008) to 14% (2009-2015) [2, 28].

Sirolimus/everolimus are agents with potent immunosuppressive properties. Sirolimus inhibits T lymphocyte activation and proliferation that occurs in response to antigenic and cytokine (Interleukin IL-2, IL-4, and IL-15) stimulation by a mechanism that is distinct from that of other immunosuppressants. Sirolimus also inhibits antibody production. In cells, sirolimus binds to the immunophilin FK Binding Protein-12 (FKBP-12) to generate an immunosuppressive complex. The sirolimus-FKBP-12 complex has no effect on calcineurin activity, instead it binds to and inhibits the activation of the mammalian Target Of Rapamycin (mTOR), a key regulatory kinase.

This inhibition suppresses cytokine-driven T-cell proliferation, preventing the progression from the G1 to the S phase of the cell cycle. The use of this drug is uncommon at the time of hospital discharge, used in approximately 2% of patients. However, by 5 years after transplantation, nearly 20% of patients are treated with either sirolimus or everolimus. Tacrolimus and mycophenolate mofetil / mycophenolic acid continue to be the most common combination of immunosuppressive agents utilized (Figure 4) [2].

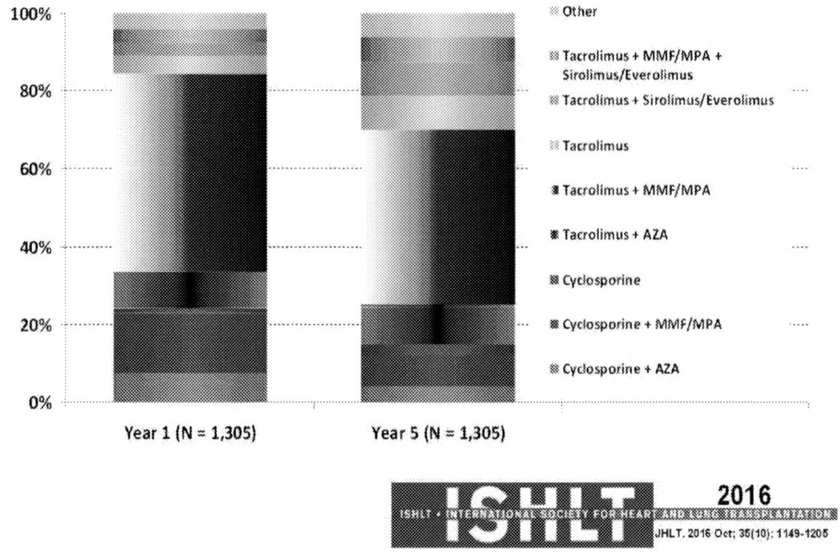

Figure 4. Maintenance immunosuppression at time of follow-up for same patients at each time-point (January 2004 to June 2015). AZA, azathioprine; MMF; mycophenolate mofetil; MPA, mycophenolic acid. (Data from ISHLT. 2016. *Pediatric Heart Transplantation Statistics.* Accessed 15 Dec 2021. https://ishltregistries.org/registries/slides.asp).

All the currently available immunosuppressive medications have known side effects or toxicities. Side effects of cyclosporine include nephrotoxicity, hypertension, neurotoxicity, electrolyte imbalance, hirsutism, and gingival hyperplasia. Tacrolimus has similar side effects excluding the hirsutism and gingival hyperplasia but has the added risk of causing hyperglycemia.

The use of sirolimus is associated with hyperlipidemia, bone marrow suppression and impaired or delayed wound healing. Mycophenolate mofetil or mycophenolic acid can produce myelosuppression and gastrointestinal side effects. The latter is reduced with mycophenolic acid. The side effects of corticosteroids are well known and include Cushingoid habitus, increased appetite, hypertension, diabetes, gastritis and gastric ulceration, growth retardation and osteoporosis.

Complications after Heart Transplantation

Acute Cellular Rejection

Acute failure of the transplanted heart is the most common cause of death in the first 30 days after transplantation and occurs more frequently in infant recipients. During the first 5 years after transplantation, acute cellular rejection and infection are the most common causes of death. Beyond 5 years, chronic rejection becomes the dominant cause of graft or even patient loss (Figure 5) [29].

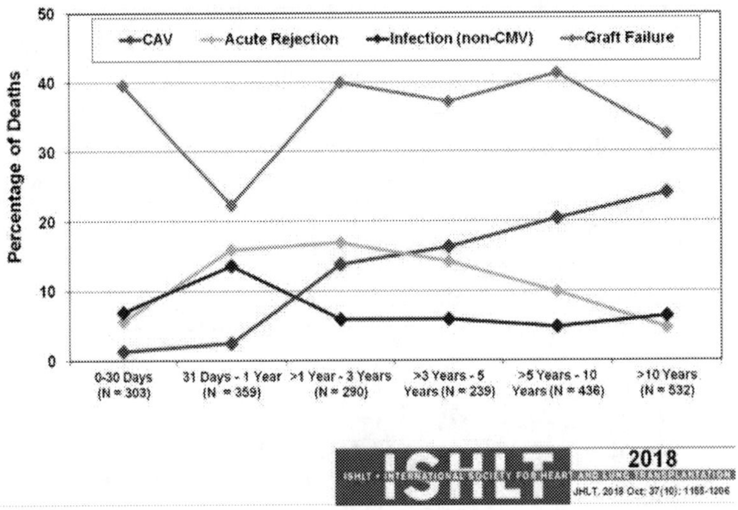

Figure 5. Pediatric heart transplants. Relative incidence of leading causes of death (January 2004–June 2017). CAV, cardiac allograft vasculopathy; CMV, cytomegalovirus. (Data from ISHLT. 2018. *Pediatric Heart Transplantation Statistics.* Accessed 15 Dec 2021. https://ishltregistries.org/registries/slides.asp).

Understanding the timing of and risk factors for acute rejection is vital for designing logical strategies for surveillance and prevention. It is also important to distinguish acute rejection from acute heart dysfunction, as the two terms are not synonymous. Most acute rejections are not associated with overt dysfunction, although subtle subclinical abnormalities of diastolic function are common.

When heart failure occurs in the first years after transplantation, acute cellular rejection is the most likely diagnosis, although other conditions should be considered, such as humoral (antibody mediated) rejection, acute presentation of chronic rejection secondary to cardiac allograft vasculopathy and viral myocarditis [30].

The overall incidence of treated rejection from hospital discharge to 1-year post-transplant continues to decrease. In the most recent era (January 2010–June 2018), 13% of recipients were treated for rejection between hospital discharge and 1-year post-transplant compared with 24% in the prior era (January 2005–December 2009). This finding was observed in all age groups and was similar in males and females. This is important, as an episode of treated rejection within the first year post-transplant is associated with worse survival, a finding observed in all age groups whether tacrolimus or cyclosporine were used at the time of hospital discharge [31].

Induction therapy was not associated with higher risk of treated rejection between hospital discharge and 1-year post-transplant (Figure 6). Furthermore, the type of induction therapy used was not associated with an increased risk of rejection.

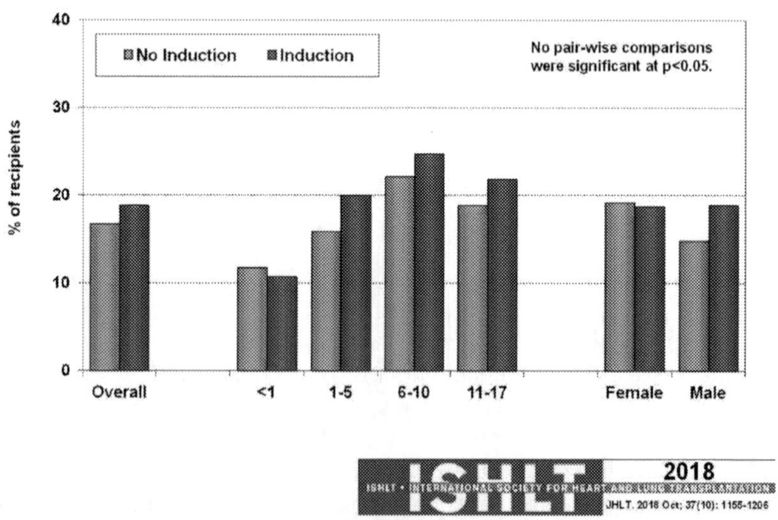

Figure 6. Percentage of recipients experiencing treated rejection between discharge and 1-year follow-up by use of induction therapy (January 2005–June 2018). NS, not significant. (Data from ISHLT. 2018. *Pediatric Heart Transplantation Statistics.* Accessed 15 Dec 2021. https://ishltregistries.org/registries/slides.asp).

Cyclosporine use at discharge was associated with a higher risk of rejection compared with tacrolimus, and this was observed regardless of the use of induction therapy and other maintenance immunosuppressive medications [31].

Episodes of acute rejection occurring late after transplantation were diagnosed in a quarter of recipients, with a probability of freedom from late rejection of 82% at 2 years and 73% at 3 years after transplantation [32]. In contrast to the first episodes of rejection occurring early after transplantation, the hazard for late rejection is more constant, with an ongoing risk for as long as the cohort has been followed. This ongoing risk for acute rejection correlates with the clinical observation that recipients do not tolerate discontinuation of immunosuppression, which at this time must be considered a lifelong therapy. Risk factors for rejection in children include older age at transplant, African American race, CMV infection, gender mismatch and previous episodes of rejection [32-35]. Hemodynamically significant rejection episodes predict a particularly poor outcome in the first year after the episode [35].

Rejection in pediatric recipients is often not associated with symptoms. However, they may present with a history of poor feeding, irritability, malaise, fever, nausea, and abdominal pain. Accompanying physical findings may include tachycardia, a gallop rhythm, rales, hepatomegaly, and new-onset arrhythmias. Although electrocardiographic evidence of low QRS voltages is a suggestive finding, the specificity and sensitivity are poor. Numerous noninvasive tools have been used to diagnose cellular rejection with conflicting results. Although echocardiography has been widely used to diagnose cellular rejection, moderate acute cellular rejection is frequently associated with a normal or stable echocardiogram [36].

Many centers, including ours, still use rejection surveillance programs based on endomyocardial biopsies. Their usefulness and safety are well established, but there is significant variation in practices between institutions. This is mainly due to its usefulness when there are no clinical signs to suspect rejection [37-39]. Taking all of this into consideration, endomyocardial biopsy remains as the gold standard method for detecting rejection and initiating treatment before a clinically significant graft dysfunction. An adequate biopsy sample should contain four to six pieces of endomyocardium. These specimens are stained with hematoxylin and eosin, and a standard biopsy grading system developed by the ISHLT is used to classify the severity of rejection and guide treatment (See Chapter 11) [40].

Episodes of moderate to severe acute cellular rejection are treated with intravenous methyl-prednisolone at 10 to 20 mg/kg in 3 doses and basal immunosuppression is adjusted, whereas episodes that are refractory to corticosteroids are treated with antithymocyte globulin.

Humoral Rejection

Humoral rejection is less common than cellular rejection and generally occurs when a patient with preformed anti-HLA antibodies receives an organ that contains antigens to which the recipient has been previously sensitized. This allosensitization is generally due to previous transfusions of blood products or homograft materials used during previous surgical palliations for congenital heart defects or associated with mechanical ventricular support. Most centers prospectively screen each transplant recipient for the presence of preformed anti-HLA panel reactive antibodies on their serum. These antibodies are detected by testing the recipient's serum against a panel of lymphocytes from numerous donors selected to represent all common HLA antigens.

The management of an outpatient candidate with an elevated level of panel reactive antibodies is controversial. Prospective crossmatching of candidate serum with potential donor lymphocytes can be attempted, but this is often not feasible because most child donor hearts are procured from distant sites where recipient serum is not available. Attempts can be made to reduce the level of recipient anti-HLA antibodies. Strategies that have been used to achieve this reduction of anti-HLA antibodies include the use of intravenous pooled immunoglobulin, plasmapheresis, and agents that may inhibit production of antibodies by B cells like the anti-B cell monoclonal antibody rituximab, a human/mouse chimeric monoclonal antibody directed against the CD 20 antigen carried on almost all B cells. There are other therapies such as obinutuzumab, a humanized anti-CD20 monoclonal antibody, proteasome inhibition with bortezomib or carfilzomib, complement inhibition with the C5 terminal complement inhibitor eculizumab or T-B cell co-stimulation inhibition with belatacept or abatacept. Additional protocols use desensitization with induction therapy at the time of solid organ transplantation [41, 42].

Cardiac Allograft Vasculopathy

Coronary artery disease subsequent to transplantation is an accelerated vasculopathy that constitutes one of the leading causes of death in the late stage of heart transplantation (Figure 5). The pathology differs from that of ischemic heart disease in the normal adult population. Typically, cardiac allograft vasculopathy (CAV) consists of myointimal proliferation that is concentric and affects the entire length of the vessel including intramyocardial branches with eventual luminal occlusion [43]. Nearly 50% of all transplant recipients have developed CAV by 15 years post-transplantation, but freedom from it has improved in the recent era. Interestingly, on univariate analysis, the use of induction therapy is associated with increased freedom from CAV. However, it is not associated with graft ischemic time or type of calcineurin inhibitor used at discharge among patients who survived beyond the first year. Age is an important risk factor, as the risk of CAV increases with age. In addition, and consistent with prior reports, an episode of rejection in the first year after heart transplantation is associated with a higher frequency of CAV at 3 years after transplantation. There is a high mortality rate in all age groups within 5 years of the diagnosis of CAV [31].

The diagnosis of CAV is difficult. Patients are often asymptomatic until they present with sudden death. As the heart of the transplant recipient is denervated patients usually do not experience typical ischemic chest pain. A symptom complex of atypical chest or abdominal pain along with other gastrointestinal complaints, heart failure or syncope may often be the initial presentation [44].

Angiography has traditionally been the gold standard for the detection of coronary artery disease in children and adults. However, angiography has serious limitations beyond the obvious fact that it is invasive an expensive as a screening tool. Angiography is a relatively insensitive marker of mild CAV due to the diffuse nature of the disease process and the propensity to affect small vessels. Despite its limitations, it is used worldwide to assess the presence and severity of CAV in heart transplant patients. On the other hand, intravascular ultrasound (IVUS) has a greater sensitivity for detection of CAV than angiography. Studies in adults have report the frequent occurrence of abnormalities on IVUS, despite angiographically normal appearance of the coronary arteries [45]. This has also been observed in large studies of heart transplant patients, including children, showing discrepancies between the findings from coronary angiography and IVUS, with better sensitivity of the latter [46-49].

Once CAV is moderate or severe, prognosis is poor with a 4-year freedom from graft loss of 30% [50]. Studies of pediatric heart transplant recipients have shown IVUS-detectable CAV in patients with normal coronary angiograms; therefore, the use of IVUS may allow earlier intervention in the disease process in order to slow progression [46, 47, 49]. IVUS detection of increasing maximal intimal thickness predicts cardiac events in adults but similar studies have not been performed in children. The frequency of complications attributed to IVUS during coronary artery surveillance in pediatric heart transplant patients is similar to that reported for coronary angiography. Adverse events of moderate or greater severity are rare. In the hands of experienced practitioners, IVUS can safely be performed in pediatric heart transplant recipients with a very low complication rate [51]. In our center, we do it annually in children over 15 kg.

Beyond retransplantation no effective treatment exists for established CAV because bypass grafting and coronary angioplasty have limited utility as a result of the diffuse nature of the disease. Similarly, stenting is of limited use because of intimal proliferation through the stent and because of progression of the disease in other areas. Even retransplantation represents a limited option. As a result of the redo nature of the procedure many patients experience greater preoperative morbidity. Existing end organ toxicities from the first transplant also can render immunosuppression more difficult. Several pharmacologic approaches have been used for prevention of CAV after transplantation. Anecdotal reports, small clinical trials in adults and experimental models in animals suggest that many agents may be potentially useful in the prevention of CAV, including angiotensin-converting enzyme inhibitors, statins, aspirin, and antiproliferative agents such as mycophenolate mofetil and sirolimus. However, it is unlikely that large multicenter clinical trials of most of these therapies, especially in children, will be conducted.

Infectious Complications

The spectrum of infections after heart transplantation in children and their prevention and treatment have been the focus of many reviews [52-56]. Most infections are caused by pathogens that also cause infection in non-immunocompromised children. Examples include respiratory viruses, streptococcus pneumonia and varicella zoster virus. All infections that may be seen in non-immunocompromised patients can cause greater disease severity in heart transplant recipients, and strategies to achieve prevention and early treatment are imperative. A particular situation is infections caused by CMV and EBV, which rarely cause severe disease in immunocompetent hosts. More rarely, opportunistic infections are seen such as those due to *Pneumocystis Jirovecii.* Although most infections are well tolerated, infection ranks comparable with early graft failure and rejection as main causes of death after heart transplantation in children [57].

Infections occur in a generally predictable time pattern after solid organ transplantation. The development of infection is delayed by prophylaxis and accelerated by intensified immunosuppression, drug toxic effects that may cause leukopenia or by immunomodulatory viral infections such as infection by the herpes virus group, mainly CMV or EBV. At the time of transplantation, a patient's short-term and long-term risk of infection can be stratified according to donor and recipient screening, the technical outcome of surgery, and the intensity of immunosuppression required to prevent graft rejection. Subsequently, an ongoing assessment of the risk of infection is used to adjust both prophylaxis and immunosuppressive therapy (Figure 7) [57].

CMV is an important cause of morbidity after solid organ transplantation, but symptomatic disease in children is relatively unusual [58]. Primary CMV infection, typically acquired from an infected organ donor, is associated with the highest morbidity and mortality rates, whereas secondary infection tends to result in milder disease. High doses of immunosuppressive agents, especially anti-thymocyte/anti-lymphocyte globulin products, are associated with higher rates of CMV disease, regardless of previous immunity. Symptomatic disease typically manifests during the intermediate time period after transplantation. However, the time of onset can be later if antiviral chemoprophylaxis is used [59]. Furthermore, some groups have suggested that CMV virus infection is a risk factor for the development of CAV [60]. Whether this is true in children is unknown but in an IVUS study from Loma Linda, CA increases in maximal intimal thickness and intimal index correlated with CMV seropositivity [46]. Consensus on the establishment of risk groups, diagnostics tools, prevention and treatment strategies was established at a recent international meeting of experts [61].

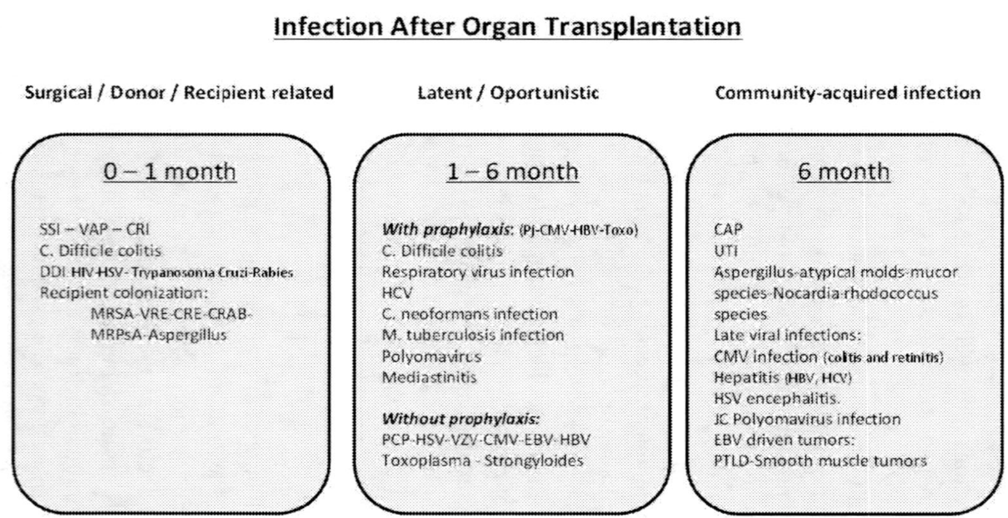

Figure 7. Infection after heart transplantation. C, Clostridium; C, Criptococcus; AP, Community-acquired pneumonia; CMV Cytomegalovirus; CRAB, Carbapenem resistant Acinetobacter Baumannii; CRE, Carbapenem-resistant Enterobacteriaceae; CRI, Catheter related infection; DDI, Donor derived infection; EBV, Epstein Barr Virus; HBV, Hepatitis B Virus; HCV, Hepatitis C virus; HIV, Human immunodeficiency virus; HSV, Herpes simplex virus; M, Mycobacterium; MRPsA, Multidrug resistant Pseudomona Aeruginosa; MRSA, Methicillin-resistant Staphylococcus aureus; PCP, Pneumocystis Jirovecii pneumonia; PJ, Pneumocystis Jirovecii; PTLD, Post-transplantation lymphoproliferative disorder. SSI, Surgical site infection; Toxo, Toxoplasmosis; UTI, Urinary tract infection; VAP, Ventilator associated pneumonia; VRE, Vancomycin resistant enterococcus; VZV, Varicella-zoster virus. (Data from Fishman JA. Infection in solid-organ transplant recipients. *N Engl J Med*. 2007 Dec 20;357(25):2601-14).

EBV infection is another major cause of concern in pediatric solid organ transplantation, mainly due to the relationship between infection and the development of post-transplant lymphoproliferative disorder (PTLD). For example, a review of the Pediatric Heart Transplant Study database identified 56 cases of PTLD among 1184 primary transplants (4.7%) at 19 North American centers, more than 80% were associated with EBV [62]. There is a bimodal presentation of PTLD disease with the early-onset disease usually possessing a less aggressive polymorphic histology and an almost invariable association with primary infection by EBV. Late-onset PTLD, usually presenting after three years of heart transplantation, can have highly variable histology and is often monomorphic with histology resembling aggressive B cell lymphoma.

The clinical manifestations of PTLD are protean. Fever, malaise, weight loss, abdominal pain, vomiting and diarrhea are common presenting clinical features. Unlike other solid organ transplantation, the disease rarely affects the allograft. Most children who develop these disorders are diagnosed with lung nodules, mediastinal or abdominal adenopathies, or both. Gastrointestinal involvement is common, and hemorrhagic obstruction or perforation can occur. Central nervous system involvement is rare. Monitoring of EBV viral load in peripheral blood of post- transplant patients by serial quantitative polymerase chain reaction shows promise for early detecting EBV disease and allows the possibility of rapid therapeutic intervention. Furthermore, the development of very high viral loads should alert the physician to look for signs or symptoms of disease, even in asymptomatic patients. In our center, we routinely monitor patients at risk by monthly polymerase chain reaction for the first six to twelve months after transplantation and at the time of symptoms suggestive of disease. The main treatment of PTLD in children is the reduction or temporary interruption of immunosuppression. In some institutions, this course of action has been associated with cure in approximately four fifths of cases with polymorphic histology [62]. However, rebound rejection is common and must be sought by increased echocardiographic and endomyocardial biopsy surveillance.

Monomorphic forms are less likely to respond to reduced immunosuppression, but this is typically attempted as first-line therapy because complete remission has been observed in some cases. However, monomorphic disease may require treatment with conventional chemotherapy agents, as do overtly malignant lymphomas such as Burkitt's lymphoma. More than nine tenths of PTLD are of recipient B cell origin so anti-B cell monoclonal antibodies such as Rituximab have been used as another line of treatment with or without chemotherapy. Adoptive immunotherapy using donor-derived cloned EBV-specific cytotoxic T cells has been used successfully for the treatment of PTLD in allogeneic bone marrow transplant recipients, but in the solid organ transplantation setting experience is more limited [63].

EBV-associated smooth muscle tumors are a rare complication of solid organ transplantation, and incidence data are limited. EBV DNA is universally present in these tumors. It is still unknown how these cells become infected with EBV, whether this is the result of primary EBV infection or reactivation, and how persistent active EBV infection after transplantation influences tumor pathogenesis [64].

Immunizations in Heart Transplant Recipients

Post-transplant immunization is routinely indicated after 3-6 months of transplantation when immunosuppression declines, except for the influenza vaccine which can be given as early as 1 month [65]. Vaccination status should be reviewed, and a vaccination plan developed in all transplant candidates and recipients. Transplant candidates should be up to date on their routine vaccinations as per national guidelines. Inactivated vaccines should be given at least 2 weeks before transplantation, when possible, for an adequate immune response. Live attenuated vaccines should be administered at least 4 weeks prior to transplantation to ensure that vaccine-related viral replication has resolved prior to transplantation and they should be avoided after heart transplantation until more information exists. In the post-transplant setting, inactivated preparation against diphtheria, pertussis, tetanus, hepatitis B virus, hepatitis A virus, haemophilus influenza, pneumococcus, meningococcus, polio (Salk), HPV are indicated. COVID-19 ARN vaccine is indicated in children from 5 years of age in the context of the pandemic [65].

Non-Immune Complications

Non-immunological complications associated with immunosuppressive drugs are systemic hypertension, hyperlipidemia, diabetes mellitus, neurological and renal dysfunction.

Systemic hypertension is a common complication, especially in patients receiving calcineurin inhibitors and steroid-based immunosuppression.

Hypertension generally responds to standard antihypertensive agents, but can sometimes be quite resistant to treatment. The addition of an angiotensin converting enzyme inhibitor has been shown to have some renal protective effects.

Hyperlipidemia is also common in children after heart transplantation. Children treated with cyclosporine experience more adverse lipid profiles compared with children treated with tacrolimus, and this effect occurs independent of the effects of corticosteroids [66]. Statin treatment is usually quite effective.

The idiosyncratic and dose-related neurological complications of current immunosuppressive regimens include seizures, tremors, paresthesias, and encephalopathies [67].

Common metabolic complications include hyperkalemia, hyperuricemia, hypomagnesemia, and most importantly, diabetes mellitus. The relative diabetogenic effect of cyclosporine and tacrolimus is the subject of considerable controversy, but the development of diabetes is rare after transplantation in preadolescents. Adolescent age, obesity, and the need for high doses of corticosteroids have been identified as the main risk factors for the development of diabetes mellitus.

Kidney dysfunction is a common long-term morbidity among heart transplant recipients. This is because they have a history of repeated acute kidney injury due to episodes of hemodynamic instability, exposures to cardiopulmonary bypass, and nephrotoxic drugs. Calcineurin inhibitors are nephrotoxic and one of the main contributors to chronic kidney dysfunction. Some children eventually require dialysis or kidney transplantation, although this is relatively uncommon, as 86-98% of recipients do not have severe kidney dysfunction at 10 years after transplantation [27]. Minimizing repeated kidney injury by avoiding dehydration and closely monitoring nephrotoxic drugs such as vancomycin are important in the long-term prognosis of kidney function in cardiac recipients. Increased use of adjuvant therapies without renal toxicity (Sirolimus/Everolimus, Mycophenolic Acid /Mycophenolate mofetil) should allow a reduced dose of nephrotoxic calcineurin inhibitors.

Survival and Quality of Life

Recent data from the International Society of Heart and Lung Transplantation show that survival of pediatric heart transplant recipients continues to improve over the 20-years interval followed by this registry. Overall, 1-year post-transplant survival improved from 87% during 2000 to 2005 to 92% during 2012 to 2017 (Figure 8) [68].

Stratified by recipient age, 1-year survival in recipients transplanted during 2012 to 2017 was 89% in infants <1-year old, 92% in children 1 to 10 years old, and 94% in children 11 to 17 years old. Recipients transplanted for dilated cardiomyopathy and congenital heart disease in 2012 to 2017 had higher survival compared to those transplanted in previous eras. Recipients of re-transplantation in the 2012 to 2017 era had a similar improvement in survival, although the difference with previous eras did not reach statistical significance, probably due to a smaller sample.

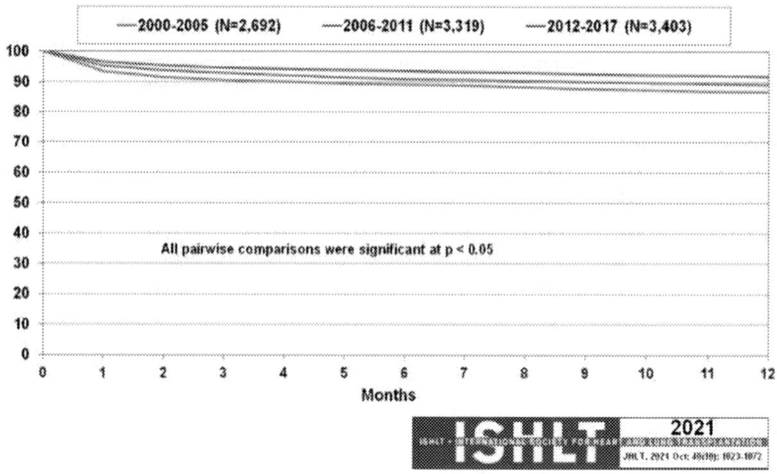

Figure 8. Pediatric Heart Transplants Kaplan-Meier Survival within 12 Months by Era (January 2000 – June 2017). (Data from ISHLT. 2021. *Pediatric Heart Transplantation Focus Theme.* Accessed 15 Dec 2021. https://ishltregistries.org/registries/slides.asp).

One-year survival among transplant recipients between 2012 to 2017 was 95%, 88% and 91% in recipients with a diagnosis of dilated cardiomyopathy, congenital heart disease and retransplantation, respectively. In an analysis stratified by mechanical circulatory support at transplant, 1-year survival improved significantly in recipients supported with a durable ventricular assist device/total artificial heart, and in those not requiring any mechanical circulatory support, but not among those supported on ECMO. When stratified by kidney function, a significant improvement in 1-year survival was only demonstrated among children with an estimated glomerular filtration rate >60 ml/min/1.73 m^2. Although recent recipients with chronic kidney disease (those with estimated glomerular filtration rate <30 and 30-60 ml/min/1.73 m^2) appeared to have better outcomes compared to recipients from the earlier era, this improvement did not reach statistical significance. One-year survival was lower among transplant recipients on dialysis at the time of transplantation than among those not on dialysis, and higher among those who received a transplant with a history of malignancy (versus the remaining recipients), probably because recipients with a history of malignancy had chemotherapy-induced cardiomyopathy whereas the remaining patients were a heterogeneous group that included higher-risk recipients with congenital heart disease.

There were no differences in 5-year conditional survival between recipients who were transplanted during 1996 to 2001 (87%) and 2002 to 2007 (88%); however, 5-year conditional survival in pediatric recipients transplanted during 2008 to 2013 (90.5%) was significantly higher (Figure 9) [68].

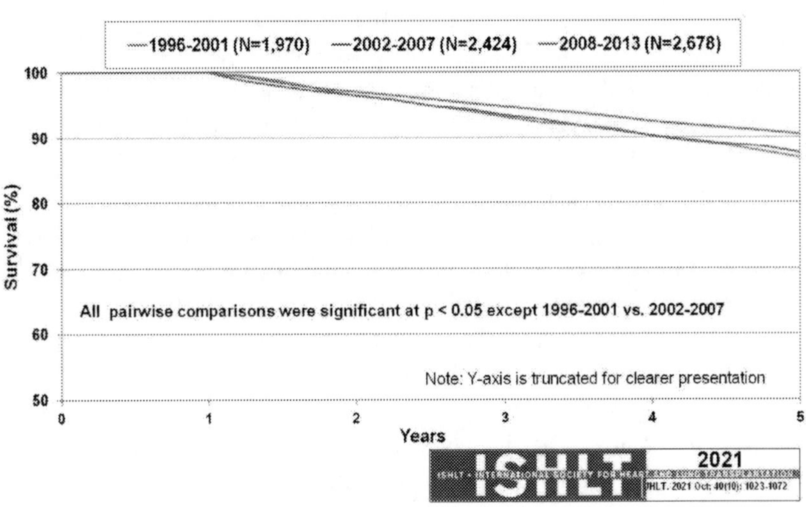

Figure 9. Pediatric Heart Transplants Kaplan-Meier Survival within 5 Years Conditional on Survival to 1 Year by Era (January 1996 - June 2013). (Data from ISHLT. 2021. *Pediatric Heart Transplantation Focus Theme.* Accessed 15 Dec 2021. https://ishltregistries.org/registries/slides.asp).

Among transplant recipients in the most recently evaluated era (2008-2013), 5-year conditional survival was 91.2% in recipients with infants <1 year, 92.3% in recipients aged 1 to 10 years and 88% in recipients aged 11 to

17 at the time of transplantation. The lower conditional survival in adolescent recipients may be explained by a potentially higher prevalence of medication non-compliance in this age group. Interestingly, 5-year conditional survival improved over time in recipients with a diagnosis of dilated cardiomyopathy but not in those with a diagnosis of congenital heart disease.

Most recipients are well rehabilitated and are in New York Heart Association class 1. Full time attendance at school is achieved in almost all patients within a few months of transplantation. Because the transplanted heart is denervated, heart transplant patients rely on catecholamine stimulation to increase heart rate and cardiac output. It has been reported that the maximum capacity for physical work and maximum heart rate are only about 2/3 of what is expected, and that the maximum volume of oxygen use is only 50% of that of normal controls [69, 70].

Although pediatric heart transplant patients are generally reported to return to a good quality of life, many recipients experience difficulties in psychosocial adjustment, with adolescents being the most vulnerable [70-73]. School performance is significantly lower than that of healthy children and the prevalence of behavior problems increases from 8% at six months to 29% at three and five years after transplantation.

At 4.5 years of age, children who received a heart transplant earlier in life had significantly lower health-related quality of life scores, as reported by their parents, than the normal population, children with chronic conditions and children with congenital heart disease who underwent surgery early in infancy. Children with kidney dysfunction pre-transplantation and those with indirect signs of low cardiac output beyond the initial postoperative days seem to be at a higher risk for a lower health-related quality of life [74].

Normal adolescent development combined with the complex psychological issues surrounding heart transplantation creates a large population of recipients at risk. Non-adherence has been linked to late rejection and high mortality rates in the adolescent age group and has been a source of immense frustration for all those who care for these individuals. Coordinated efforts among pediatricians, psychologists, and transplant teams are necessary to help identify patients at risk and design interventions that serve to prevent unnecessary morbidity and mortality in this challenging group of patients [75, 76].

Conclusion

In recent decades there have been great improvements in outcomes after heart transplantation in children. Surgeons have faced the challenge of transplanting recipients with complex anatomy and have achieved great success in reducing early mortality. Ventricular assist devices have made it possible to stabilize patients who previously would not have been able to access heart transplantation.

There have also been important advances in recent years in understanding the immune response to solid organ allografts. Better patient care is the result of these advances.

Understanding of risk factors that impact on individual outcomes is also improving, including new knowledge about genetic factors. A better understanding of the immune response to EBV infection, combined with new monitoring and treatment strategies, suggests that lymphoproliferative disorders can be prevented after transplantation or that they can be treated more successfully in the years to come. ABO incompatible heart transplantation and the development of tolerance induction strategies can improve transplantation chances and outcomes, potentially transforming transplantation from palliative to curative therapy.

Children deserve the effort.

References

[1] Kantrowitz A, Haller JD, Joos H, Cerruti MM, Carstensen HE. Transplantation of the heart in an infant and an adult. *Am J Cardiol.* 1968 Dec;22(6):782-90.

[2] Rossano JW, Dipchand AI, Edwards LB, Goldfarb S, Kucheryavaya AY, Levvey Rn BJ, Lund LH, Meiser B, Yusen RD, Stehlik J; International Society for Heart and Lung Transplantation. The Registry of the International Society for Heart and Lung Transplantation: Nineteenth Pediatric Heart Transplantation Report-2016; Focus Theme: Primary Diagnostic Indications for Transplant. *J Heart Lung Transplant.* 2016 Oct;35(10):1185-1195.

[3] Michels VV, Moll PP, Miller FA, Tajik AJ, Chu JS, Driscoll DJ, Burnett JC, Rodeheffer RJ, Chesebro JH, Tazelaar HD. The frequency of familial dilated cardiomyopathy in a series of patients with idiopathic dilated cardiomyopathy. *N Engl J Med.* 1992 Jan 9;326(2):77-82.

[4] Bowles NE, Ni J, Kearney DL, Pauschinger M, Schultheiss HP, McCarthy R, Hare J, Bricker JT, Bowles KR, Towbin JA. Detection of viruses in myocardial tissues by

polymerase chain reaction. evidence of adenovirus as a common cause of myocarditis in children and adults. *J Am Coll Cardiol.* 2003 Aug 6;42(3):466-72.

[5] Maron BJ, Shirani J, Poliac LC, Mathenge R, Roberts WC, Mueller FO. Sudden death in young competitive athletes. Clinical, demographic, and pathological profiles. *JAMA.* 1996 Jul 17;276(3):199-204.

[6] Canter CE, Shaddy RE, Bernstein D, Hsu DT, Chrisant MR, Kirklin JK, Kanter KR, Higgins RS, Blume ED, Rosenthal DN, Boucek MM, Uzark KC, Friedman AH, Young JK; American Heart Association Council on Cardiovascular Disease in the Young; American Heart Association Council on Clinical Cardiology; American Heart Association Council on Cardiovascular Nursing; American Heart Association Council on Cardiovascular Surgery and Anesthesia; Quality of Care and Outcomes Research Interdisciplinary Working Group. Indications for heart transplantation in pediatric heart disease: a scientific statement from the American Heart Association Council on Cardiovascular Disease in the Young; the Councils on Clinical Cardiology, Cardiovascular Nursing, and Cardiovascular Surgery and Anesthesia; and the Quality of Care and Outcomes Research Interdisciplinary Working Group. *Circulation.* 2007 Feb 6;115(5):658-76.

[7] Lipshultz SE, Sleeper LA, Towbin JA, Lowe AM, Orav EJ, Cox GF, Lurie PR, McCoy KL, McDonald MA, Messere JE, Colan SD. The incidence of pediatric cardiomyopathy in two regions of the United States. *N Engl J Med.* 2003 Apr 24;348(17):1647-55.

[8] Russo LM, Webber SA. Idiopathic restrictive cardiomyopathy in children. *Heart.* 2005 Sep;91(9):1199-202.

[9] Murali S, Kormos RL, Uretsky BF, Schechter D, Reddy PS, Denys BG, Armitage JM, Hardesty RL, Griffith BP. Preoperative pulmonary hemodynamics and early mortality after orthotopic cardiac transplantation: the Pittsburgh experience. *Am Heart J.* 1993 Oct;126(4):896-904.

[10] Gajarski RJ, Towbin JA, Bricker JT, Radovancevic B, Frazier OH, Price JK, Schowengerdt KO, Denfield SW. Intermediate follow-up of pediatric heart transplant recipients with elevated pulmonary vascular resistance index. *J Am Coll Cardiol.* 1994 Jun;23(7):1682-7.

[11] Chiu P, Russo MJ, Davies RR, Addonizio LJ, Richmond ME, Chen JM. What is high risk? Redefining elevated pulmonary vascular resistance index in pediatric heart transplantation. *J Heart Lung Transplant.* 2012 Jan;31(1):61-6.

[12] Weiss ES, Nwakanma LU, Russell SB, Conte JV, Shah AS. Outcomes in bicaval versus biatrial techniques in heart transplantation: an analysis of the UNOS database. *J Heart Lung Transplant.* 2008 Feb;27(2):178-83.

[13] el Gamel A, Yonan NA, Grant S, Deiraniya AK, Rahman AN, Sarsam MA, Campbell CS. Orthotopic cardiac transplantation: a comparison of standard and bicaval Wythenshawe techniques. *J Thorac Cardiovasc Surg.* 1995 Apr;109(4):721-9; discussion 729-30.

[14] Trento A, Czer LS, Blanche C. Surgical techniques for cardiac transplantation. *Semin Thorac Cardiovasc Surg.* 1996 Apr;8(2):126-32.

[15] Sachdeva R, Seib PM, Burns SA, Fontenot EE, Frazier EA. Stenting for superior vena cava obstruction in pediatric heart transplant recipients. *Catheter Cardiovasc Interv.* 2007 Nov 15;70(6):888-92.

[16] Webber SA, Fricker FJ, Michaels M, Pickering RM, del Nido PJ, Griffith BP, Armitage JM. Orthotopic heart transplantation in children with congenital heart disease. *Ann Thorac Surg.* 1994 Dec;58(6):1664-9.

[17] Hsu DT, Quaegebeur JM, Michler RE, Smith CR, Rose EA, Kichuk MR, Gersony WM, Douglas JF, Addonizio LJ. Heart transplantation in children with congenital heart disease. *J Am Coll Cardiol.* 1995 Sep;26(3):743-9.

[18] Kirklin JK. Current challenges in pediatric heart transplantation for congenital heart disease. *Curr Opin Organ Transplant.* 2015 Oct;20(5):577-83.

[19] Krishnan US, Lamour JM, Hsu DT, Kichuk MR, Donnelly CM, Addonizio LJ. Management of aortopulmonary collaterals in children following cardiac transplantation for complex congenital heart disease. *J Heart Lung Transplant.* 2004 May;23(5):564-9.

[20] Dori Y, Glatz AC, Hanna BD, Gillespie MJ, Harris MA, Keller MS, Fogel MA, Rome JJ, Whitehead KK. Acute effects of embolizing systemic-to-pulmonary arterial collaterals on blood flow in patients with superior cavopulmonary connections: a pilot study. *Circ Cardiovasc Interv.* 2013 Feb;6(1):101-6.

[21] Jayakumar KA, Addonizio LJ, Kichuk-Chrisant MR, Galantowicz ME, Lamour JM, Quaegebeur JM, Hsu DT. Cardiac transplantation after the Fontan or Glenn procedure. *J Am Coll Cardiol.* 2004 Nov 16;44(10):2065-72.

[22] Lamour JM, Kanter KR, Naftel DC, Chrisant MR, Morrow WR, Clemson BS, Kirklin JK; Cardiac Transplant Registry Database; Pediatric Heart Transplant Study. The effect of age, diagnosis, and previous surgery in children and adults undergoing heart transplantation for congenital heart disease. *J Am Coll Cardiol.* 2009 Jul 7;54(2):160-5.

[23] Michielon G, Parisi F, Squitieri C, Carotti A, Gagliardi G, Pasquini L, Di Donato RM. Orthotopic heart transplantation for congenital heart disease: an alternative for high-risk fontan candidates? *Circulation.* 2003 Sep 9;108 Suppl 1:II140-9.

[24] Simpson KE, Pruitt E, Kirklin JK, Naftel DC, Singh RK, Edens RE, Barnes AP, Canter CE. Fontan Patient Survival After Pediatric Heart Transplantation Has Improved in the Current Era. *Ann Thorac Surg.* 2017 Apr;103(4):1315-1320.

[25] Kanter KR. Heart Transplantation in Children after a Fontan Procedure: Better than People Think. *Semin Thorac Cardiovasc Surg Pediatr Card Surg Annu.* 2016;19(1):44-9.

[26] Miller JR, Simpson KE, Epstein DJ, Lancaster TS, Henn MC, Schuessler RB, Balzer DT, Shahanavaz S, Murphy JJ, Canter CE, Eghtesady P, Boston US. Improved survival after heart transplant for failed Fontan patients with preserved ventricular function. *J Heart Lung Transplant.* 2016 Jul;35(7):877-83.

[27] Rossano JW, Cherikh WS, Chambers DC, Goldfarb S, Hayes D Jr, Khush KK, Kucheryavaya AY, Toll AE, Levvey BJ, Meiser B, Stehlik J. The International Thoracic Organ Transplant Registry of the International Society for Heart and Lung Transplantation: Twenty-first pediatric heart transplantation report-2018; Focus

theme: Multiorgan Transplantation. *J Heart Lung Transplant.* 2018 Oct;37(10):1184-1195.

[28] D'Addese L, Joong A, Burch M, Pahl E. Pediatric heart transplantation in the current era. *Curr Opin Pediatr.* 2019 Oct;31(5):583-591.

[29] Reinhardt Z. Paediatric heart transplantation: an update. *Arch Dis Child.* 2019 Dec;104(12):1216-1222.

[30] Colvin MM, Cook JL, Chang P, Francis G, Hsu DT, Kiernan MS, Kobashigawa JA, Lindenfeld J, Masri SC, Miller D, O'Connell J, Rodriguez ER, Rosengard B, Self S, White-Williams C, Zeevi A; American Heart Association Heart Failure and Transplantation Committee of the Council on Clinical Cardiology; American Heart Association Heart Failure and Transplantation Committee of the Council on Cardiopulmonary Critical Care, Perioperative and Resuscitation; American Heart Association Heart Failure and Transplantation Committee of the Council on Cardiovascular Disease in the Young; American Heart Association Heart Failure and Transplantation Committee of the Council on Clinical Cardiology, Council on Cardiovascular and Stroke Nursing; American Heart Association Heart Failure and Transplantation Committee of the Council on Cardiovascular Radiology and Intervention; American Heart Association Heart Failure and Transplantation Committee of the Council on Cardiovascular Surgery and Anesthesia. Antibody-mediated rejection in cardiac transplantation: emerging knowledge in diagnosis and management: a scientific statement from the American Heart Association. *Circulation.* 2015 May 5;131(18):1608-39.

[31] Rossano JW, Singh TP, Cherikh WS, Chambers DC, Harhay MO, Hayes D Jr, Hsich E, Khush KK, Meiser B, Potena L, Toll AE, Sadavarte A, Zuckermann A, Stehlik J; International Society for Heart and Lung Transplantation. The International Thoracic Organ Transplant Registry of the International Society for Heart and Lung Transplantation: Twenty-second pediatric heart transplantation report - 2019; Focus theme: Donor and recipient size match. *J Heart Lung Transplant.* 2019 Oct;38(10):1028-1041.

[32] Webber SA, Naftel DC, Parker J, Mulla N, Balfour I, Kirklin JK, Morrow R; Pediatric Heart Transplant Study Group. Late rejection episodes more than 1 year after pediatric heart transplantation: risk factors and outcomes. *J Heart Lung Transplant.* 2003 Aug;22(8):869-75.

[33] Westbrook TC, Morales DLS, Khan MS, Bryant R, Castleberry C, Chin C, Zafar F. Interaction of older donor age and survival after weight-matched pediatric heart transplantation. *J Heart Lung Transplant.* 2017 May;36(5):554-558.

[34] Kawauchi M, Gundry SR, de Begona JA, Fullerton DA, Razzouk AJ, Boucek MM, Nehlsen-Cannarella S, Bailey LL. Male donor into female recipient increases the risk of pediatric heart allograft rejection. *Ann Thorac Surg.* 1993 Mar;55(3):716-8.

[35] Pahl E, Naftel DC, Canter CE, Frazier EA, Kirklin JK, Morrow WR; Pediatric Heart Transplant Study. Death after rejection with severe hemodynamic compromise in pediatric heart transplant recipients: a multi-institutional study. *J Heart Lung Transplant.* 2001 Mar;20(3):279-87.

[36] Badano LP, Miglioranza MH, Edvardsen T, Colafranceschi AS, Muraru D, Bacal F, Nieman K, Zoppellaro G, Marcondes Braga FG, Binder T, Habib G, Lancellotti P;

Document reviewers. European Association of Cardiovascular Imaging/Cardiovascular Imaging Department of the Brazilian Society of Cardiology recommendations for the use of cardiac imaging to assess and follow patients after heart transplantation. *Eur Heart J Cardiovasc Imaging*. 2015 Sep;16(9):919-48.

[37] Wagner K, Oliver MC, Boyle GJ, Miller SA, Law YM, Pigula F, Webber SA. Endomyocardial biopsy in pediatric heart transplant recipients: a useful exercise? (Analysis of 1,169 biopsies). *Pediatr Transplant*. 2000 Aug;4(3):186-92.

[38] Duong SQ, Zhang Y, Hall M, Hollander SA, Thurm CW, Bernstein D, Feingold B, Godown J, Almond C. Impact of institutional routine surveillance endomyocardial biopsy frequency in the first year on rejection and graft survival in pediatric heart transplantation. *Pediatr Transplant.* 2021 Sep;25(6):e14035.

[39] Zinn MD. Is it time to change the routine for surveillance endomyocardial biopsy after pediatric heart transplantation? *Pediatr Transplant*. 2021 Nov;25(7):e14080.

[40] Stewart S, Winters GL, Fishbein MC, Tazelaar HD, Kobashigawa J, Abrams J, Andersen CB, Angelini A, Berry GJ, Burke MM, Demetris AJ, Hammond E, Itescu S, Marboe CC, McManus B, Reed EF, Reinsmoen NL, Rodriguez ER, Rose AG, Rose M, Suciu-Focia N, Zeevi A, Billingham ME. Revision of the 1990 working formulation for the standardization of nomenclature in the diagnosis of heart rejection. *J Heart Lung Transplant.* 2005 Nov;24(11):1710-20.

[41] Chang DH, Kobashigawa JA. Desensitization strategies in the patient awaiting heart transplantation. *Curr Opin Cardiol*. 2017 May;32(3):301-307.

[42] Asante-Korang A, Amankwah EK, Lopez-Cepero M, Ringewald J, Carapellucci J, Krasnopero D, Berg A, Quintessenza J, Jacobs JP. Outcomes in highly sensitized pediatric heart transplant patients using current management strategies. *J Heart Lung Transplant.* 2015 Feb;34(2):175-81.

[43] Billingham ME. Histopathology of graft coronary disease. *J Heart Lung Transplant.* 1992 May-Jun;11(3 Pt 2):S38-44.

[44] Pahl E, Zales VR, Fricker FJ, Addonizio LJ. Posttransplant coronary artery disease in children. A multicenter national survey. *Circulation*. 1994 Nov;90(5 Pt 2):II56-60. PMID: 7955283.

[45] St Goar FG, Pinto FJ, Alderman EL, Valantine HA, Schroeder JS, Gao SZ, Stinson EB, Popp RL. Intracoronary ultrasound in cardiac transplant recipients. In vivo evidence of "angiographically silent" intimal thickening. *Circulation.* 1992 Mar;85(3):979-87.

[46] Kuhn MA, Jutzy KR, Deming DD, Cephus CE, Chinnock RE, Johnston J, Bailey LL, Larsen RL. The medium-term findings in coronary arteries by intravascular ultrasound in infants and children after heart transplantation. *J Am Coll Cardiol.* 2000 Jul;36(1):250-4

[47] Dent CL, Canter CE, Hirsch R, Balzer DT. Transplant coronary artery disease in pediatric heart transplant recipients. *J Heart Lung Transplant.* 2000 Mar;19(3):240-8.

[48] Schratz LM, Meyer RA, Schwartz DC. Serial intracoronary ultrasound in children: feasibility, reproducibility, limitations, and safety. *J Am Soc Echocardiogr*. 2002 Aug;15(8):782-90.

[49] Costello JM, Wax DF, Binns HJ, Backer CL, Mavroudis C, Pahl E. A comparison of intravascular ultrasound with coronary angiography for evaluation of transplant coronary disease in pediatric heart transplant recipients. *J Heart Lung Transplant.* 2003 Jan;22(1):44-9.
[50] Pahl E, Naftel DC, Kuhn MA, Shaddy RE, Morrow WR, Canter CE, Kirklin J; Pediatric Heart Transplant Study. The impact and outcome of transplant coronary artery disease in a pediatric population: a 9-year multi-institutional study. *J Heart Lung Transplant.* 2005 Jun;24(6):645-51.
[51] Auerbach SR, Fenton MJ, Grutter G, Albert DC, Di-Filippo S, Burch M, Kuhn MA. The complication rate of intravascular ultrasound (IVUS) in a multicenter pediatric heart transplant population: A study of the international pediatric IVUS consortium. *Clin Transplant.* 2020 Sep;34(9):e13981.
[52] Knackstedt ED, Danziger-Isakov L. Infections in pediatric solid-organ transplant recipients. *Semin Pediatr Surg.* 2017 Aug;26(4):199-205.
[53] Towbin JA, Ware SM, Jefferies JL. Heart transplants in pediatric patients: viral infection as a loss predictor. *Future Cardiol.* 2010 Nov;6(6):735-41.
[54] Rostad CA, Wehrheim K, Kirklin JK, Naftel D, Pruitt E, Hoffman TM, L'Ecuyer T, Berkowitz K, Mahle WT, Scheel JN. Bacterial infections after pediatric heart transplantation: Epidemiology, risk factors and outcomes. *J Heart Lung Transplant.* 2017 Sep;36(9):996-1003.
[55] Keough WL, Michaels MG. Infectious complications in pediatric solid organ transplantation. *Pediatr Clin North Am.* 2003 Dec;50(6):1451-69, x.
[56] Green M, Michaels MG. Infections in Pediatric Solid Organ Transplant Recipients. *J Pediatric Infect Dis Soc.* 2012 Jun;1(2):144-51.
[57] Fishman JA. Infection in solid-organ transplant recipients. *N Engl J Med.* 2007 Dec 20;357(25):2601-14.
[58] Das BB, Prusty BK, Niu J, Sue PK. Cytomegalovirus infection and allograft rejection among pediatric heart transplant recipients in the era of valganciclovir prophylaxis. *Pediatr Transplant.* 2020 Dec;24(8):e13750.
[59] Paya C, Humar A, Dominguez E, Washburn K, Blumberg E, Alexander B, Freeman R, Heaton N, Pescovitz MD; Valganciclovir Solid Organ Transplant Study Group. Efficacy and safety of valganciclovir vs. oral ganciclovir for prevention of cytomegalovirus disease in solid organ transplant recipients. *Am J Transplant.* 2004 Apr;4(4):611-20.
[60] Koskinen PK, Nieminen MS, Krogerus LA, Lemström KB, Mattila SP, Häyry PJ, Lautenschlager IT. Cytomegalovirus infection and accelerated cardiac allograft vasculopathy in human cardiac allografts. *J Heart Lung Transplant.* 1993 Sep-Oct;12(5):724-9.
[61] Kotton CN, Kumar D, Caliendo AM, Huprikar S, Chou S, Danziger-Isakov L, Humar A; The Transplantation Society International CMV Consensus Group. The Third International Consensus Guidelines on the Management of Cytomegalovirus in Solid-organ Transplantation. *Transplantation.* 2018 Jun;102(6):900-931.
[62] Webber SA, Naftel DC, Fricker FJ, Olesnevich P, Blume ED, Addonizio L, Kirklin JK, Canter CE; Pediatric Heart Transplant Study. Lymphoproliferative disorders

after paediatric heart transplantation: a multi-institutional study. *Lancet.* 2006 Jan 21;367(9506):233-9.

[63] Allen UD, Preiksaitis JK; AST Infectious Diseases Community of Practice. Post-transplant lymphoproliferative disorders, Epstein-Barr virus infection, and disease in solid organ transplantation: Guidelines from the American Society of Transplantation Infectious Diseases Community of Practice. *Clin Transplant.* 2019 Sep;33(9):e13652.

[64] Stubbins RJ, Alami Laroussi N, Peters AC, Urschel S, Dicke F, Lai RL, Zhu J, Mabilangan C, Preiksaitis JK. Epstein-Barr virus associated smooth muscle tumors in solid organ transplant recipients: Incidence over 31 years at a single institution and review of the literature. *Transpl Infect Dis.* 2019 Feb;21(1):e13010.

[65] Danziger-Isakov L, Kumar D; AST ID Community of Practice. Vaccination of solid organ transplant candidates and recipients: Guidelines from the American society of transplantation infectious diseases community of practice. *Clin Transplant.* 2019 Sep;33(9):e13563.

[66] Law YM, Yim R, Agatisa P, Boyle GJ, Miller SA, Lawrence K, Webber SA. Lipid profiles in pediatric thoracic transplant recipients are determined by their immunosuppressive regimens. *J Heart Lung Transplant.* 2006 Mar;25(3):276-82.

[67] Walker RW, Brochstein JA. Neurologic complications of immunosuppressive agents. *Neurol Clin.* 1988 May;6(2):261-78.

[68] Singh TP, Cherikh WS, Hsich E, Chambers DC, Harhay MO, Hayes D Jr, Khush KK, Perch M, Potena L, Sadavarte A, Toll AE, Zuckermann A, Stehlik J; International Society for Heart and Lung Transplantation. The International Thoracic Organ Transplant Registry of the International Society for Heart and Lung Transplantation: Twenty-fourth pediatric heart transplantation report - 2021; focus on recipient characteristics. *J Heart Lung Transplant.* 2021 Oct;40(10):1050-1059.

[69] Nytrøen K, Gullestad L. Exercise after heart transplantation: An overview. *World J Transplant.* 2013 Dec 24;3(4):78-90.

[70] Hsu DT, Garofano RP, Douglas JM, Michler RE, Quaegebeur JM, Gersony WM, Addonizio LJ. Exercise performance after pediatric heart transplantation. *Circulation.* 1993 Nov;88(5 Pt 2):II238-42.

[71] Uzark KC, Sauer SN, Lawrence KS, Miller J, Addonizio L, Crowley DC. The psychosocial impact of pediatric heart transplantation. *J Heart Lung Transplant.* 1992 Nov-Dec;11(6):1160-7.

[72] Wray J, Pot-Mees C, Zeitlin H, Radley-Smith R, Yacoub M. Cognitive function and behavioural status in paediatric heart and heart-lung transplant recipients: the Harefield experience. *BMJ.* 1994 Oct 1;309(6958):837-41.

[73] Wray J, Long T, Radley-Smith R, Yacoub M. Returning to school after heart or heart-lung transplantation: how well do children adjust? *Transplantation.* 2001 Jul 15;72(1):100-6.

[74] Garcia Guerra G, Bond GY, Joffe AR, Dinu IA, Hajihosseini M, Al-Aklabi M, Robertson CMT, Urschel S; Western Canadian Complex Pediatric Therapies Follow-up Program. Health-related quality of life after pediatric heart transplantation in early childhood. *Pediatr Transplant.* 2020 Nov;24(7):e13822.

[75] Mintzer LL, Stuber ML, Seacord D, Castaneda M, Mesrkhani V, Glover D. Traumatic stress symptoms in adolescent organ transplant recipients. *Pediatrics.* 2005 Jun;115(6):1640-4.

[76] Green A, Meaux J, Huett A, Ainley K. "It has its ups and downs": adolescents' quality of life after heart transplantation *Prog Transplant* 2011 Jun;21(2):115-20.

Chapter 16

Heart Transplantation in Chagas Cardiomyopathy

Carlos Vigliano[1,*] and Liliana Favaloro[2]
[1]Pathology Department, Favaloro Foundation University Hospital, Buenos Aires, Argentina
[2]Heart Failure and Heart Transplantation, Favaloro Foundation University Hospital, Buenos Aires, Argentina

Abstract

Heart transplantation modifies the natural history of end-stage chronic Chagas cardiomyopathy and is currently established as a valuable therapeutic option.

Patients with Chagas disease and heart transplantation require close and multidisciplinary follow-up, since reactivation can occur after heart transplantation. The most frequent clinical manifestations of reactivation are fever, panniculitis and myocarditis. In order to prevent reactivation after heart transplantation, it is recommended to reduce the immunosuppression regimen by avoiding induction and the use of mycophenolate mofetil, as well as early reduction or suspension of steroids.

Only blood or tissue parasitological methods have diagnostic value for reactivation. Positive PCR results anticipate the Strout test and the clinical manifestations of reactivation. When it occurs, Benznidazole is the safest and most effective treatment.

Heart transplantation is a safe and effective treatment in patients with Chagas cardiomyopathy, since it is associated with a survival

* Corresponding Author's E-mail: cavigliano@ffavaloro.org.

In: Heart Transplantation
Editor: Elian Facundo Giordanino
ISBN: 978-1-68507-759-4

similar to those transplanted for other causes, and reactivation of the disease is not associated with higher mortality.

Keywords: Chagas cardiomyopathy, heart transplantation, latent infection, polymerase chain reaction, Benznidazole

Introduction

Chagas disease or American trypanosomiasis is a parasitic zoonosis, endemic in 21 Latin-America's countries, constituting a serious public health problem. It is caused by the protozoan *Trypanosoma cruzi* and transmitted by infected Triatominae insects [1].

Chagas disease has spread from rural to urban areas, and from endemic to non-endemic regions [2]. In fact, it is estimated that between six and eight million people are infected with *T. cruzi*, and another 65 million are at risk of acquiring the disease through vector-borne transmission, blood or congenital transmission, infected organ donors or food-borne transmission [3].

The incidence of Chagas disease in the Americas has been substantially reduced through efforts in vector control and systematic blood screening. The estimated number of new cases has decreased by 32%, from 41,000 in 2006 to 28,000 in 2010, and the mortality from 45,000 deaths per year to the current 12,000 [4].

Phases of Chagas Disease and Clinical Evolution

Three phases are described in the course of the disease: acute, indeterminate and chronic. The acute phase of *T. cruzi* infection lasts 6 to 8 weeks. Longitudinal studies reveal that between 20 to 30% of those infected patients progress to the chronic phase of the disease. The chronic phase is characterized mainly by neurological, gastrointestinal and cardiac involvement, with the latter being the most frequent clinical manifestation. Cardiac compromise has been linked to ventricular arrhythmias, conduction disorders, embolisms, formation of apical or posterobasal ventricular aneurysms, and progression to dilated cardiomyopathy with severe heart failure, which has the greatest impact on morbidity and mortality [5]. Although the pathogenesis of chronic Chagas disease is not yet fully understood, evidence indicates that inflammatory processes related to parasite persistence and immunological response are the main effectors of cardiac tissue damage [6, 7].

Chagasic heart disease represents a model of cardiac remodeling different from that of other human cardiomyopathies, since the presence of a causal infectious agent is observed in the lesions with the persistence of an inflammatory cardiac infiltrate for years [8]. These lead to cardiac remodeling and heart failure, with a histopathological substrate of cell death, fibrosis, and hypertrophy that characterize chronic Chagas cardiomyopathy [9].

The eradication of the parasite in the organism using antiparasitic drugs could have a role in selected patients, especially newly infected children, women of childbearing age for the prevention of vertical transmission of *T. cruzi* infection, and adults in the early stages of infection [10-13].

There have been a number of studies evaluating pharmacological treatment of heart failure in patients with chronic Chagas cardiomyopathy [14]. Antiarrhythmic therapy is based on limited observational data and extrapolated from results for other etiologies, and implantable cardioverter-defibrillators are indicated for the prevention of sudden cardiac death [15, 16].

Chagas disease was formerly considered a potential contraindication for heart transplantation due to the risk of reactivation with immunosuppression; however, heart transplantation is currently established as a valuable therapeutic option in end-stage heart failure secondary to Chagas cardiomyopathy and it is becoming an increasingly frequent indication, especially in Latin America [17, 18].

Heart Transplantation as Treatment for Chagasic Cardiomyopathy

Organ transplantation in patients with chronic Chagas disease and the use of organs from infected donors has been a topic of debate for many years [19]. The increasing number of infected people now living in non-endemic regions has increased the possibility that they might become transplant candidates or organ donors [20, 21]. In Argentina, data from the Instituto Nacional Central Único Coordinador de Ablación e Implante (INCUCAI) showed that 9% of all heart candidates on the waiting list were infected (data not published).

It should be noted that Chagas disease is an important cause of end-stage dilated cardiomyopathy in Latin America. Furthermore, Chagas cardiomyopathy is an independent predictor of mortality in patients with advanced heart failure compared to other etiologies [22-24].

The first heart transplant for a recipient with Chagas cardiomyopathy was performed in 1985 in Brazil [25]. The first data were published by Bocchi and Fiorelli in 2001, with an experience of 117 recipients with Chagas cardiomyopathy of 720 heart transplants in Brazil. The authors reported a survival of 71% and 57% at one and four years, respectively, slightly higher than that of heart transplant recipients from other causes [26]. Furthermore, a good response to 30-60 days of treatment with benznidazole has been described for reactivation episodes, with adequate graft and patient survival after long-term follow-up. Mortality related to Chagas disease reactivation has been reported to be 0.3%, and the survival rates are no different from those of other heart transplant recipients [26, 27].

Currently, heart transplantation is established as an effective and safe therapeutic option in those patients who evolve with progressive Chagas cardiomyopathy and advanced heart failure [18, 28, 29]. Over time, this condition has become the third leading cause of heart transplantation in Brazil and Argentina [18, 30].

Donors with *Trypanosoma Cruzi* Infection

Donor-derived transmission of *Trypanosoma cruzi* has emerged as a problem in non-endemic regions in recent years. Programs may consider transplantation of kidneys and livers from *T. cruzi*-infected donors with informed consent from recipients but heart transplantation from infected donors is not recommended [20].

In endemic regions, Chagas serology is performed at the time of ablation by enzyme-linked immunosorbent assay (ELISA), indirect hemagglutination assay (IHA), and immunofluorescence test (IFT). Serologic tests are quick and easy to perform and are widely available; therefore, this does not cause delays in the distribution of organs. Some of the recommendations for pre-transplant evaluation and post-transplant follow-up in heart transplant recipients with Chagas disease are summarized in the multidisciplinary Argentine Consensus on Transplantation in Chagas Disease, published in 2010, which is based on the experience accumulated in different centers in Argentina [31].

Reactivation Diagnosis

Since Chagas disease is a chronic infection, it was long considered a potential contraindication for transplantation due to the risk of infection reactivation with immunosuppression. For patients undergoing heart transplantation, a structured clinical and laboratory monitoring protocol is necessary to detect *T. cruzi* reactivation. In our center, Strout and PCR tests are performed on each endomyocardial biopsy, and patients are examined for clinical manifestations of reactivation (See Chapter 14).

The diagnosis of Chagas reactivation is made by detecting the parasite in blood or tissues, since serology lacks diagnostic value to confirm reactivation. A follow-up strategy with specific diagnostic methods that anticipate the onset of symptoms is essential, because if reactivation is treated early and adequately, it has a relatively benign clinical course. In addition, the patient should be instructed to be aware of the appearance of skin lesions in order to quickly inform the treating medical team.

Reactivation has been reported to occur in 20% to 61% of patients [28, 32-34]. In a study by Campos et al, multivariate analysis showed that number of rejection episodes, neoplasms, and the use of mycophenolate mofetil were independent determinants for reactivation after transplantation (Table 1) [35]. In addition, reactivation can be completely asymptomatic, and be diagnosed solely by the detection of parasitemia.

When clinical manifestations appear, there are signs of subcutaneous involvement -reminiscent of erythema nodosum- and panniculitis, with tenderness and characteristic limb involvement. Tissue samples should always be obtained from suspicious lesions. Skin and subcutaneous tissue biopsies show a nonspecific inflammatory infiltrate and numerous nests of amastigote (Figure 1). Myocardial reactivation may correspond to a focal or diffuse location. Symptoms are usually overlapping with those of acute graft rejection, and include dyspnea, fatigue, peripheral edema and/or palpitations. Acute myocarditis is characterized by an intense inflammatory infiltrate, consisting of mononuclear and polymorphonuclear cells, edema and numerous amastigote nests in cardiomyocytes.

Differential diagnosis with acute cellular graft rejection may be challenging in this situation, as both present with inflammatory infiltrates. However, the presence of multiple amastigote nests in the case of Chagas reactivation allows the correct diagnosis to be established (Figure 2) [36].

Table 1. Diagnosis of reactivation and / or primary infection by *T. cruzi.*

Risk factors for reactivation	• High Level of Immunosuppression • High Number of Rejections • Methylprednisolone Pulses • Mycophenolate mofetil
Parasitological diagnosis	• PCR (DNA) • Strout
Clinical diagnosis	• Fever • Panniculitis • Myocarditis • Encephalitis
Treatment	• Benznidazole 5 mg/kg/day (30-60 days) • Nifurtimox 8-10mg/kg/day (90 Days)
Follow-up	• Clinical • Strout • PCR (DNA)

PCR, Polymerase chain reaction. (Data from Campos SV et al. Risk factors for Chagas' disease reactivation after heart transplantation. J Heart Lung Transplant. 2008 Jun;27(6):597-602 and Diez M et al. Usefulness of PCR strategies for early diagnosis of Chagas' disease reactivation and treatment follow-up in heart transplantation. *Am J Transplant.* 2007 Jun;7(6):1633-40.)

Monitoring for *T. cruzi* reactivation is recommended so that treatment can be initiated before the development of clinically significant disease. Polymerase chain reaction (PCR) of blood and tissue fragments has become a very important tool for detecting early infection, showing positive results days to weeks before circulating trypomastigotes are detected by the Strout method [37].

The available tissue samples (skin biopsy in case of panniculitis, or endomyocardial biopsies as part of heart transplant follow-up) should be evaluated to determine the presence of amastigote nests. Myocarditis can present with or without symptoms of heart failure. In fact, when it is detected, it is usually a finding of routine endomyocardial biopsies.

Regarding molecular diagnosis, parasite DNA can be detected by PCR techniques [38]. The PCR products are electrophoresed in 2% agarose gels and stained with ethidium bromide and are then analyzed on a UV transilluminator. Blood collection, sample DNA purification, assembly of reagent mixtures, cycling, and gel electrophoresis procedures should be performed in separate laboratory working areas to avoid contamination by amplicon carryover [29].

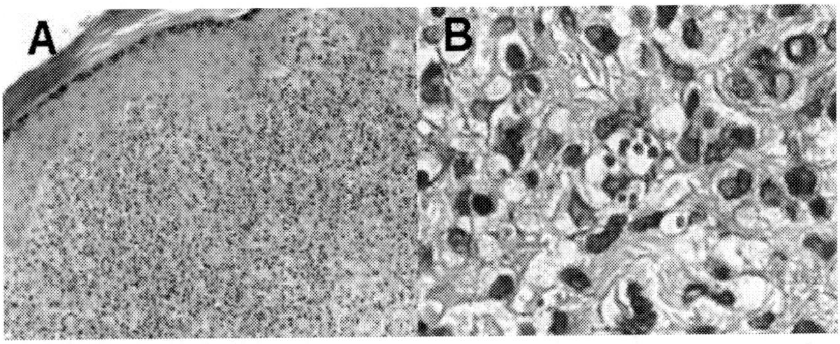

Figure 1. Skin biopsy of a nodular lesion (*"chagoma"*). A. Nonspecific inflammatory infiltrate. B. Nests of amastigote.

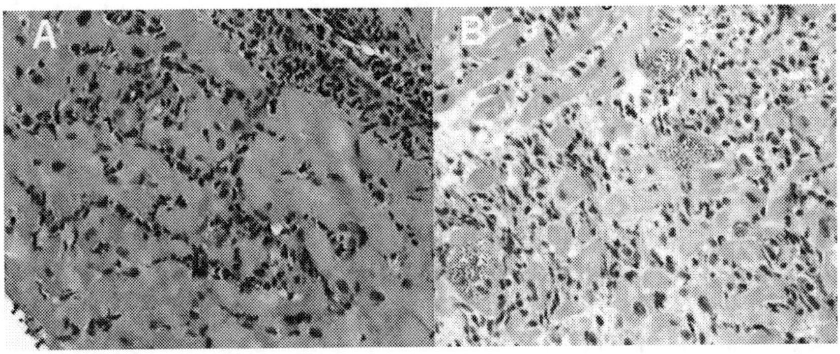

Figure 2. Differential diagnosis between acute cellular rejection and Chagas reactivation. A. Acute cellular rejection grade 2R with inflammatory infiltrates. B. Myocarditis due to Chagas reactivation, with inflammatory infiltrates and multiples amastigote nests.

Analysis of Heart Explants

Analysis of cardiac explant samples provides additional evidence of the involvement of parasite persistence in the pathogenesis of myocarditis and chronic Chagas heart disease, in agreement with other immunochemical and molecular studies [39-44]. Genetic characterization of parasite populations involved in reactivation may shed more light on the role of parasitic factors in this phenomenon. *T. cruzi* strains cluster into 6 discrete typing units associated with different geographical distribution, transmission cycles and varying disease symptoms. In the southern cone of South America, a study by Burgos et al., revealed that *T. cruzi* II, V, and VI populations appear to be associated with Chagas disease and *T. cruzi* I to sylvatic cycles. Multiple discrete typing units may coexist in patients with Chagas disease, and *T. cruzi* I is frequently associated with cardiac damage in heart explants, revealing its possible pathogenic role in chronic Chagas heart disease in this location [41]. In our experience, reactivation was associated with myocarditis severity and parasite persistence in explanted heart samples [42]. In fact, cardiac explant samples with detectable nests (*T. cruzi* Id and *T. cruzi* VI) and with higher proportion of PCR-positive sections belonged to patients who experienced reactivation of Chagas disease.

Post-Transplant Follow-Up and Immunosuppressive Treatment

After heart transplantation in a recipient with Chagas disease, immunosuppressive treatment with steroids, calcineurin inhibitors (tacrolimus or cyclosporine) and antiproliferatives is started. Regarding the latter, azathioprine is preferred over mycophenolate mofetil, as a higher incidence of reactivation has been reported in patients receiving mycophenolate mofetil compared to those receiving azathioprine (Table 2) [45]. Prophylactic benznidazole is not indicated.

The follow-up of these patients focuses on detecting the reactivation of Chagas disease. Blood samples are collected at the time of each endomyocardial biopsy for Strout and PCR analysis. For pathology examination and parasitological diagnosis, samples from endomyocardial biopsies are fixed in 10% buffered formaldehyde and embedded in Histowax and 4 to 5 μm sections are stained with hematoxylin-eosin, Masson trichrome and Giemsa for amastigote nests detection. Chagasic myocarditis is defined by the presence of active myocarditis and *T. cruzi* parasite nests present within cardiomyocytes.

Reactivation episodes should be treated with benznidazole 5 mg per kilogram per day for 60 days. As an alternative therapy in cases of intolerance, nifurtimox can be used. Taking into account the good response to trypanocidal treatment, it is recommended to maintain a level of immunosuppression as low as possible, but without putting the patient at risk of acute graft rejection.

Table 2. Scheme and dose of immunosuppressive treatment.

Months	**1-3**	**3-6**	**6-9**	**9-12**	**>12**
Ciclosporine	250-300ng/ml	250ng/ml	200-150ng/ml		100ng/ml
Prednisone	0.5-1mg/kg/d	0.25-.5mg/kg/d	0.15-0.25mg/kg/d		0-0.15mg/kg/d
Tacrolimus	15 ng/ml		10 ng/ml		
Azathioprine	1.5-2 mg/kg/d				
Mycophenolate Mofetil	2 gr/d				
Everolimus	3-8 ng/ml				
Sirolimus	5-10 ng/ml				

Ciclosporine, Tacrolimus, Everolimus and Sirolimus values correspond to the plasma concentration of these drugs. (Data from Cochrane AB et al. 2nd. Report from the 2018 consensus conference on immunomodulating agents in thoracic transplantation: Access, formulations, generics, therapeutic drug monitoring, and special populations. *J. Heart Lung Transplant*. 2020 Oct;39(10):1050-1069.)

The diagnosis of graft rejection is made based on clinical and echocardiographic suspicion and confirmed by endomyocardial biopsy as with any other heart transplant recipient [46, 47]. Treatment of acute rejection is also similar, with methylprednisolone in isolated cellular rejection and associated with plasmapheresis, anti-thymocyte globulin, and immunoglobulin in antibody-mediated or mixed rejection (See Chapter 11).

Cardiac allograft vasculopathy is screened annually with coronary angiography and endovascular ultrasound as usually recommended [48].

In general, there is no difference in the survival of heart transplant patients due to Chagas cardiomyopathy compared to those transplanted for other causes, nor between the patients who reactivated Chagas disease and those who did not [49].

Conclusion

Over the decades, our institutional experience continues to support that heart transplantation is a safe and effective treatment in patients with Chagas cardiomyopathy, since it is associated with a survival similar to those transplanted for other causes.

Although the reactivation of *Trypanosoma Cruzi* infection is a frequent complication, currently available therapies, implemented in a timely manner, have shown a favorable evolution in the follow-up of these patients, without impact on their prognosis.

References

[1] Monteiro F A, Weirauch C, Felix M, Lazoski C, Abad-Franch F. Evolution, Systematics, and Biogeography of the Triatominae, Vectors of Chagas Disease. *Adv. Parasitol.* 2018;99:265-344.

[2] Gascon J, Bern C, Pinazo M J. Chagas disease in Spain, the United States and other non-endemic countries. *Acta Trop*. 2010 Jul-Aug;115(1-2):22-7.

[3] Chagas disease in Latin America: an epidemiological update based on 2010 estimates. *Wkly Epidemiol. Rec.* 2015 Feb 6;90(6):33-43.

[4] Pan American Health Organization, *Guidelines for the diagnosis and treatment of Chagas disease [online].* 2019 [cited 2022-Jan-20]. Available from: https://iris.paho.org/bitstream/handle/10665.2/49653/9789275120439_eng.pdf

[5] Prata A. Clinical and epidemiological aspects of Chagas disease. *Lancet Infect. Dis.* 2001 Sep;1(2):92-100.

[6] Zhang L, Tarleton R L. Parasite persistence correlates with disease severity and localization in chronic Chagas' disease. *J. Infect. Dis*. 1999 Aug;180(2):480-6.

[7] Rassi A Jr, Rassi A, Marin-Neto J A. Chagas disease. *Lancet.* 2010 Apr 17;375(9723):1388-402.

[8] Laguens R P, Cabeza Meckert P M, Vigliano C. Patogenia, In Viotti R, Vigliano C. Enfermedad de Chagas. Un enfoque práctico basado en la investigación médica. [*Pathogeny, In Chagas disease. A practical approach based on medical research*] Buenos Aires: Panamericana, 2015, 81-102.

[9] Chao C, Leone J L, Vigliano C A. Chagas disease: Historic perspective. *Biochim. Biophys. Acta Mol. Basis Dis.* 2020 May 1;1866(5):165689.

[10] de Andrade A L, Zicker F, de Oliveira R M, Almeida Silva S, Luquetti A, Travassos LR, Almeida IC, de Andrade SS, de Andrade J G, Martelli C M. Randomised trial of efficacy of benznidazole in treatment of early Trypanosoma cruzi infection. *Lancet.* 1996 Nov 23;348(9039):1407-13.

[11] Fabbro D L, Danesi E, Olivera V, Codebó M O, Denner S, Heredia C, Streiger M, Sosa-Estani S. Trypanocide treatment of women infected with Trypanosoma cruzi and its effect on preventing congenital Chagas. *PLoS Negl. Trop. Dis*. 2014 Nov 20;8(11):e3312.

[12] Álvarez M G, Vigliano C, Lococo B, Bertocchi G, Viotti R. Prevention of congenital Chagas disease by Benznidazole treatment in reproductive-age women. An observational study. *Acta Trop.* 2017 Oct;174:149-152.

[13] Viotti R, Vigliano C, Lococo B, Bertocchi G, Petti M, Alvarez M G, Postan M, Armenti A. Long-term cardiac outcomes of treating chronic Chagas disease with benznidazole versus no treatment: a nonrandomized trial. *Ann. Intern. Med.* 2006 May 16;144(10):724-34.

[14] Bocchi E A, Bestetti R B, Scanavacca M I, Cunha Neto E, Issa V S. Chronic Chagas Heart Disease Management: From Etiology to Cardiomyopathy Treatment. *J. Am. Coll. Cardiol.* 2017 Sep 19;70(12):1510-1524.

[15] Malik L H, Singh G D, Amsterdam E A. The Epidemiology, Clinical Manifestations, and Management of Chagas Heart Disease. *Clin. Cardiol.* 2015 Sep;38(9):565-9.

[16] Romero J, Velasco A, Pisani C F, Alviz I, Briceno D, Díaz J C, Della Rocca D G, Natale A, de Lourdes Higuchi M, Scanavacca M, Di Biase L. Advanced Therapies for Ventricular Arrhythmias in Patients With Chagasic Cardiomyopathy: JACC State-of-the-Art Review. *J. Am. Coll. Cardiol.* 2021 Mar 9;77(9):1225-1242.

[17] Kirchhoff L V. American trypanosomiasis (Chagas' disease)--a tropical disease now in the United States. *N. Engl. J. Med.* 1993 Aug 26;329(9):639-44.

[18] Benatti R D, Oliveira G H, Bacal F. Heart Transplantation for Chagas Cardiomyopathy. *J. Heart Lung Transplant.* 2017 Jun;36(6):597-603.

[19] Cura C I, Lattes R, Nagel C, Gimenez M J, Blanes M, Calabuig E, Iranzo A, Barcan LA, Anders M, Schijman AG. Early molecular diagnosis of acute Chagas disease after transplantation with organs from *Trypanosoma cruzi*-infected donors. *Am. J. Transplant.* 2013 Dec;13(12):3253-61.

[20] Chin-Hong P V, Schwartz B S, Bern C, Montgomery S P, Kontak S, Kubak B, Morris M I, Nowicki M, Wright C, Ison M G. Screening and treatment of chagas disease in organ transplant recipients in the United States: recommendations from the chagas in transplant working group. *Am. J. Transplant*. 2011 Apr;11(4):672-80.

[21] Salvador F, Sánchez-Montalvá A, Sulleiro E, Moreso F, Berastegui C, Caralt M, Pinazo MJ, Moure Z, Los-Arcos I, Len O, Gavaldà J, Molina I. Prevalence of Chagas Disease among Solid Organ-Transplanted Patients in a Nonendemic Country. *Am. J. Trop. Med. Hyg.* 2018 Mar;98(3):742-746.

[22] Bertolino N D, Villafanha D F, Cardinalli-Neto A, Cordeiro J A, Arcanjo M J, Theodoropoulos T A, Bestetti R B. Prognostic impact of Chagas' disease in patients awaiting heart transplantation. *J. Heart Lung Transplant.* 2010 Apr;29(4):449-53.

[23] Pereira Nunes Mdo C, Barbosa M M, Ribeiro A L, Amorim Fenelon L M, Rocha MO. Predictors of mortality in patients with dilated cardiomyopathy: relevance of Chagas disease as an etiological factor. *Rev. Esp. Cardiol.* 2010 Jul;63(7):788-97.

[24] Ciapponi A, Alcaraz A, Calderón M, Matta M G, Chaparro M, Soto N, Bardach A. Burden of Heart Failure in Latin America: A Systematic Review and Meta-analysis. *Rev. Esp. Cardiol. (Engl Ed).* 2016 Nov;69(11):1051-1060.

[25] Stolf N A, Higushi L, Bocchi E, Bellotti G, Auler J O, Uip D, Amato Neto V, Pileggi F, Jatene A D. Heart transplantation in patients with Chagas' disease cardiomyopathy. *J. Heart Transplant.* 1987;6:307-12.

[26] Bocchi E A, Fiorelli A. The paradox of survival results after heart transplantation for cardiomyopathy caused by Trypanosoma cruzi. First Guidelines Group for Heart

Transplantation of the Brazilian Society of Cardiology. *Ann. Thorac. Surg.* 2001;71:1833–1838.

[27] Fiorelli A I, Stolf N A, Honorato R, Bocchi E, Bacal F, Uip D, Strabelli T, Issa V, Amato V A, Fiorelli L R, Oliveira S A. Later evolution after cardiac transplantation in Chagas' disease. *Transplant. Proc.* 2005 Jul-Aug;37(6):2793-8.

[28] Diez M, Favaloro L, Bertolotti A, Burgos J M, Vigliano C, Lastra M P, Levin M J, Arnedo A, Nagel C, Schijman A G, Favaloro RR. Usefulness of PCR strategies for early diagnosis of Chagas' disease reactivation and treatment follow-up in heart transplantation. *Am. J. Transplant.* 2007 Jun;7(6):1633-40.

[29] Favaloro L, Peradejordi Lastra M, Nagel C. Enfermedad de Chagas y trasplante de órganos, In Viotti R, Vigliano C. Enfermedad de Chagas. Un enfoque práctico basado en la investigación médica. [*Chagas disease and organ transplant, In Chagas disease. A practical approach based on medical research*] Buenos Aires: Panamericana, 2015, 303-320.

[30] Peradejordi Lastras M A, Favaloro L E, Vigliano C, Renedo M F, Martínez L, Moscoloni SE, Abud J, Absi DO, Favaloro RR, Bertolotti AM. Outcomes of Heart Transplantation Based on Recipient's Clinical Profile: 21-Year Experience. *Rev. Argent. Cardiol.* 2016 Jun;84(3):235-241

[31] Chagas' Disease Argentine Collaborative Transplant Consortium, Casadei D. Chagas' disease and solid organ transplantation. *Transplant. Proc.* 2010 Nov;42(9):3354-9.

[32] Bestetti R B, Theodoropoulos T A. A systematic review of studies on heart transplantation for patients with end-stage Chagas' heart disease. *J. Card. Fail.* 2009 Apr;15(3):249-55.

[33] Fiorelli A I, Santos R H, Oliveira J L Jr, Lourenço-Filho D D, Dias R R, Oliveira AS, da Silva MF, Ayoub FL, Bacal F, Souza GE, Bocchi EA, Stolf NA. Heart transplantation in 107 cases of Chagas' disease. *Transplant. Proc.* 2011 Jan-Feb;43(1):220-4.

[34] Gray E B, La Hoz R M, Green J S, Vikram H R, Benedict T, Rivera H, Montgomery SP. Reactivation of Chagas disease among heart transplant recipients in the United States, 2012-2016. *Transpl. Infect. Dis.* 2018 Dec;20(6):e12996.

[35] Campos S V, Strabelli T M, Amato Neto V, Silva C P, Bacal F, Bocchi E A, Stolf NA. Risk factors for Chagas' disease reactivation after heart transplantation. *J. Heart Lung Transplant.* 2008 Jun;27(6):597-602.

[36] Vigliano C A, González P H, Viotti R J Pathology of cardiac complications and reactivation, In Viotti R, Vigliano C. Enfermedad de Chagas. Un enfoque práctico basado en la investigación médica. [*Chagas disease and organ transplant, In Chagas disease. A practical approach based on medical research*] Buenos Aires: Panamericana, 2015, 209-222.

[37] Strout R G. A method for concentrating hemoflagellates. *J. Parasitol.* 1962 Feb;48:100.

[38] Schijman A G, Vigliano C, Burgos J, Favaloro R, Perrone S, Laguens R, Levin M J. Early diagnosis of recurrence of Trypanosoma cruzi infection by polymerase chain reaction after heart transplantation of a chronic Chagas' heart disease patient. *J. Heart Lung Transplant.* 2000 Nov;19(11):1114-7.

[39] Edwards W D, Tajik A J, Seward J B. Standardized nomenclature and anatomic basis for regional tomographic analysis of the heart. *Mayo Clin. Proc.* 1981 Aug;56(8):479-97.

[40] Brandariz S, Schijman A, Vigliano C, Arteman P, Viotti R, Beldjord C, Levin M J. Detection of parasite DNA in Chagas' heart disease. *Lancet.* 1995 Nov 18;346(8986):1370-1.

[41] Burgos J M, Diez M, Vigliano C, Bisio M, Risso M, Duffy T, Cura C, Brusses B, Favaloro L, Leguizamon M S, Lucero R H, Laguens R, Levin M J, Favaloro R, Schijman A G. Molecular identification of Trypanosoma cruzi discrete typing units in end-stage chronic Chagas heart disease and reactivation after heart transplantation. *Clin. Infect. Dis.* 2010 Sep 1;51(5):485-95.

[42] Schijman A G, Vigliano C A, Viotti R J, Burgos J M, Brandariz S, Lococo B E, Leze M I, Armenti H A, Levin M J. Trypanosoma cruzi DNA in cardiac lesions of Argentinean patients with end-stage chronic Chagas heart disease. *Am. J. Trop. Med. Hyg.* 2004 Feb;70(2):210-20.

[43] Benvenuti L A, Roggério A, Freitas H F, Mansur A J, Fiorelli A, Higuchi M L. Chronic American trypanosomiasis: parasite persistence in endomyocardial biopsies is associated with high-grade myocarditis. *Ann. Trop. Med. Parasitol.* 2008 Sep; 102(6):481-7.

[44] Eberhardt N, Sanmarco L M, Bergero G, Favaloro R R, Vigliano C, Aoki M P. HIF-1α and CD73 expression in cardiac leukocytes correlates with the severity of myocarditis in end-stage Chagas disease patients. *J. Leukoc. Biol.* 2021 Jan;109(1):233-244.

[45] Bacal F, Silva C P, Bocchi E A, Pires P V, Moreira L F, Issa V S, Moreira S A, das Dores Cruz F, Strabelli T, Stolf N A, Ramires J A. Mychophenolate mofetil increased chagas disease reactivation in heart transplanted patients: comparison between two different protocols. *Am. J. Transplant.* 2005 Aug;5(8):2017-21.

[46] Stewart S, Winters G L, Fishbein M C, Tazelaar H D, Kobashigawa J, Abrams J, Andersen C B, Angelini A, Berry G J, Burke M M, Demetris A J, Hammond E, Itescu S, Marboe C C, McManus B, Reed E F, Reinsmoen N L, Rodriguez E R, Rose A G, Rose M, Suciu-Focia N, Zeevi A, Billingham M E. Revision of the 1990 working formulation for the standardization of nomenclature in the diagnosis of heart rejection. *J. Heart Lung Transplant.* 2005 Nov;24(11):1710-20.

[47] Berry G J, Burke M M, Andersen C, Bruneval P, Fedrigo M, Fishbein M C, Goddard M, Hammond E H, Leone O, Marboe C, Miller D, Neil D, Rassl D, Revelo M P, Rice A, Rene Rodriguez E, Stewart S, Tan C D, Winters G L, West L, Mehra M R, Angelini A. The 2013 International Society for Heart and Lung Transplantation Working Formulation for the standardization of nomenclature in the pathologic diagnosis of antibody-mediated rejection in heart transplantation. *J. Heart Lung Transplant.* 2013 Dec;32(12):1147-62.

[48] Mehra M R, Crespo-Leiro M G, Dipchand A, Ensminger S M, Hiemann N E, Kobashigawa J A, Madsen J, Parameshwar J, Starling R C, Uber P A. International Society for Heart and Lung Transplantation working formulation of a standardized

nomenclature for cardiac allograft vasculopathy-2010. *J. Heart Lung Transplant.* 2010 Jul;29(7):717-27.

[49] Echeverría L E, Figueredo A, Rodriguez M J, Salazar L, Pizarro C, Morillo C A, Rojas L Z, Gómez-Ochoa S A, Castillo V R. Survival after heart transplantation for Chagas cardiomyopathy using a conventional protocol: A 10-year experience in a single center. *Transpl. Infect. Dis.* 2021 Aug;23(4):e13549.

Chapter 17

Heart Transplantation in Congenital Heart Disease

Federico Ignacio Zeppa*
Adult Congenital Heart Disease, Favaloro Foundation University Hospital, Buenos Aires, Argentina

Abstract

Thanks to advances in surgical techniques used for the management of congenital heart disease (CHD), an increasing number of patients survive and reach adulthood. Some of these patients will develop advanced heart failure (HF), with a particular clinical presentation and prognosis as compared to other etiologies.

Apart from medical therapy, with scarce evidence available in this group of patients, heart transplant (HTx) and mechanical circulatory support (MCS) are part of the treatment armamentarium. Heart transplant is associated with a higher early mortality rate as compared to other causes of HF due to worse perioperative outcomes secondary to the anatomical characteristics of heart disease and the history of previous surgeries. However, post-transplant long term survival is longer in this group of adult congenital heart disease (ACHD) patients due to younger age and comorbidities. MCS is used less frequently as a bridge to transplant due to engraftment issues and lack of familiarity of use.

To improve the results of advanced therapies in HF a timely referral, adequate patient selection and management in centers with experience in transplantation and CHD are essential.

Keywords: congenital heart defects, heart failure, heart transplantation

---

* Corresponding Author's E-mail: fzeppa@ffavaloro.org.

In: Heart Transplantation
Editor: Elian Facundo Giordanino
ISBN: 978-1-68507-759-4

Introduction

Advances in surgical techniques and neonatal care have improved the survival of neonates with congenital heart diseases (CHD). More than 90% of these patients reach adulthood, which justifies expansion to this patient population in recent decades [1].

In spite of both medical and surgical management, many adult patients with CHD will experience progressive cardiopulmonary function impairment leading to heart failure (HF), one of the most prevalent causes of death in this population (between 25 and 50%) [2-4]. Also, the number of hospitalizations for HF in adult congenital heart disease (ACHD) patients has increased twofold in recent decades, which shows the relevance of an increasingly common issue [5]. In this setting and as drug therapy is less useful than in other HF etiologies, mechanical circulatory support (MCS) and heart transplant (HTx) appear as useful tools to improve prognosis based on adequate patient selection and a timely indication.

The aim of this chapter is to review the characteristics of both diagnosis and treatment of advanced HF in patients with ACHD.

Heart Failure in Congenital Heart Disease

Causes

Although many simple forms of CHD are not associated with a higher risk of HF in adulthood, patients with more severe lesions (systemic left ventricle and univentricular physiology) or lesions not timely treated (short circuits) may develop HF.

Heart failure is seen in up to 22% of patients with ACHD undergoing an atrial switch (Mustard or Senning procedure) for D transposition of the great arteries (d-TGA), 32% in patients with L transposition of the great arteries (l-TGA), and approximately 40% of patients with Fontan circulation [6].

From the pathophysiology standpoint, ACHD and HF (ACHD-HF) may be divided into three groups [7]. The first group includes patients with uncorrected defects due to a misdiagnosis, lack of timely intervention or inadequate access to health care. The second group includes patients diagnosed in childhood and managed with corrective or palliative surgeries, who in time develop signs of HF. An example of this condition is d-TGA after an atrial switch which will probably evolve into systemic right ventricle (RV) dysfunction or corrected Fallot's tetralogy with RV dysfunction due to progression of pulmonary insufficiency. Finally, the third group includes patients evolving into Fontan circulation dysfunction and represents the most common cause for heart transplant in CHD.

Diagnosis

Symptoms may be similar to those seen in classical HF, such as dyspnea, fatigue and exercise intolerance or specifically related to either corrective or palliative surgery, such as for example, plastic bronchitis (PB) or protein-losing enteropathy (PLE) in patients with Fontan circulation.

Some characteristics of ACHD which may contribute to the occurrence of HF symptoms are chronotropic incompetence and atrioventricular blocks commonly associated with previous surgeries, valve disease, acquired short circuits (e.g., detachment of the interventricular communication patch) or aorto-pulmonary collaterals.

It is not uncommon for ACHD patients to adapt to their functional limitations and do not complain of symptoms [8]. This may be related to the presence of heart disease since birth. Typically, when symptoms are recognized, HF related complications turn out to be severe and irreversible [9-10]. For this reason, the classification based on functional class with scores such as the New York Heart Association (NYHA) may underestimate the severity of the disease.

Restrictive pulmonary disease related to post-surgical changes in the chest wall or abnormal lung development are more common in this population, and, as they may favor the occurrence of dyspnea or intolerance to exercise, they make the diagnosis of HF more complex [11].

Brain natriuretic peptide (BNP) levels vary widely among the ACHD groups, and may not have a diagnostic value in patients with Fontan circulation or a systemic RV, so their predictive value is lower than in other HF causes.

Apart from the echocardiogram, which is a baseline study in ACHD-HF patients, a magnetic resonance and computed tomography may be necessary to understand the complex anatomies, evaluate the size and function of the cardiac cavities, and recognize complications associated with previous surgeries (Figure 1).

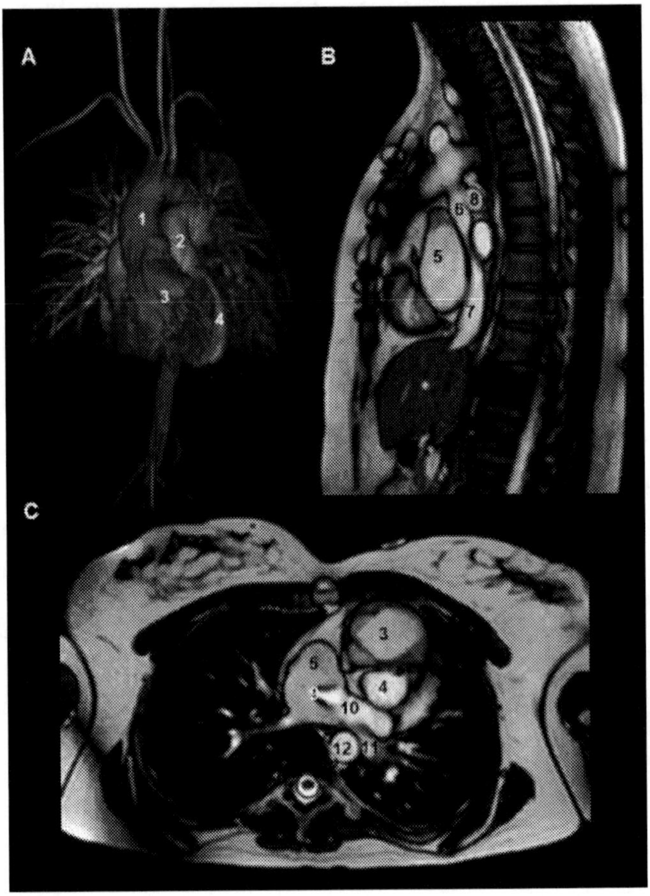

Figure 1. Cardiac magnetic resonance imaging of a 34-year-old patient with atrial switch surgery. A. 3d reconstruction. B. Sagital view. C. Axial view. 1. Aorta emerging from systemic ventricle (morphologically right ventricle). 2. Pulmonary artery emerging from pulmonary ventricle (morphologically left ventricle). 3. Systemic ventricle (morphologically right ventricle). 4. Pulmonary ventricle (morphologically left ventricle). 5. Peripheral atrium. 6. Superior vena cava. 7. Inferior vena cava. 8. Right pulmonary artery. 9. Neo interatrial septum. 10. Central atrium. 11. Lower left pulmonary vein. 12. Descending aorta.

Catheterization is a fundamental tool in the assessment of pulmonary pressures, functioning of Fontan circulation and identification of both arterial and venous collaterals, which will be later described in this chapter.

Prognosis

The prediction of prognosis in patients with ACHD-HF is more difficult than in other etiologies. This is because of the heterogeneity in presentation of HF symptoms in relation to age and the underlying anatomy. There are some markers of poor prognosis which have proved to be useful in this population, like in the case of acquired HF: hyponatremia, anemia, kidney and liver dysfunction, previous hospitalizations related to HF and pulmonary hypertension (PH) [8, 12-13].

Some parameters such as BNP, left ventricle ejection fraction, maximum oxygen consumption (VO_2max), and risk scores seem to be less useful than in other HF etiologies, and are not equally applicable to the different types of CHD [8, 14].

The risk scores designed for the general population with HF may help identify high risk patients with ACHD-HF although the evidence available is limited in this setting [13]. In patients undergoing Fontan surgery the MELD-XI score was able to independently predict the combined endpoint of sudden death, death due to heart failure or heart transplant [15]. Likewise, the cardiopulmonary exercise test has proved useful in patients undergoing Fontan surgery to predict mortality and the need for transplant. Although there are no fairly clear parameters to suggest an indication for transplant such as acquired HF, in patients with ACHD a VO_2max under 50% according to age might be an indication [8, 16].

Heart Failure in Patients with Fontan Circulation

Among CHDs possibly leading to HF, a heart with univentricular physiology deserves special attention due to its characteristics. In these patients, first line treatment is Fontan surgery, where the systemic venous flow is redirectioned to the pulmonary arteries without passing through a subpulmonary ventricular chamber. Transplant-free survival at 20 years after Fontan surgery is close to 80% whereas HF is responsible for about one third or half of the deaths in the adult population undergoing this type of surgery [2, 3, 17-19].

HF in patients undergoing Fontan surgery has a worse prognosis than in patients with a biventricular physiology: hospitalization due to dysfunction of the Fontan system is associated with an 8% mortality rate, and 4 times higher than in ACHD with biventricular physiology [20].

There are three specific associated problems in this group of patients adding to the typical clinical presentation of HF: PLE, Fontan associated liver disease (FALD) and PB.

- PLE occurs due to a lymphatic alteration secondary to chronic liver congestion resulting in loss of lymph fluid rich in proteins towards the gastrointestinal tract [21]. Morbi-mortality is high, and in most of the cases it resolves after HTx; for this reason, it is one of the specific indications to proceed to pre-transplant assessment. Diarrhea may be a clinical manifestation and hypoalbuminemia leads to a reduced oncotic vascular pressure, which results in ascites and pleural effusion, loss of coagulation factors and lymphopenia. Patients who develop PLE usually have preserved LV function and high pressures in the Fontan circuit.
- PB is characterized by the production of bronchial casts with a lymphatic origin obstructing the lumen of the respiratory airway. It is caused by the effusion of lymph rich in proteins through lymphatic-bronchial communication and occurs in <5% of the individuals with Fontan circulation. It presents with chronic coughing and hypoxemia, and is associated with higher mortality in this group of patients [22].
- Chronic liver congestion leads to some degree of FALD in all adult patients with Fontan. This may include mild lab changes and even advanced cirrhosis, liver failure or hepatocarcinoma which lead to a worse outcome [22].

Apart from PLE, PB and FALD, other manifestations of HF in this group of patients include: arrhythmias, systemic atrio-ventricular valve dysfunction, cyanosis and kidney failure [23].

Patients undergoing Fontan surgery may develop HF without ventricular function impairment or decreased cardiac output. In fact, in patients with high pressures in the Fontan system and a cardiac output over 2.5–3.0 l/min/m2 higher mortality rates have been reported [24-25]. The contradictory prognostic outcome may be explained by a higher proportion of liver disease, PLE and arterio-venous collaterals present in this group of patients [26, 27].

PVR measurement may be a great challenge due to the absence of pulsatile flow towards the pulmonary artery and the development of veno-venous collateral circulation reducing pulmonary pressure. Stenosis in one of the pulmonary branches may cause an asymmetrical flow between the lungs, and therefore differences in PVR in each lung. In patients with Fontan circulation, some vascular lung remodeling occurs as well as some small increases in PVR which may cause significant reductions in cardiac output [28].

Selection of Candidates for Advanced Therapy Assessment

Patients with complex CHD must be followed in centers with experience in both ACHD and HF.

One of the most difficult aspects in the care of patients with ACHD is the timely identification for either MSC or HTx. These patients may present more advanced disease as compared with other HTx etiologies, but they also have longer waiting-times due to the anatomical complexity, sensitization and need for multivisceral transplant [29].

There are some indicators of advanced disease orienting to the assessment of these therapies shared with other HF etiologies, as follows [30]:

- Progression to NYHA functional class III and IV.
- History of two or more hospitalizations for decompensated HF in the last year.
- VO_2max <14 mL/kg/min or <50% of the predicted value.
- Need for inotropic agents for symptomatic management or organ function maintenance.
- Worsening of right HF, diuretic resistance.
- Progressive kidney or liver failure.
- Hyponatremia.
- High mortality at one year as predicted by traditional scores (20-25%).
- Intolerance to angiotensin converting enzyme inhibitors or beta blockers.
- Recurrent or refractory ventricular tachyarrhythmia.
- Cardiac cachexia.

Particularly in patients with ACHD, some additional conditions associated to worse prognosis that should be considered for the evaluation of advanced therapies are [31]:

- Presence of PLE and/or PB refractory to medical therapy for HF.
- Progressive cyanosis with functional class deterioration which cannot be improved with palliative surgery or percutaneous treatment.

Treatments in Heart Failure due to Congenital Heart Disease

The initial approach in patients with ACHD-HF is similar to that of patients with acquired heart disease, although the evidence of both diagnostic and therapeutic management is much more limited.

In the first place, it is important to evaluate and recognize defects of the original heart disease or later surgeries that can be corrected. Such is the case of, for example, pulmonary regurgitation in adults after corrected Fallot´s tetralogy or Fontan circulation complications that are potentially treatable, such as stenosis in pulmonary branches, collaterals or new arrhythmias hemodynamically involving the circuit functioning.

The medical treatment options for patients with ACHD-HF are limited, and the supporting evidence is weak. Typically, the recommendations applied in acquired heart disease with ventricular dysfunction are extrapolated, where the benefits of medical therapy have been widely proven. For this reason, HTx and MCS devices are especially attractive options in this population and the proportion of transplants performed in patients with ACHD has increased in time. At present, CHD account for 3.3% of the total number of HF cases, with data showing a 40% increase as compared with previous figures [32, 33].

The implementation of advanced therapies in the heterogeneous population is complex. Results vary depending on the underlying congenital heart disease, the complexity and the number of previous surgeries, presence of pulmonary hypertension, kidney and liver disease, sensitization level and the experience of the transplant center among other conditioning factors [29].

Transplant in Congenital Heart Disease

Data reported by the International Society for Heart and Lung Transplantation (ISHLT) showed that between 1992 and 2003, 1.9% of the total number of HTxs were in ACHD patients, a figure that increased to as high as 3.1%, considering the data between 2009 and 2017. About 40% of ACHD patients undergoing transplantation had univentricular physiology [34]. Great vessel transposition with systemic RV dysfunction (congenitally acquired or

D-transposition with atrial switch surgery) was the next cause of CHD in the transplant group. Also, other less common HTx indications were reported such as short non-repaired circuits or Fallot´s tetralogy.

ACHD-HF patients listed for HTx are, on average, younger and present a lower percentage of obesity, smoking, kidney disease and diabetes as compared to other HF etiologies [35-36]. However, their priority is low in HTx lists as compared with other causes of HF, they spend more time on waiting list, have less probabilities of receiving an organ (considering the same allocation level), and face a higher mortality rate while listed for HTx [35-37].

Below are the characteristics differentiating ACHD patients from other causes of HT.

History of Previous Surgery

Most of the ACHD patients referred for transplant have a history of heart surgery with an average of 2.4 previous surgeries [38]. A history of 3 or more sternotomies is associated with a higher risk of death after transplant [39]. Previous surgeries favor the development of adhesions which condition a longer cold ischemia time in the donor, a higher risk of lesions in the heart and large vessels, increased extracorporeal circulation time and bleeding rate. As much as 30% of the ACHD patients require an additional procedure at the time of transplant, including reconstruction of the pulmonary arteries, systemic veins and large vessels [40].

Accesses and Vascular Anatomy

Previous catheterization and surgeries may cause thrombosis of venous accesses. This may be a hurdle in the surgical approach during transplantation. Preparation of femoral accesses may be useful in case an emergency femoro-femoral cannulation is necessary. Patients with ACHD are more likely to develop aorto-pulmonary collaterals, which increases the risk of peri-operative bleeding (Figure 2). Embolization of collaterals via catheterization before transplant may be performed but is not always successful [41].

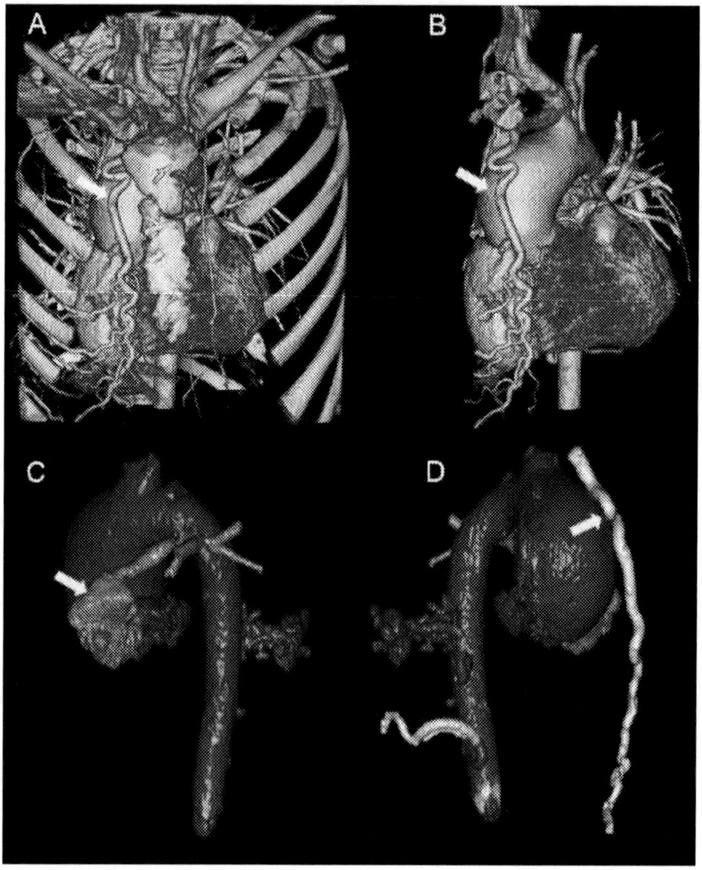

Figure 2. Angiotomography with 3D reconstruction of a 17-year-old patient with pulmonary atresia and ventricular septal defect, with palliative surgery. A and B. Tortuous and highly developed ectasic right mammary artery and intercostal branches that generate collaterals arteries to the right lung. C. Right ventricle/ Pulmonary artery conduit with left pulmonary branch (absence of right pulmonary branch). D. Relationship between aorta and right mammary artery.

Sensitization

Due to the history of heart surgeries, patients with ACHD have commonly been exposed to blood product transfusions or cadaveric grafting. This contributes to higher allosensitization rates [42-43].

Pulmonary Hypertension

High pulmonary vascular resistance (PVR) is another important factor affecting eligibility for transplant and a good outcome in patients with ACHD-HF. This is more common among ACDH patients listed for HTx as compared to other indications [44-45]. Moreover, an accurate assessment of pulmonary pressures may be difficult in certain complex physiologies where flow is not pulsatile, the flow distribution in the pulmonary beds is asymmetrical and when developmental anomalies are limited to one lung or lung segment.

Heart Transplant Outcome in Congenital Heart Disease

There is general agreement in the literature that perioperative survival and survival at one year after HTx is lower than in patients undergoing transplantation for other causes [34, 43, 45-47]. Given the higher complexity of HTx in ACHD, perioperative outcomes are expected to be worse than in non-CHD patients. Data from the ISHLT registry show that the risk in ACHD patients undergoing transplantation was twice as high within a year as compared to the group of patients with acquired heart disease [48].

Table 1 describes the factors accounting for the higher postoperative mortality and lower survival rate at one year. Surgical times and ischemia times are longer due to a more complex surgery which usually requires a prolonged sternum opening, lysis of adhesions, alternative cannulation strategies and vascular reconstruction, as previously described [45-47]. Also, the risk of bleeding is higher due to the tissue characteristics and the development of collateral circulation with a probability of rupture [12, 49]. For this reason, surgical factors account for 10% of deaths in ACHD patients as compared to 4% in patients undergoing transplantation for other causes of HF [12].

Early post-transplant death in ACHD patients is mainly due to primary graft dysfunction (most common cause of death), bleeding and cerebrovascular accident. Also, the risk of acute kidney failure (present in 50%) and the need for dialysis are higher [33, 40, 43, 45, 46].

Table 1. Factors associated with worse perioperative and 1-year survival after heart transplantation

FACTORS ASSOCIATED WITH WORSE PERIOPERATIVE AND 1-YEAR SURVIVAL AFTER HT
Prolonged surgical time and ischemia time
Higher bleeding rate and need for surgical re-exploration
Higher rates of acute kidney failure and need for dialysis
Higher post-operative cerebrovascular accident rate
Higher primary graft dysfunction rate

HT, heart transplantation. (Data from Burchill LJ et al. Heart transplantation in adult congenital heart disease. *Heart*. 2016 Dec 1; 102(23): 1871-1877 and Davies RR et al. Listing and transplanting adults with congenital heart disease. *Circulation*. 2011 Feb 22; 123(7): 759-67.)

Considering the CHD types, patients with univentricular physiology seem to justify the excess mortality probably conditioned by a larger number of previous sternotomies, PLE, presence of collateral vessels and sensitization level [33, 50]. When patients undergoing Fontan surgery are excluded, the HTx outcomes in other CHDs are similar to those of patients with acquired heart diseases [51].

High PVR seems to be a risk factor for death while listed for HTx; however, recent data show there may not be any association between a longer time on waiting list or higher post-transplant mortality rate [52].

In spite of the higher allosensitization rates among ACHD patients, a higher antibody-mediated or vascular graft disease rejection rate has not been reported [45-46]. Younger transplant recipients with ACHD are more likely to require another transplant.

Paradoxically, although survival curves in CHD transplant patients show a high early mortality rate, long term survival is higher as compared to other heart diseases: patients surviving after the first year have better long-term outcomes. Mortality at 5 years in patients with and without CHD is similar (30.8% and 29.5% respectively); but at 10 years the trend is reverted, and mortality is lower in ACHD patients (40.7% vs. 49%) [45]. Figure 3 shows survival curves in patients with and without CHD [34].

The higher long-term survival rate may be related to a lower incidence of death secondary to malignancy, infection, rejection and vascular graft disease in ACHD receptors [33, 45, 53, 54].

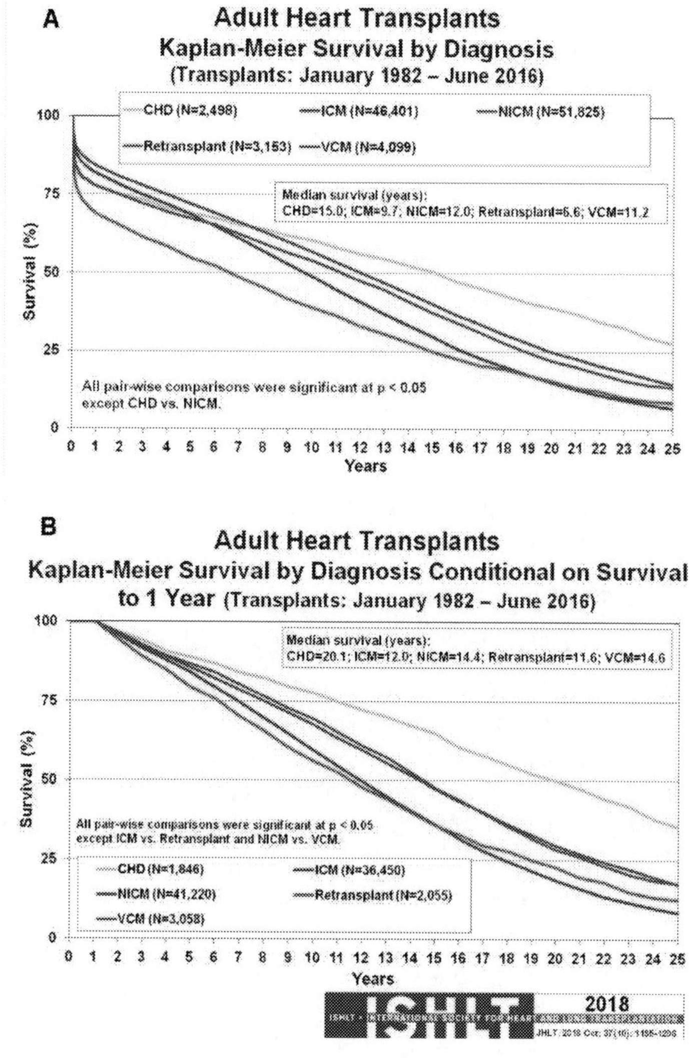

Figure 3. Survival after heart transplantation according to different etiologies. A. Survival by diagnosis. B. Survival by diagnosis conditional on survival to 1 year. CHD, congenital heart disease; ICM, ischemic cardiomyopathy; NICM, non-ischemic cardiomyopathy; VCM, valvular cardiomyopathy. (Data from ISHLT. 2018. *Adult Heart Transplantation Statistics*. Accessed 20 Dec 2021. https://ishltregistries.org/registries/slides.asp).

Thirty-day mortality after transplant was considerably lower in centers with a high and intermediate HTx volume in ACHD (9.0% y 10.2%) as compared to centers with a low volume (16.7%). Survival at one year in high volume centers was 84% as compared to 75% in low volume centers [55]. For this reason, transplants should be performed at centers with a high volume with combined experience in the management of congenital heart disease and HT. Thorough transplant planning is important, that is, using multi-images to have a clear definition of the anatomy, together with planning of the cannulation strategy and correction of residual anatomic lesions and adequate patient selection.

Special Transplant Situations in ACHD-HF

Two groups of ACHD patients deserve a specific discussion: Fontan physiology and Eisenmenger syndrome (ES):

Transplant in Patients with Fontan Circulation

Patients who are candidates for transplant may be divided into two categories: Patients with impaired ventricular function and patients with preserved ventricular function. Patients with Fontan circulation dysfunction typically present higher ventricular telediastolic pressure and PVR, lower systemic vascular resistance and higher aorto-pulmonary collaterals, and more organ dysfunction. Also, PLE and PB are expected to be more common in this population [26].

As mentioned before in this chapter, patients with Fontan circulation have a history of previous sternotomies and have received either blood transfusions or allografts. Their complex anatomies require reconstruction of pulmonary arteries and vena cava, factors associated with prolonged ischemia times, sensitization and surgical bleeding at the time of HTx [42, 43, 56]. The identification and embolization of collaterals before transplant may favor surgical outcomes [41].

As FALD progresses and heart failure occurs, multiorgan transplant should be considered. Some data in pediatric patients with Fontan suggest that fibrosis may resolve with HTx alone, which would then avoid the need of a liver transplant [57]. However, similar results, and even better results than in heart transplant alone have been reported in combined heart-liver transplantation which may be justified due to the improved liver synthesis function and induced immune tolerance seen after liver transplant [58-59]. This might play an important role in highly sensitized patients [60].

The decision to perform a combined transplant or heart transplant alone in this group of patients will depend on the experience of the center and expert opinion.

Fontan patients represent a population with a worse outcome associated to HT. In fact, as mentioned before, some studies suggest that this group of patients justifies most of the excess risk associated with heart transplant in ACHD-HF [45, 61].

Survival described in patients with Fontan undergoing transplantation is higher in those with impaired ventricular function as compared to those with preserved function [26, 27]. In this group, about 80% of patients develop PLE, a prognostic marker of a more advanced stage of the disease and possible justification of adverse outcome [27]. PLE and PB resolve after transplant in most of the cases [62]. Like other subtypes of ACHD, after the early phase, survival is good and mortality is mainly associated with rejection episodes.

Transplant in Patients with Eisenmenger Syndrome

ES is the result of a hemodynamically significant unrepaired left-right short circuit, which leads to PH in the late stage, with the consequent inversion of the short circuit from right to left and presence of cyanosis. It is difficult to determine the correct time for transplant due to the prolonged life expectancy as compared to other causes of PH [16]. Mortality in patients with ES treated with pulmonary vasodilators seems to be under 5% annually [63]. Therefore, transplantation must be reserved only for those patients who do not benefit from pulmonary vasodilators.

Transplant options include cardiopulmonary transplant, bilateral lung transplant or unipulmonary transplant. Patients with CHD and associated PH account for more than 50% of combined cardio-pulmonary transplant cases [64].

In ES patients, the outcome of the different types of transplants (bipulmonary vs cardiopulmonary transplant) seems to be different according to the underlying congenital heart disease. Sertic F. et al. showed that patients with atrial septum defect (ASD) have longer survival after bipulmonary transplant and closure of the defect as compared to cardiopulmonary transplant, and that patients with ventricular septum defect (VSD) had longer survival with cardiopulmonary transplant as compared to bipulmonary transplant [65]. RV function is expected to improve after lung transplant as it occurs with other etiologies of PH.

The difference in outcome considering the different types of transplants according to the underlying heart disease might be related to several factors. The most common cause of death in patients with VSD and bipulmonary transplant is ventricular failure (more expected even in patients with LV volume overload due to VSD as compared to ASD). Post-operative hemorrhage is the most common cause of death in patients undergoing cardiopulmonary transplant, and is less probable in patients undergoing bipulmonary transplant. Therefore, in patients with ES and ASD, bipulmonary transplant and closure of the defect might seem to be the first option whenever feasible (vs. cardiopulmonary transplant) and in patients with ES and VSD or more complex congenital heart disease, cardiopulmonary transplant is the strategy of choice.

Cardiac Transplant Allocation in Congenital Heart Disease

In 2018, the United Network for Organ Sharing (UNOS) modified the HTX allocation system for adults, with significant consequences for listed ACHD patients.

The new UNOS criteria try to reflect the level of risk more accurately. The most significant change for this population is that patients with ACHD-HF were included in Stage 4, with a priority equivalent to non-CHD patients who are stable and managed with a left ventricle assist device (LVAD), or on inotropic agents in the ambulatory setting. This represents a priority over most of the non-CHD stable patients included in Stage 6. However, the stages with more priority in terms of allocation indicate that patients must be on high doses of inotropic agents or mechanic circulatory support, which is less common in ACHD patients who are less likely to meet these criteria [66].

Mechanical Circulatory Support in Congenital Heart Disease

Data provided by INTERMACS (Interagency Registry for Mechanically Assisted Circulatory Support) show that only 0.8% of MCS patients presented a history of CHD [67, 68]. Of those patients, 45% received the device as a bridge to transplant, 38% as a bridge to candidacy and 16% as destination therapy. As for the type of CHD most patients presented a systemic LV, followed by those with a systemic RV and less commonly recipients had a univentricular physiology.

Although patients with CHD on MCS had higher mortality as compared to non-ACHD patients, in the first group the use of biventricular assist devices or total artificial hearts is more common. In the case of total artificial hearts, this is because in some patients with ACHD (e.g., Fontan) the anatomy prevents placement of a ventricular assist device [69].

The limited use of MCS in ACHD patients is due to several factors. One of them is heterogeneity in the cardiac anatomy and physiology, which makes placement difficult. For example, a systemic RV may present a different location from the typical location or present trabeculae requiring an additional procedure for placement. Moreover, the common history of a previous sternotomy is related to an unfavorable anatomy of the chest wall, with more difficult access and increased possibility of bleeding at the time of placement [37, 66, 70]. PLE may increase the risk of infection, bleeding or thrombosis and affect surgical wound healing. Another reason for the limited use as compared to other heart diseases is the lack of familiarity with the use of MCS in this group of patients.

As to the outcome after MCS, ACHD patients usually develop kidney failure, liver dysfunction and respiratory failure, arrhythmias, infection and device malfunctioning as compared to patients on MCS without ACHD [68]. The largest proportion of excess mortality seems to occur in the perioperative period.

When comparing ACHD patients undergoing transplantation with and without previous MCS as a bridge to transplant, no differences were observed in terms of mortality at 30 days or long-term survival [71].

Because of all these factors, MCS may be used as the last option in ACHD patients, which leads to worse outcomes, since these patients are more critically ill at the time of device placement. It may be advisable to reduce the threshold for MCS use in ACHD patients as bridge to transplant. With better training in MCS placement in ACHD patients and using this tool in early stages of the disease, results might improve.

Conclusion

Advanced HF is an important cause of death in ACHD and due to this increasing patient population, the prevalence will become more and more common. The clinical presentation is oftentimes different from that of acquired HF, and a history of cardiac surgery is especially relevant for the associated complications and the complexity of treatment with advanced therapies such as HTx and MSC.

An important challenge to continue improving the life expectancy of this group of patients is early and timely referral to centers with experience in ACHD and HF.

HTx has become a treatment option with good long-term outcomes. As experience grows, perioperative transplant outcomes in ACHD are expected to get close to those seen in the general population, mainly in high volume centers where surgical planning to reduce ischemia time and bleeding risk is essential. Advances in changing specific organ allocation systems for CHD patients and increased use of MSC will be the key to improve outcomes for these patients listed for transplant.

References

[1] Moons P, Bovijn L, Budts W, Belmans A, Gewillig M. Temporal trends in survival to adulthood among patients born with congenital heart disease from 1970 to 1992 in Belgium. *Circulation.*, 2010 Nov 30; 122(22): 2264-72.

[2] Verheugt CL, Uiterwaal CS, van der Velde ET, Meijboom FJ, Pieper PG, van Dijk AP, Vliegen HW, Grobbee DE, Mulder BJ. Mortality in adult congenital heart disease. *Eur Heart J.*, 2010 May; 31(10): 1220-9.

[3] Diller GP, Kempny A, Alonso-Gonzalez R, Swan L, Uebing A, Li W, Babu-Narayan S, Wort SJ, Dimopoulos K, Gatzoulis MA. Survival Prospects and Circumstances of Death in Contemporary Adult Congenital Heart Disease Patients Under Follow-Up at a Large Tertiary Centre. *Circulation.*, 2015 Dec 1; 132(22): 2118-25.

[4] Yu C, Moore BM, Kotchetkova I, Cordina RL, Celermajer DS. Causes of death in a contemporary adult congenital heart disease cohort. *Heart.*, 2018 Oct; 104(20): 1678-1682.

[5] Opotowsky AR, Siddiqi OK, Webb GD. Trends in hospitalizations for adults with congenital heart disease in the U.S. *J Am Coll Cardiol.*, 2009 Jul 28; 54(5): 460-7.

[6] Budts W, Roos-Hesselink J, Rädle-Hurst T, Eicken A, McDonagh TA, Lambrinou E, Crespo-Leiro MG, Walker F, Frogoudaki AA. Treatment of heart failure in adult congenital heart disease: a position paper of the Working Group of Grown-Up Congenital Heart Disease and the Heart Failure Association of the European Society of Cardiology. *Eur Heart J.*, 2016 May 7; 37(18): 1419-27.

[7] Hosseinpour AR, Cullen S, Tsang VT. Transplantation for adults with congenital heart disease. *Eur J Cardiothorac Surg.*, 2006 Sep; 30(3): 508-14.

[8] Stout KK, Broberg CS, Book WM, Cecchin F, Chen JM, Dimopoulos K, Everitt MD, Gatzoulis M, Harris L, Hsu DT, Kuvin JT, Law Y, Martin CM, Murphy AM,

Ross HJ, Singh G, Spray TL; American Heart Association Council on Clinical Cardiology, Council on Functional Genomics and Translational Biology, and Council on Cardiovascular Radiology and Imaging. Chronic Heart Failure in Congenital Heart Disease: A Scientific Statement From the American Heart Association. *Circulation.*, 2016 Feb 23; 133(8): 770-801.

[9] Warnes CA. The adult with congenital heart disease: born to be bad? *J Am Coll Cardiol.*, 2005 Jul 5; 46(1): 1-8.

[10] Diller GP, Dimopoulos K, Okonko D, Li W, Babu-Narayan SV, Broberg CS, Johansson B, Bouzas B, Mullen MJ, Poole-Wilson PA, Francis DP, Gatzoulis MA. Exercise intolerance in adult congenital heart disease: comparative severity, correlates, and prognostic implication. *Circulation.*, 2005 Aug 9; 112(6): 828-35.

[11] Müller J, Ewert P, Hager A. Number of thoracotomies predicts impairment in lung function and exercise capacity in patients with congenital heart disease. *J Cardiol.*, 2018 Jan; 71(1): 88-92.

[12] Burchill LJ. Heart transplantation in adult congenital heart disease. *Heart.*, 2016 Dec 1; 102(23): 1871-1877.

[13] Stefanescu A, Macklin EA, Lin E, Dudzinski DM, Johnson J, Kennedy KF, Jacoby D, DeFaria Yeh D, Lewis GD, Yeh RW, Liberthson R, Lui G, Bhatt AB. Usefulness of the Seattle Heart Failure Model to identify adults with congenital heart disease at high risk of poor outcome. *Am J Cardiol.*, 2014 Mar 1; 113(5): 865-70.

[14] Van De Bruaene A, Hickey EJ, Kovacs AH, Crean AM, Wald RM, Silversides CK, Redington AN, Ross HJ, Alba AC, Billia F, Nair K, Benson L, Horlick E, Osten M, Colman J, Heggie J, Oechslin EN, Roche SL. Phenotype, management and predictors of outcome in a large cohort of adult congenital heart disease patients with heart failure. *Int J Cardiol.*, 2018 Feb 1; 252: 80-87.

[15] Assenza GE, Graham DA, Landzberg MJ, Valente AM, Singh MN, Bashir A, Fernandes S, Mortele KJ, Ukomadu C, Volpe M, Wu F. MELD-XI score and cardiac mortality or transplantation in patients after Fontan surgery. *Heart.*, 2013 Apr; 99(7): 491-6.

[16] Houyel L, To-Dumortier NT, Lepers Y, Petit J, Roussin R, Ly M, Lebret E, Fadel E, Hörer J, Hascoët S. Heart transplantation in adults with congenital heart disease. *Arch Cardiovasc Dis.*, 2017 May; 110(5): 346-353.

[17] Pundi KN, Johnson JN, Dearani JA, Pundi KN, Li Z, Hinck CA, Dahl SH, Cannon BC, O'Leary PW, Driscoll DJ, Cetta F. 40-Year Follow-Up After the Fontan Operation: Long-Term Outcomes of 1,052 Patients. *J Am Coll Cardiol.*, 2015 Oct 13; 66(15): 1700-10.

[18] Downing TE, Allen KY, Glatz AC, Rogers LS, Ravishankar C, Rychik J, Faerber JA, Fuller S, Montenegro LM, Steven JM, Spray TL, Nicolson SC, Gaynor JW, Goldberg DJ. Long-term survival after the Fontan operation: Twenty years of experience at a single center. *J Thorac Cardiovasc Surg.*, 2017 Jul; 154(1): 243-253.e2.

[19] Ohuchi H, Inai K, Nakamura M, Park IS, Watanabe M, Hiroshi O, Kim KS, Sakazaki H, Waki K, Yamagishi H, Yamamura K, Kuraishi K, Miura M, Nakai M, Nishimura K, Niwa K; JSACHD Fontan Investigators. Mode of death and predictors

of mortality in adult Fontan survivors: A Japanese multicenter observational study. *Int J Cardiol.*, 2019 Feb 1; 276: 74-80.

[20] Egbe AC, Connolly HM, Miranda WR, Ammash NM, Hagler DJ, Veldtman GR, Borlaug BA. Hemodynamics of Fontan Failure: The Role of Pulmonary Vascular Disease. *Circ Heart Fail.*, 2017 Dec; 10(12): e004515.

[21] Itkin M, Piccoli DA, Nadolski G, Rychik J, DeWitt A, Pinto E, Rome J, Dori Y. Protein-Losing Enteropathy in Patients With Congenital Heart Disease. *J Am Coll Cardiol.*, 2017 Jun 20; 69(24): 2929-2937.

[22] Rychik J, Atz AM, Celermajer DS, Deal BJ, Gatzoulis MA, Gewillig MH, Hsia TY, Hsu DT, Kovacs AH, McCrindle BW, Newburger JW, Pike NA, Rodefeld M, Rosenthal DN, Schumacher KR, Marino BS, Stout K, Veldtman G, Younoszai AK, d'Udekem Y; American Heart Association Council on Cardiovascular Disease in the Young and Council on Cardiovascular and Stroke Nursing. Evaluation and Management of the Child and Adult With Fontan Circulation: A Scientific Statement From the American Heart Association. *Circulation.*, 2019 Jul 1: CIR0000000000000696.

[23] Backer CL, Russell HM, Pahl E, Mongé MC, Gambetta K, Kindel SJ, Gossett JG, Hardy C, Costello JM, Deal BJ. Heart transplantation for the failing Fontan. *Ann Thorac Surg.*, 2013 Oct; 96(4): 1413-1419.

[24] Miranda WR, Borlaug BA, Hagler DJ, Connolly HM, Egbe AC. Haemodynamic profiles in adult Fontan patients: associated haemodynamics and prognosis. *Eur J Heart Fail.*, 2019 Jun; 21(6): 803-809.

[25] Ohuchi H, Miyazaki A, Negishi J, Hayama Y, Nakai M, Nishimura K, Ichikawa H, Shiraishi I, Yamada O. Hemodynamic determinants of mortality after Fontan operation. *Am Heart J.*, 2017 Jul; 189: 9-18.

[26] Murtuza B, Hermuzi A, Crossland DS, Parry G, Lord S, Hudson M, Chaudhari MP, Haynes S, O'Sullivan JJ, Hasan A. Impact of mode of failure and end-organ dysfunction on the survival of adult Fontan patients undergoing cardiac transplantation. *Eur J Cardiothorac Surg.*, 2017 Jan; 51(1): 135-141.

[27] Griffiths ER, Kaza AK, Wyler von Ballmoos MC, Loyola H, Valente AM, Blume ED, del Nido P. Evaluating failing Fontans for heart transplantation: predictors of death. *Ann Thorac Surg.*, 2009 Aug; 88(2): 558-63; discussion 563-4.

[28] Ridderbos FJ, Wolff D, Timmer A, van Melle JP, Ebels T, Dickinson MG, Timens W, Berger RM. Adverse pulmonary vascular remodeling in the Fontan circulation. *J Heart Lung Transplant.*, 2015 Mar; 34(3): 404-13.

[29] Menachem JN, Schlendorf KH, Mazurek JA, Bichell DP, Brinkley DM, Frischhertz BP, Mettler BA, Shah AS, Zalawadiya S, Book W, Lindenfeld J. Advanced Heart Failure in Adults With Congenital Heart Disease. *JACC Heart Fail.*, 2020 Feb; 8(2): 87-99.

[30] Fang JC, Ewald GA, Allen LA, Butler J, Westlake Canary CA, Colvin-Adams M, Dickinson MG, Levy P, Stough WG, Sweitzer NK, Teerlink JR, Whellan DJ, Albert NM, Krishnamani R, Rich MW, Walsh MN, Bonnell MR, Carson PE, Chan MC, Dries DL, Hernandez AF, Hershberger RE, Katz SD, Moore S, Rodgers JE, Rogers JG, Vest AR, Givertz MM; Heart Failure Society of America Guidelines Committee.

Advanced (stage D) heart failure: a statement from the Heart Failure Society of America Guidelines Committee. *J Card Fail.*, 2015 Jun; 21(6): 519-34.

[31] Ross HJ, Law Y, Book WM, Broberg CS, Burchill L, Cecchin F, Chen JM, Delgado D, Dimopoulos K, Everitt MD, Gatzoulis M, Harris L, Hsu DT, Kuvin JT, Martin CM, Murphy AM, Singh G, Spray TL, Stout KK; American Heart Association Adults With Congenital Heart Disease Committee of the Council on Clinical Cardiology and Council on Cardiovascular Disease in the Young, the Council on Cardiovascular Radiology and Intervention, and the Council on Functional Genomics and Translational Biology. Transplantation and Mechanical Circulatory Support in Congenital Heart Disease: A Scientific Statement From the American Heart Association. *Circulation.*, 2016 Feb 23; 133(8): 802-20.

[32] Lund LH, Edwards LB, Kucheryavaya AY, Benden C, Dipchand AI, Goldfarb S, Levvey BJ, Meiser B, Rossano JW, Yusen RD, Stehlik J. The Registry of the International Society for Heart and Lung Transplantation: Thirty-second Official Adult Heart Transplantation Report--2015; Focus Theme: Early Graft Failure. *J Heart Lung Transplant.*, 2015 Oct; 34(10): 1244-54.

[33] Karamlou T, Hirsch J, Welke K, Ohye RG, Bove EL, Devaney EJ, Gajarski RJ. A United Network for Organ Sharing analysis of heart transplantation in adults with congenital heart disease: outcomes and factors associated with mortality and retransplantation. *J Thorac Cardiovasc Surg.*, 2010 Jul; 140(1): 161-8.

[34] Khush KK, Cherikh WS, Chambers DC, Goldfarb S, Hayes D Jr,, Kucheryavaya AY, Levvey BJ, Meiser B, Rossano JW, Stehlik J; International Society for Heart and Lung Transplantation. The International Thoracic Organ Transplant Registry of the International Society for Heart and Lung Transplantation: Thirty-fifth Adult Heart Transplantation Report-2018; Focus Theme: Multiorgan Transplantation. *J Heart Lung Transplant.*, 2018 Oct; 37(10): 1155-1168.

[35] Alshawabkeh LI, Hu N, Carter KD, Opotowsky AR, Light-McGroary K, Cavanaugh JE, Bartlett HL. Wait-List Outcomes for Adults With Congenital Heart Disease Listed for Heart Transplantation in the U.S. *J Am Coll Cardiol.*, 2016 Aug 30; 68(9): 908-17.

[36] Hsich EM, Rogers JG, McNamara DM, Taylor DO, Starling RC, Blackstone EH, Schold JD. Does Survival on the Heart Transplant Waiting List Depend on the Underlying Heart Disease? *JACC Heart Fail.*, 2016 Sep; 4(9): 689-97.

[37] Everitt MD, Donaldson AE, Stehlik J, Kaza AK, Budge D, Alharethi R, Bullock EA, Kfoury AG, Yetman AT. Would access to device therapies improve transplant outcomes for adults with congenital heart disease? Analysis of the United Network for Organ Sharing (UNOS). *J Heart Lung Transplant.*, 2011 Apr; 30(4): 395-401.

[38] Cohen S, Houyel L, Guillemain R, Varnous S, Jannot AS, Ladouceur M, Boudjemline Y, Bonnet D, Iserin L. Temporal trends and changing profile of adults with congenital heart disease undergoing heart transplantation. *Eur Heart J.*, 2016 Mar 1; 37(9): 783-9.

[39] Lewis M, Ginns J, Schulze C, Lippel M, Chai P, Bacha E, Mancini D, Rosenbaum M, Farr M. Outcomes of Adult Patients With Congenital Heart Disease After Heart

Transplantation: Impact of Disease Type, Previous Thoracic Surgeries, and Bystander Organ Dysfunction. *J Card Fail.*, 2016 Jul; 22(7): 578-82.

[40] Irving C, Parry G, O'Sullivan J, Dark JH, Kirk R, Crossland DS, Chaudhari M, Griselli M, Hamilton JR, Hasan A. Cardiac transplantation in adults with congenital heart disease. *Heart.*, 2010 Aug; 96(15): 1217-22.

[41] Miller JR, Simpson KE, Epstein DJ, Lancaster TS, Henn MC, Schuessler RB, Balzer DT, Shahanavaz S, Murphy JJ, Canter CE, Eghtesady P, Boston US. Improved survival after heart transplant for failed Fontan patients with preserved ventricular function. *J Heart Lung Transplant.*, 2016 Jul; 35(7): 877-83.

[42] O'Connor MJ, Lind C, Tang X, Gossett J, Weber J, Monos D, Shaddy RE. Persistence of anti-human leukocyte antibodies in congenital heart disease late after surgery using allografts and whole blood. *J Heart Lung Transplant.*, 2013 Apr; 32(4): 390-7.

[43] Patel ND, Weiss ES, Allen JG, Russell SD, Shah AS, Vricella LA, Conte JV. Heart transplantation for adults with congenital heart disease: analysis of the United network for organ sharing database. *Ann Thorac Surg.*, 2009 Sep; 88(3): 814-21; discussion 821-2.

[44] Mehra MR, Canter CE, Hannan MM, Semigran MJ, Uber PA, Baran DA, Danziger-Isakov L, Kirklin JK, Kirk R, Kushwaha SS, Lund LH, Potena L, Ross HJ, Taylor DO, Verschuuren EAM, Zuckermann A; International Society for Heart Lung Transplantation (ISHLT) Infectious Diseases, Pediatric and Heart Failure and Transplantation Councils. The 2016 International Society for Heart Lung Transplantation listing criteria for heart transplantation: A 10-year update. *J Heart Lung Transplant.*, 2016 Jan; 35(1): 1-23.

[45] Doumouras BS, Alba AC, Foroutan F, Burchill LJ, Dipchand AI, Ross HJ. Outcomes in adult congenital heart disease patients undergoing heart transplantation: A systematic review and meta-analysis. *J Heart Lung Transplant.*, 2016 Nov; 35(11): 1337-1347.

[46] Burchill LJ, Edwards LB, Dipchand AI, Stehlik J, Ross HJ. Impact of adult congenital heart disease on survival and mortality after heart transplantation. *J Heart Lung Transplant.*, 2014 Nov; 33(11): 1157-63.

[47] Davies RR, Russo MJ, Yang J, Quaegebeur JM, Mosca RS, Chen JM. Listing and transplanting adults with congenital heart disease. *Circulation.*, 2011 Feb 22; 123(7): 759-67.

[48] Lund LH, Edwards LB, Kucheryavaya AY, Dipchand AI, Benden C, Christie JD, Dobbels F, Kirk R, Rahmel AO, Yusen RD, Stehlik J; International Society for Heart and Lung Transplantation. The Registry of the International Society for Heart and Lung Transplantation: Thirtieth Official Adult Heart Transplant Report--2013; focus theme: age. *J Heart Lung Transplant.*, 2013 Oct; 32(10): 951-64.

[49] Sandeep N, Uchida Y, Ratnayaka K, McCarter R, Hanumanthaiah S, Bangoura A, Zhao Z, Oliver-Danna J, Leatherbury L, Kanter J, Mukouyama YS. Characterizing the angiogenic activity of patients with single ventricle physiology and aortopulmonary collateral vessels. *J Thorac Cardiovasc Surg.*, 2016 Apr; 151(4): 1126-35.e2.

[50] Lamour JM, Kanter KR, Naftel DC, Chrisant MR, Morrow WR, Clemson BS, Kirklin JK; Cardiac Transplant Registry Database; Pediatric Heart Transplant Study. The effect of age, diagnosis, and previous surgery in children and adults undergoing heart transplantation for congenital heart disease. *J Am Coll Cardiol*. 2009 Jul 7; 54(2): 160-5.

[51] Besik J, Szarszoi O, Hegarova M, Konarik M, Smetana M, Netuka I, Pirk J, Maly J. Non-Fontan Adult Congenital Heart Disease Transplantation Survival Is Equivalent to Acquired Heart Disease Transplantation Survival. *Ann Thorac Surg*. 2016 May; 101(5): 1768-73.

[52] Krishnamurthy Y, Cooper LB, Lu D, Schroder JN, Daneshmand MA, Rogers JG, Milano CA, Hernandez AF, Patel CB. Trends and outcomes of patients with adult congenital heart disease and pulmonary hypertension listed for orthotopic heart transplantation in the United States. *J Heart Lung Transplant.*, 2016 May; 35(5): 619-24.

[53] Menachem JN, Golbus JR, Molina M, Mazurek JA, Hornsby N, Atluri P, Fuller S, Birati EY, Kim YY, Goldberg LR, Wald JW. Successful cardiac transplantation outcomes in patients with adult congenital heart disease. *Heart.*, 2017 Sep; 103(18): 1449-1454.

[54] Shah DK, Deo SV, Althouse AD, Teuteberg JJ, Park SJ, Kormos RL, Burkhart HM, Morell VO. Perioperative mortality is the Achilles heel for cardiac transplantation in adults with congenital heart disease: Evidence from analysis of the UNOS registry. *J Card Surg.*, 2016 Dec; 31(12): 755-764.

[55] Menachem JN, Lindenfeld J, Schlendorf K, Shah AS, Bichell DP, Book W, Brinkley DM, Danter M, Frischhertz B, Keebler M, Kogon B, Mettler B, Rossano J, Sacks SB, Young T, Wigger M, Zalawadiya S. Center volume and post-transplant survival among adults with congenital heart disease. *J Heart Lung Transplant.*, 2018 Nov; 37(11): 1351-1360.

[56] Bryant R 3rd, Morales D. Overview of adult congenital heart transplants. *Ann Cardiothorac Surg.*, 2018 Jan; 7(1): 143-151.

[57] Simpson KE, Esmaeeli A, Khanna G, White F, Turnmelle Y, Eghtesady P, Boston U, Canter CE. Liver cirrhosis in Fontan patients does not affect 1-year post-heart transplant mortality or markers of liver function. *J Heart Lung Transplant.*, 2014 Feb; 33(2): 170-7.

[58] Bradley EA, Pinyoluksana KO, Moore-Clingenpeel M, Miao Y, Daniels C. Isolated heart transplant and combined heart-liver transplant in adult congenital heart disease patients: Insights from the united network of organ sharing. *Int J Cardiol.*, 2017 Feb 1; 228: 790-795.

[59] Bryant R 3rd, Rizwan R, Zafar F, Shah SA, Chin C, Tweddell JS, Morales DL. Contemporary Outcomes of Combined Heart-Liver Transplant in Patients With Congenital Heart Disease. *Transplantation.*, 2018 Feb; 102(2): e67-e73.

[60] Padegimas A, Molina M, Korwin A, Birati E, Kamoun M. Successful long-term outcomes in combined heart-liver transplants across pre-formed high levels of donor-specific antibodies in highly sensitized patients. *J Heart Lung Transplant.*, 2016 Nov; 35(11): 1382-1384.

[61] Karamlou T, Diggs BS, Welke K, Tibayan F, Gelow J, Guyton SW, Slater MS, Broberg C, Song HK. Impact of single-ventricle physiology on death after heart transplantation in adults with congenital heart disease. *Ann Thorac Surg.*, 2012 Oct; 94(4): 1281-7; discussion 1287-8.

[62] Gamba A, Merlo M, Fiocchi R, Terzi A, Mammana C, Sebastiani R, Ferrazzi P. Heart transplantation in patients with previous Fontan operations. *J Thorac Cardiovasc Surg.*, 2004 Feb; 127(2): 555-62.

[63] Arnott C, Strange G, Bullock A, Kirby AC, O'Donnell C, Radford DJ, Grigg LE, Celermajer DS. Pulmonary vasodilator therapy is associated with greater survival in Eisenmenger syndrome. *Heart.*, 2017 Aug 9: heartjnl-2017-311876.

[64] Chambers DC, Cherikh WS, Goldfarb SB, Hayes D Jr, Kucheryavaya AY, Toll AE, Khush KK, Levvey BJ, Meiser B, Rossano JW, Stehlik J; International Society for Heart and Lung Transplantation. The International Thoracic Organ Transplant Registry of the International Society for Heart and Lung Transplantation: Thirty-fifth adult lung and heart-lung transplant report-2018; Focus theme: Multiorgan Transplantation. *J Heart Lung Transplant.*, 2018 Oct; 37(10): 1169-1183.

[65] Sertic F, Han J, Diagne D, Richards T, Chavez L, Berg A, Wald J, Rame JE, Crespo MM, Bermudez CA. Not All Septal Defects Are Equal: Outcomes of Bilateral Lung Transplant With Cardiac Defect Repair vs Combined Heart-Lung Transplant in Patients With Eisenmenger Syndrome in the United States. *Chest.*, 2020 Nov; 158(5): 2097-2106.

[66] Monaco J, Khanna A, Khazanie P. Transplant and mechanical circulatory support in patients with adult congenital heart disease. *Heart Fail Rev.*, 2020 Jul; 25(4): 671-683.

[67] VanderPluym CJ, Cedars A, Eghtesady P, Maxwell BG, Gelow JM, Burchill LJ, Maltais S, Koehl DA, Cantor RS, Blume ED. Outcomes following implantation of mechanical circulatory support in adults with congenital heart disease: An analysis of the Interagency Registry for Mechanically Assisted Circulatory Support (INTERMACS). *J Heart Lung Transplant.*, 2018 Jan; 37(1): 89-99.

[68] Cedars A, Vanderpluym C, Koehl D, Cantor R, Kutty S, Kirklin JK. An Interagency Registry for Mechanically Assisted Circulatory Support (INTERMACS) analysis of hospitalization, functional status, and mortality after mechanical circulatory support in adults with congenital heart disease. *J Heart Lung Transplant.*, 2018 May; 37(5): 619-630.

[69] Ryan TD, Jefferies JL, Zafar F, Lorts A, Morales DL. The evolving role of the total artificial heart in the management of end-stage congenital heart disease and adolescents. *ASAIO J.*, 2015 Jan-Feb; 61(1): 8-14.

[70] Bryant R Rd, Morales DLS. Regarding mechanical circulatory support in adults with congenital heart disease: Is it time to lower the threshold for use? *J Heart Lung Transplant.*, 2018 Jan; 37(1): 141-142.

[71] Maxwell BG, Wong JK, Sheikh AY, Lee PH, Lobato RL. Heart transplantation with or without prior mechanical circulatory support in adults with congenital heart disease. *Eur J Cardiothorac Surg.*, 2014 May; 45(5): 842-6.

Chapter 18

Heart Transplantation in Familial Hypertrophic/Restrictive Cardiomyopathy

Adrián Fernández* and Alejandro Quiroga
Familial Cardiomyopathies Working Group, Clinical Cardiology Service, Favaloro Foundation University Hospital, Buenos Aires, Argentina

Abstract

Familial cardiomyopathies comprise a large group of hereditary diseases, characterized by structural and functional abnormalities of the myocardium that are not explained by coronary artery disease or abnormal loading conditions. These cardiomyopathies have often an autosomal dominant inheritance pattern caused by mutations in genes that encode different proteins of the cardiac sarcomere. Sarcomere dysfunction can lead to hypertrophic cardiomyopathy (HCM), restrictive cardiomyopathy (RCM), among others, and sometimes overlapping phenotypes. Familial forms of RCM are currently considered to be a part of the phenotypic spectrum of HCM and not a distinct genetic cardiomyopathy. HCM and RCM can occasionally be caused by other genetic disorders including inherited metabolic disorders (e.g., Anderson-Fabry disease), glycogen storage diseases, genetic syndromes (e.g., Noonan syndrome), genetic neuromuscular diseases, chromosomal abnormalities, genetics infiltrative diseases (e.g., hereditary transthyretin amyloidosis) and non-genetic disorders (e.g., wild type transthyretin and light chain amyloidosis) which mimic genetic forms of these entities. In this chapter we will focus on the main causes of familial HCM/RCM that can lead to heart transplantation.

---

* Corresponding Author's E-mail: afernandez@ffavaloro.org.

In: Heart Transplantation
Editor: Elian Facundo Giordanino
ISBN: 978-1-68507-759-4

Keywords: hypertrophic cardiomyopathy, restrictive cardiomyopathy, heart transplantation

Introduction

Patients with hypertrophic cardiomyopathy (HCM) and restrictive cardiomyopathy (RCM) may exhibit different clinical manifestations ranging from no symptoms to sudden cardiac death (SCD) or severe heart failure (HF) [1-4]. Decreased left ventricular systolic function in HCM and RCM occurs in a small number of patients, and the mechanisms involved in its progression are poorly understood [5-8]. Heart transplantation (HT) is the treatment of choice for patients who progress to HF, and remain severely symptomatic despite optimal medical therapy [2-8]. Referral of patients with HCM or RCM for HT is not indicated only in systolic dysfunction, because patients with preserved ejection fraction (EF) can also develop advanced HF with restrictive physiology or refractory recurrent ventricular arrhythmias [2-4].

Systolic Dysfunction in Hypertrophic Cardiomyopathy

HCM is defined as the presence of increased thickness of the left ventricular wall of at least 15 mm (or 13 mm in patients who have familial history of the disease) that is not explained solely by abnormal loading conditions [2-4]. It is a myocardial disorder with marked heterogeneous expression of clinical, morphologic, and functional features. HCM is usually associated with left ventricular (LV) diastolic dysfunction, however, a few patients (ranging from 4% to 9% in different series) have progressive LV systolic dysfunction (HCM-LVSD), which in HCM is defined by convention as an EF < 50% [2-4]. In HCM patients, EF usually overestimates LV systolic function and for this reason an EF < 50% is considered a significant reduction hence referred to as HCM-LVSD since it is associated with a worse prognosis [5-13].

Although these patients show left ventricular remodeling with dilation of the cavity, in some, this process is less evident and includes non-dilated and hypertrophied left ventricles, thus having HCM-LVSD, which often occurs before the appearance of other signs of classical remodeling [12-15].

The clinical course of HCM-LVSD is variable but generally unfavorable and usually takes an aggressive course with profound clinical deterioration [5-11]. Mechanisms involved in the progression from typical HCM to HCM-LVSD remain unclear [14-16]. In some patients, this progression may be genetically determined and HCM-LVSD can be seen in members of the same family [17-20]. Presence of marked fibrosis suggests that myocyte death may be one of the main factors responsible for HCM-LVSD [5-12].

In these patients, it is important to rule out concomitant epicardial coronary artery disease (CAD), heart valve disease and metabolic disorders as possible causes of HCM-LVSD [2-4, 12, 13]. The incidence of epicardial CAD and coronary myocardial bridging was similar in patients who developed LV impairment and those who did not. This observation led to the suggestion that coronary microvascular dysfunction may be involved in the development of fibrosis [8-12]. Progression to advanced disease would then be related to myocardial loss due to replacement fibrosis [21-24]. Maron et al. found that in HCM, arterioles are dysplastic and feature a narrow lumen and thickened wall [25]. In addition to the presence of arteries with morphologic abnormalities, in a series of patients from our center, we observed a selected decrease in the number and length densities of medium sized arterioles measuring <50 μm in diameter. However, larger vessels measuring >50 μm did not exhibit changes compared to controls. Our results indicate that in HCM-LVSD, large vessels can remodel along with an increase in myocardial mass, but median and smaller vessels appear to be unable to do so [8]. This observation confirms reports of decreased arteriolar density but indicates that the decrease in the number and length of the smaller arteries is selective, sparing the larger vessels, thus supporting the finding of decreased coronary flow reserve in these patients [25-27]. The magnitude of microvascular dysfunction and the extent of fibrosis are predictors of adverse remodeling leading to systolic dysfunction, clinical deterioration, and death [8-13]. Cecchi et al. used positron emission tomography to evaluate vasodilator response to dipyridamole and proved that the degree of microvascular dysfunction is an independent predictor of clinical deterioration and death [9]. Olivotto et al. confirmed that severe microvascular dysfunction is a robust long-term predictor of LV adverse remodeling and HCM-LVSD [11]. This microvascular dysfunction may occur years before actual clinical deterioration [9, 11]. A minority of patients with HCM-LVSD exhibit a very slight increase in LV cavity size. Probably in these cases fibrous replacement of the myocardium leads to a loss of contractile function without apparent remodeling of the left ventricle [5, 10]. Patients with dilated HCM may develop more fibrosis and apparently less disarray because of myocyte loss and replacement fibrosis [28]. Varnava et al. found that disarray probably occurs as a direct response to functional or structural alterations of the mutated sarcomeric protein; in contrast, fibrosis and small-vessel disease is a secondary manifestation that is not related to disarray [28].

Patients with HCM-LVSD should receive pharmacological treatment according to evidence-based medicine for adults with other forms of HF with reduced EF, including angiotensin converting enzyme inhibitors (ACEI) or angiotensin II receptor blockers (ARB II) if ACEI are not tolerated, beta-blockers and mineralocorticoid receptor antagonists to improve symptoms, reduce hospitalizations for HF and premature death (See Chapter 1) [29]. On the other hand, negative inotropic agents such as verapamil, diltiazem or disopyramide are contraindicated. In patients with atrial fibrillation, it is important to achieve reversion to sinus rhythm or perform rate control [29].

Cardiac resynchronization therapy (CRT) for symptomatic improvement can be considered in patients with HCM-LVSD who present left bundle branch block with QRS duration > 120 ms and New York Heart Association (NYHA) class II-IV symptoms refractory to drug treatment [30-33]. For patients with severe HCM-LVSD, the indication of CRT is based on the recommendations for patients with EF ≤ 35% who have HF from other causes, although the criteria to identify possible responders in HCM have not been defined and are presumably different from classic systolic HF [30-33].

HCM-LVSD is currently considered as a risk factor for SCD [4, 34]. We must also take into account that the finding of extensive myocardial fibrosis, which is revealed by the presence of extensive late gadolinium enhancement by cardiac magnetic resonance imaging, is associated with increased risk for potentially life-threatening ventricular arrhythmias [4, 35, 36]. In our series, SCD or syncope with documented sustained ventricular tachycardia or ventricular fibrillation was more frequent in patients with HCM-LVSD, and three patients waiting for HT underwent appropriate defibrillator therapies [8]. Currently, in HCM-LVSD patients, an implantable cardioverter defibrillator should be considered for primary prevention of SCD (recommendation class IIa, level of evidence B-NR) (Table 1) [4].

Table 1. Main differences between non-obstructive Hypertrophic/Restrictive Cardiomyopathy patients who evolve with Heart Failure due to Severe Systolic dysfunction or Severe Diastolic Dysfunction

	noHCM/RCM LV Systolic Dysfunction	**noHCM/RCM LV Diastolic Dysfunction**
Ejection Fraction	<50%	≥50%
There may be LV dilation	Yes	No
LV wall thickness regression	Yes	No
Progressive Increase in LV wall thickness	No	Yes
Restrictive physiology	Usually not	Yes
LV chamber remodeling	Yes	No
Extensive Late Gadolinium Enhancement	Yes	No
Risk factor for Sudden Cardiac Death	Yes	No
Primary Prevention ICD	Yes	Consider at risk of SCD according to the Guidelines
Commonly develop severe symptoms	Yes	No (only 10%)
CRT if Left Bundle Branch Block	Yes	No
We can consider inotropes in ES	Yes	Usually not
We can consider VAD if LVED >55 mm in ES	Yes	Not indicated

CRT, cardiac resynchronization therapy; ES, end stage; ICD, implantable cardioverter defibrillator; LV, left ventricle; LVED, left ventricle end diastolic diameter, noHCM, non-obstructive hypertrophic cardiomyopathy; RCM, restrictive cardiomyopathy; SCD, sudden cardiac death, VAD, ventricular assist device.

Heart Failure with Preserved Systolic Function in Non-Obstructive Hypertrophic Cardiomyopathy

Patients with non-obstructive HCM and EF ≥ 50% who evolve with HF should be treated with beta-blockers, verapamil or diltiazem, to improve ventricular filling and decrease LV diastolic pressures [2-4]. Atrial fibrillation is also usually very poorly tolerated, but in these cases the use of digoxin is not recommended in order to avoid the harmful effects of the positive inotropic effect in this group of patients [37]. The prospective, multicenter, open-label, randomized, phase II controlled three-arm SILICOFCM clinical trial is designed to assess the effect of a 4-month pharmacological (sacubitril/valsartan) versus lifestyle intervention (physical activity and dietary nitrate) on functional capacity, clinical phenotype, and quality of life in patients with non-obstructive HCM [38]. In appropriately selected non-obstructive HCM patients with preserved EF and small LV cavity size who have severe symptoms due to diastolic HF despite maximal medical therapy, apical myectomy may be considered by experienced surgeons at centers of excellence. This is to augment LV cavity size in order to increase systolic volume, decrease LV end-diastolic pressure and, therefore, reduce symptoms. (Class IIb recommendation, level of evidence C-LD) [4, 39].

Heart Failure Due to Familial Restrictive Cardiomyopathy

RCM is an entity that includes different diseases characterized by a rigid myocardium, in the presence of near normal-sized LV, with normal or reduced diastolic or systolic volumes (of one or both ventricles) and normal or near normal ventricular wall thickness. Myocardial rigidity determines a restrictive LV physiology, characterized by an abnormal filling pattern that causes a sudden elevation in ventricular pressure with small increases in volume. For this reason, atria enlarge due to increased end-diastolic pressure in the ventricles [1, 40, 41].

At the beginning of the disease, systolic function in RCM can be near normal and, sometimes, it can be overestimated as it occurs in HCM (it is rare for contractility to be really normal), but systolic function might be reduced in advanced stages of the disease and in some patients it can evolve with severe systolic dysfunction and need for HT (Table 1) [1, 40, 41].

In clinical practice, the initial diagnosis of RCM is based on morphological and functional criteria. However, we know that RCM, like HCM, is more than a disease. It is a group of diseases with different etiologies. Therefore, it has great heterogeneity in its clinical presentation, prognosis and therapeutic management [1, 40, 41]. Differential diagnosis between RCM and HCM can be difficult, especially when hypertrophy is mild and, on occasions, there may be a phenotypic overlap between these two entities [42, 43]. There was a time when the cardiologist's task was limited to the morph-functional diagnosis of HCM/RCM. Today, this task has been expanded and requires cardiologists to focus on reaching an etiological diagnosis as well. This becomes essential since new therapies are currently available for some causes of HCM/RCM that, if early applied, can significantly improve the prognosis and quality of life of patients [44].

During patient's anamnesis, it is important to collect as much information as possible about the patient's family history, since there are a large number of causes of HCM/RCM that have a hereditary genetic origin and we must differentiate them from non-familiar causes of HCM/RCM such as non-inherited infiltrative and/or storage disease as light chain (AL) or wild type transthyretin (ATTRwt) amyloidosis, sarcoidosis, fatty infiltration; non-infiltrative, non-hereditary diseases (e.g., acromegaly, cardiac lipomatosis, hypothyroidism); non-familiar myocardial diseases (e.g., radiation, metastatic cancer, carcinoid, anthracycline toxicity) and drugs causing fibrous endocarditis, among others [1, 41, 45].

Genetic-based RCM is a condition with high mortality and is caused by mutations in genes that encode sarcomere and non-sarcomeric proteins [1, 40, 46-48]. Individual clinical manifestations and prognosis depend on many factors in addition to the primary causal mutation, and for that reason any genetic variant will have variable clinical presentations in different individuals, even within members of the same family. In this sense, we have to bear in mind that sometimes, in the same family, some individuals may be affected by either RCM or HCM with the same genetic variant (e.g., mutations in the genes that encodes cardiac troponin T - TNNT2, troponin I -TNNI3, MYL2, among others.) [43, 46-48]. This leads us to the hypothesis that familial forms of RCM represent a part of the phenotypic spectrum of HCM and not a different genetic cardiomyopathy [42, 46]. Therefore, we must investigate if there is a history of a relative with evidence of structural heart disease, regardless of whether it was phenotypically expressed as HCM or RCM [46-48].

Differential Diagnosis of Familial Cardiomyopathies with Systemic Manifestations

The age at which RCM manifests is the first variable that we must consider in the evaluation of these patients. A HCM/RCM that is diagnosed very early in life can be the consequence of inherited metabolic diseases, whereas a HCM/RCM that manifests after 65 years of age can be caused, for example, by the entity once termed "senile systemic amyloidosis" now known as ATTRwt (Figure 1) [1-4].

We must also consider the "extracardiac" personal and family history, especially when there is the possibility of a syndromic or metabolic cause of HCM/RCM [45, 49-51]. The inheritance pattern can also guide the diagnosis. For example, there are causes of RCM such as hemochromatosis caused by mutations in the HFE gene associated with an autosomal recessive inheritance [1, 52]. Anderson-Fabry disease has an X-linked pattern of inheritance and can be the cause of either HCM or RCM depending on the stage of the disease [49-51].

When familial RCM is associated with conduction defects, it can sometimes be caused by mutations in the desmin gene that are often associated with skeletal myopathy [53]. In the presence of conduction disorders, we must also rule out HCM/RCM due to infiltrative or deposit diseases [52, 54, 55].

Taking into account that many causes of HCM/RCM can have multisystemic manifestations, we must carefully investigate the presence of cardiac signs and symptoms related to the involvement of other organs and systems. Sometimes, the manifestations in other organs precede the cardiovascular ones. For instance, the presence of carpal tunnel syndrome can guide us to ATTR amyloidosis (especially if it is bilateral) [55]. The presence of paresthesias and neuropathic pain can orient hereditary transthyretin amyloidosis (ATTRh) or Fabry disease type 1 [45, 50, 55]. Angiokeratomas, hypohidrosis, hearing loss (tinnitus), gastrointestinal disorders, kidney failure, among others are also observed in classic Fabry disease [49-51]. In patients who manifest progressive muscle weakness, we must consider as possible differential diagnoses a group of muscular dystrophies included within the so-called myofibrillary myopathies (DES, FLNC, BAG3, CRYAB; FHL1, etc.) and glycogenosis (PRKAG2; LAMP2/Danon) [45, 53, 56]. From this, it follows that many of these diseases require management and monitoring by a multidisciplinary team made up of cardiologists, neurologists, nephrologists, ophthalmologists, dermatologists, among others (Figure 1).

In the electrocardiogram, the presence of low voltage, an antero-septal pseudoinfarction pattern, atrioventricular and bundle branch blocks should suggest an infiltrative process or sarcoidosis. The presence of pre-excitation syndrome can lead us to the diagnosis of glycogenosis [54]. The finding of atrial fibrillation is nonspecific since it is frequent to find in the different causes of RCM [51-54].

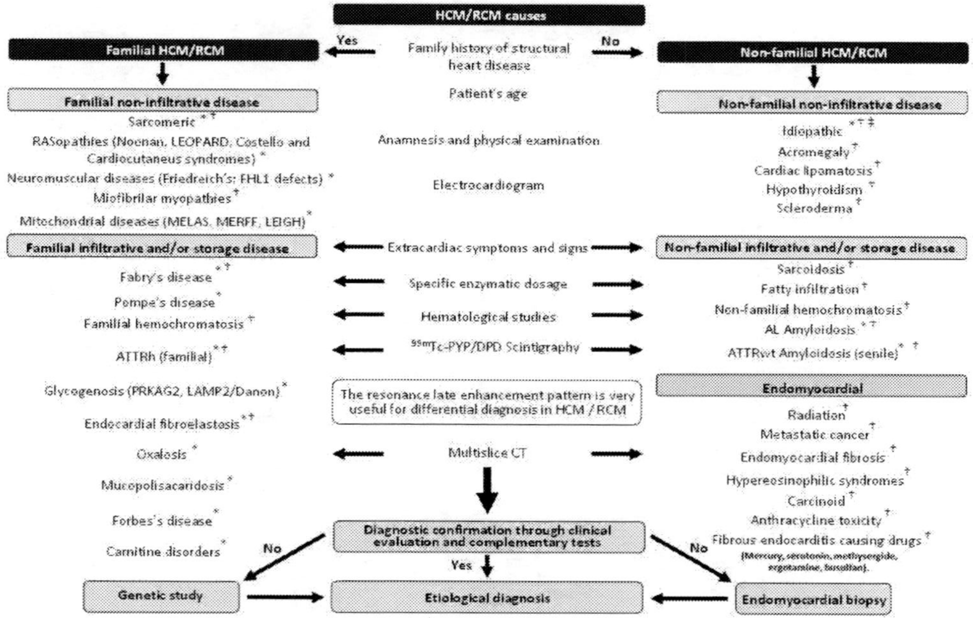

Figure 1. Etiological diagnosis of HCM/RCM. * Most common phenotype: HCM (LVMWT ≥ 15 mm); † Most common phenotype: RCM (LVMWT < 15 mm + Restrictive physiology); ‡ A "negative" family history does not exclude a genetic etiology. AL, light chain amyloidosis; ATTRh, hereditary transthyretin amyloidosis; ATTRwt, wild type transthyretin amyloidosis; HCM, hypertrophic cardiomyopathy; LVMWT, Left ventricular maximum wall thickness; RCM, restrictive cardiomyopathy; ^{99m}Tc-PYP/DPD, technetium-99m pyrophosphate/diphosphono-propanodicarboxylic acid; CT, computed tomography. (Data from Fernández A et al. Argentine Consensus on the diagnosis and treatment of hypertrophic cardiomyopathy 2016. *Rev Argent Cardiol* 2017 May;85 (2):1-78).

Some laboratory tests can be of great help. For example, when lysosomal diseases such as Fabry or Pompe are suspected, the measurement of the specific enzymatic activity can be very useful to arrive at the diagnosis [57, 58].

Routine laboratory tests, together with determinations of some specific hematological parameters, are very important tools when there is suspicion of RCM caused by hemochromatosis or other hematological diseases such as AL [52, 59-63]. Phosphonate scintigraphy currently allows us to noninvasively identify patients with transthyretin cardiac amyloidosis [45, 55, 64, 65]. The pattern of fibrosis distribution observed in cardiac magnetic resonance imaging can guide us towards the diagnosis of certain entities that produce RCM [66].

On the other hand, multislice computed tomography (CT) allows for better visualization of thrombi and subendocardial calcification, reasons that make multislice CT the method of choice when endomyocardial fibrosis is suspected [67].In patients with familial HCM/RCM, the identification of the specific genetic defect will help have a better understanding of the mechanisms involved in the expression of the disease, allow us to complete the familial genetic screening, and have direct implications in treating patients who require specific therapies that improve prognosis [68]. Finally, endomyocardial biopsy (EMB) is reasonable in the context of HF associated with HCM/RCM of unexplained cause (Class IIa recommendation, level of evidence C) [69] (Figure 1).

Unfortunately, cardiologists often make a diagnosis when these hereditary genetic causes of cardiomyopathies are in very advanced stages, often irreversible, and in which we no longer have therapeutic options. One of the most important contributions that cardiologists can make is to perform genetic screening to identify relatives with early cardiac involvement who will benefit from specific therapies which, administered early, will significantly improve the prognosis of these patients [44-50, 64]. It is essential to make a family tree/pedigree of three to four generations that will help determine the pattern and probability of inheritance, and identify other family members who are at risk [2-4].

Indications for Heart Transplantation in Familial Hypertrophic/Restrictive Cardiomyopathy

In a low percentage of patients with HCM/RCM, HT is the only therapeutic alternative. Among the candidates for HT are patients with non-obstructive HCM-LVSD or RCM with systolic dysfunction (EF <50%) who evolve with rapid clinical worsening to advanced HF (NYHA class III to class IV) and do not achieve improvement with optimal pharmacological treatment or other advanced treatment options such as CRT [1-10, 70, 71]. The referral for HT should be made according to the recommendations of the guidelines (Figure 2) [4, 72-74].

Cardiopulmonary exercise testing (CPET) should be performed to objectively evaluate the functional capacity of these patients and to help select candidates for HT [4, 75-76].

Referral of patients with HCM/RCM for HT is not indicated only in systolic dysfunction, because patients with preserved EF with restrictive physiology can also develop advanced HF [70, 77]. Therefore, the indication for HT is currently recommended for selected patients with non-obstructive HCM or RCM with normal EF (≥ 50%) who present severe symptoms of HF caused by diastolic dysfunction (NYHA class III-IV) refractory to pharmacological treatment [2-4, 70, 71, 77]. However, this subgroup of HCM/RCM patients may have symptoms of progressive and advanced HF despite CPET or echocardiography not reflecting the severity of the disease, leading to an inadequate estimation of risk [73-75].

In addition, HCM/RCM patients, due to the small left ventricular chamber size and restrictive biventricular physiology, are often less tolerant to inotropes and are not considered good candidates for mechanical circulatory support devices [78, 79]. For this reason, the revised 2018 United Network for Organ Sharing Heart Transplant Allocation considered an increase in priority for HT in the HCM/RCM according to clinical parameters and without specific hemodynamic or pharmacological/mechanical support criteria [73, 74, 79]. This new allocation policy has proven to be effective for HCM/RCM patients, which has led to an increase in HT in this subgroup and a reduction in mortality on the waiting list [73, 74, 79].

HCM/RCM patients with systemic diseases have a higher risk of frailty and renal dysfunction, which are predictors of waitlist death or delisting due to worsening of the clinical status [4, 79, 80].

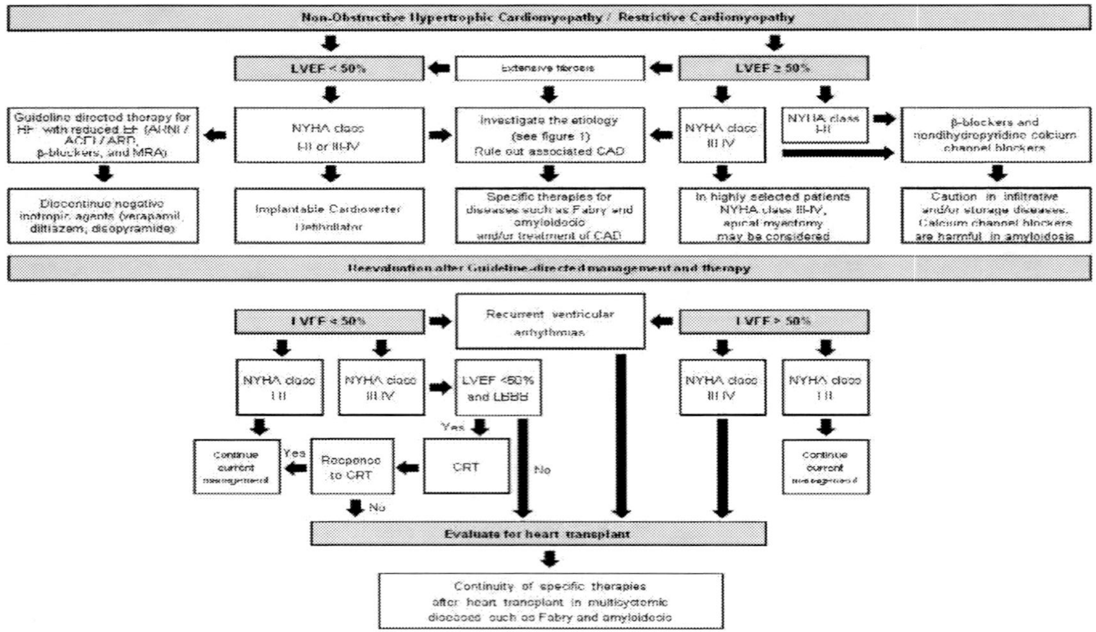

Figure 2. Management of Hypertrophic/Restrictive Cardiomyopathy. ACE, angiotensin-converting enzyme; ARB, angiotensin receptor blocker; ARNI, angiotensin receptor-neprilysin inhibitors; CAD, coronary artery disease, CRT, cardiac resynchronization therapy; LBBB, left bundle branch block; LVEF, left ventricular ejection fraction; MRA, mineralocorticoid receptor antagonist; NYHA, New York Heart Association. (Data from Fernández A et al. Argentine Consensus on the diagnosis and treatment of hypertrophic cardiomyopathy 2016. *Rev Argent Cardiol* 2017 May;85 (2):1-78).

HCM patients with LV outflow tract obstruction who respond to surgical treatment, alcohol septal ablation, or dual-chamber pacemaker, would not justify evaluation for HT [2-4].

Current recommendations for HT in HCM/RCM also extend to patients with refractory recurrent ventricular arrhythmias that cause hemodynamic decompensation and are life-threatening [4, 70, 78] (Figure 2).

Children with HCM should also be considered for HT if they evolve with refractory HF or recurrent ventricular arrhythmias that do not respond to different therapeutic alternatives [4, 81, 82].

Multisystemic Diseases with Continuity of Specific Therapies After Heart Transplantation

Fabry's Disease

Fabry disease (FD) is an X-linked lysosomal sphingolipidosis caused by pathogenic variants in the α-galactosidase A (GLA) gene which cause a reduction or absence of activity of the enzyme hydrolase α-galactosidase A (αGal A). This leads to the progressive accumulation of glycosphingolipids having galactose α-glycosidic terminal, especially globotriaosylceramide (GL-3; also abbreviated as Gb3) and the deacylated GL-3 (lyso-globotriaosylceramide [lyso-GL3]), which therefore accumulates mainly at the cardiovascular system (including cardiomyocytes, cells of the conduction system, valvular fibroblasts, vascular endothelial cells and arterial smooth muscle cells) but also in skin, kidneys, peripheral nerves and central nervous system [49-51].

The main manifestation of cardiac involvement in FD is the progressive thickening of the myocardial walls. Therefore, it can be expressed morphologically as an RCM or as an HCM depending on the moment in which the disease is diagnosed [49-51]. Cardiac involvement, kidney dysfunction and stroke are the most serious complications and become evident from the third decade of life in men and approximately from the fourth decade in women.

The forms of presentation are divided into a "classic" phenotype with pediatric onset and multisystem involvement (type 1 FD), and a late-onset or adult phenotype (type 2 FD) with predominantly cardiac or renal manifestations [49-51].

For the treatment of FD, we have specific therapies such as enzyme replacement therapies (ERT) and pharmacological chaperones, which must be administered in conjunction with the measures and treatments necessary to relieve symptoms [49-51]. Since 2001, ERT with recombinant human αGAL (rhαGAL, recombinant human α-galactosidase A) has been available to treat FD. There are currently two ERTs available for specific therapies, agalsidase alfa and agalsidase beta, both administered intravenously every two weeks [49-51]. A new therapy based on pharmacological chaperones was recently approved for patients with FD older than 16 years, with a glomerular filtration rate ≥ 30 ml/min and that present certain "responder" pathogenic variants [49-51]. Furthermore, several treatments are under development that includes substrate reduction therapy, modified enzymes, and gene therapy [49-51].

In classic or type 1 FD, it is important that we make a differential diagnosis with other causes of HCM/RCM through the clinical manifestations previously described.

The most common detection method for FD is the measurement of αGAL activity in dried blood on filter paper (DBS) [57, 58]. However, any positive result on a DBS should be confirmed by direct methods, such as the activity dosage of αGAL in leukocytes, plasma, cultured fibroblasts or by genotyping [57, 58]. Although a decrease in αGal A activity in DBS can make the diagnosis of FD in hemizygous men, it is not the most reliable diagnostic method in women, in whom levels of enzyme activity may be within the normal range in a percentage close to 40% due to the random inactivation of the X chromosome [49-51]. For this reason, in women with high clinical suspicion, the identification of a pathogenic variant by means of studying the GLA gene is necessary to confirm the diagnosis [49-51, 57, 58]. Molecular study is also indicated in men to identify the specific genetic variant in the GLA gene [49-51]. To date, there have been more than 1000 variants identified in the GLA gene, with great variation in residual enzyme activity, which allows us to understand why patients with FD have different phenotypic expressions, with differences both in clinical presentation and in evolution and prognosis [49-51]. It should be noted that most of the laboratories around the world that perform genetic studies to investigate the causes of HCM/RCM currently include the GLA gene in their panels using the method of next-generation sequencing which makes it possible to have a greater diagnosis of variants with predominantly cardiac involvement such as p.N215S or IVS4+919G > A [49-51]. If a genetic variant is not reported or is considered to be of uncertain significance, the presence of symptoms associated with FD, added to decreased enzymatic activity and high levels of lyso-GL3 are sufficient to confirm the FD diagnosis [49-51, 58]. EMB is the confirmatory tool for the diagnosis of cardiac involvement in cases in which doubts arise, demonstrating vacuolization and typical lysosomal inclusions or "zebra" bodies in electron microscopy [49-51]. However, its interpretation must be very cautious since certain medications such as amiodarone, chloroquine, and tamoxifen have a storage pattern similar to FD, so this history should be ruled out [49-51, 58].

Most FD patients have preserved systolic function and symptoms are due to LV diastolic dysfunction, but in very few patients with advanced disease, there may be systolic dysfunction [49-51, 83, 84].

ERT for FD has more benefits when administered early, but unfortunately, we diagnose FD in advanced stages when cardiac involvement is severe, the main cause of the substantial increase in morbidity and mortality in these patients [49-51].

In advanced stages of the disease, patients can develop conduction disorders, arrhythmias, and progressive deterioration of ventricular function, leading to an increased risk of stroke due to atrial fibrillation, death from heart failure, and SCD [49-51]. Patients who develop systolic dysfunction have extensive replacement by fibrosis caused by ischemia secondary to severe microvascular dysfunction and accumulation of metabolites identified as profibrotic [49-51, 83, 84]. In patients with severe cardiac involvement, especially if they have extensive fibrosis, ERT has not shown an improvement in LV function [83, 84].

A model for the evolution of myocardial involvement in FD has been proposed, consisting of a subclinical phase I of "silent" deposition of GL3 and an increase in trophic factors (lyso-GL3), which begins in childhood and progresses faster in men. This is followed by a phase II marked by hypertrophy and inflammation where fibrosis is limited to the inferolateral basal region (the presence of fibrosis can occur before LVH in women and in the IVS4 variant), neurohumoral activation and elevation of high-sensitivity cardiac troponin T (hs-TNT). Finally, a phase III characterized by clinical HF, extensive fibrosis with parietal thinning and deterioration of ventricular function, with very high levels of hs-TNT and N-terminal pro b-type natriuretic peptide [83, 84].

In patients with conduction disorders and progressive systolic dysfunction, signs of asynchrony should be assessed [50]. CRT should be considered in symptomatic patients with pacing indication and an

LVEF <50% and a QRS duration >120 ms (Class IIa recommendation, level of evidence C) and CRT may be considered in symptomatic patients with pacing indication and an LVEF ≥50% irrespective of QRS duration (Class IIb recommendation, level of evidence C) [50].

A low percentage of patients with FD evolve with rapid clinical worsening to advanced heart failure (NYHA class III to class IV) and do not achieve improvement with optimal pharmacological treatment or other advanced treatment options such as CRT. HT may be considered in these patients and in some cases combined HT and kidney transplantation may be recommended for patients with associated severe renal failure who do not respond to late-onset ERT [85]. ERT can prevent the recurrence of glycosphingolipids accumulation in transplanted organs, and prevent the progression of involvement in other organs [50, 85, 86].

Cardiac Amyloidosis

Over the last decade the number of articles being published on cardiac amyloidosis (CA) has grown exponentially [87]. This was driven by several factors. Firstly, advances have been made regarding the diagnostic algorithm providing the clinician with a non-biopsy diagnosis for a specific type of CA; and secondly new therapeutic approaches are available for the two most common causes of CA [59, 60, 64, 88]. This has fueled a revolution in the field which has helped raise awareness of a not so uncommon disease and providing patients with better outcomes.

Amyloidosis refers to the disease caused by the deposition of amyloid fibrils in the extracellular matrix [89]. Over 30 types of amyloidosis exist. Each type is named after the precursor protein that, due to different causes, aggregates into protofilaments and then fibrils, hence producing amyloid. Each type of amyloidosis will have its own clinical presentation but still, patients might differ among the same type of amyloidosis. The disease may be systemic or localized. When cardiac involvement is present the former is frequently the case. Furthermore, in most patients with CA the underlying disease will be one of two possible types: AL or ATTR [90, 91]. These two entities will have a similar cardiac phenotype but will differ in the extracardiac extent of the disease. It is important to correctly assess a patient with suspected CA for these two types of amyloidosis as they carry markedly different prognosis and treatments. Moreover, in both types of amyloidosis, the fact that the patient has reached cardiac involvement portends a worse prognosis than if the patient did not have cardiac infiltration [92].

AL is characterized by the overproduction of light chains by a clone causing them to circulate freely from their pair, the heavy chain. These free light chains misfold, and then aggregate into dimers and oligomers building up in tissue as amyloid. Cardiac involvement is frequent and rates ranging from 40-70% have been reported [93]. The clinical profile of these patients at diagnosis has been described as being 57% NYHA class ≥ III [94]. Preserved left ventricular EF is more frequent and an EF < 30% was seen in 22% of AL patients [94]. Even though AL should be thought of as a systemic disease, there are 5% of patients who present themselves with only cardiac involvement [61].

ATTR arises due to the disaggregation of the soluble TTR tetramer. The cause for this may either be due to a specific mutation as it is the case in the ATTRh, also referred to as variant ATTR or mutant ATTR, or due to an imbalance in proteostasis as it happens in ATTRwt. In ATTRh the spectrum of the phenotype will be set by the underlying mutation. It can range from a predominantly neurologic phenotype to a predominantly cardiac phenotype having mixed phenotypes in between [55]. To date there are more than 140 known mutations [95]. Conversely, in ATTRwt cardiac involvement will be the norm. When ATTR-CA takes place, the main clinical profile is HF ranging from 53% to 86% as the cause leading to a diagnosis. Most patients will be at a NYHA class II or III (II: 26-50%, III: 25-31%). Not many patients will be in class IV at time of diagnosis (0.9-6%) [55]. Moreover, the reported EF in the literature shows that 36.8% will have an EF < 50% and that only 10% will have an EF < 36% [55, 65].

When considering HT for CA different scenarios may arise:

Advanced HF due to AL Cardiac Amyloidosis

In this setting, if the clinical hemodynamics of the patient cannot tolerate autologous stem cells transplantation (ASCT) by itself then a sequential approach of HT and ASCT within a year should be followed. The main criteria to rule patients in or out for HT will be the extent of organ damage by the disease. Different series following this selective strategy have reported up to a 60% 5-year survival [62, 63, 72, 96]. As treatment options continue being developed newer combination therapies may surpass ASCT with better outcomes.

Advanced HF in the Context of ATTRwt Cardiac Amyloidosis

As this disease is characterized by its late onset the time needed to reach the hemodynamic compromise to require transplantation often renders a patient well outside the age bracket considered for HT. Given an earlier onset, the management and evaluation does not differ from other etiologies that lead to HT.

Advanced HF in the Context of ATTRh Cardiac Amyloidosis

A different approach is taken when treating patient with ATTRh, specifically early onset Val50Met mutations. In these patients orthotopic liver transplantation (OLT) is an established therapeutic option given its use to reduce the progression of the neuropathy [97]. Val50Met with OLT has better outcomes when compared with other forms of Familial Amyloid Neuropathy FAP [98]. Although this approach has its benefits it does not come without its own set of complications. Ranging from the classical complications of a transplant recipient one adds the possibility of the phenomena known as seeding [99]. This is the process by which deposits of the misfolded variant TTR "set up the way" for the continued polymerization of native TTR synthetized by the transplanted liver, perpetuating the organic compromise despite OLT. Presently, there are no approved and adopted treatments adjunctive to immunosuppression directed to stop this process. This renders the possibility of a slow but progressive cardiac infiltration post-OLT. If this takes place, when the patients have reached advanced HF management should be the same as with HT for other etiologies and determine if the age and organ damage is not excessive to perform HT. On the contrary, in the case of a mixed phenotype with advanced HF the decision will likely be a combined heart and liver transplantation.

Currently, HT remains a valuable therapeutic option in the setting of CA. Survival is similar between transplant recipients with amyloid cardiomyopathy and non-amyloid forms of restrictive cardiomyopathies [100]. Its role in the future is unclear as newer therapies are being developed and may change the way we see the disease today.

Conclusion

Familial RCM and HCM have in common that they are caused by mutations in genes that encode sarcomeric proteins and, in some cases, by storage and infiltrative diseases, which can present a restrictive or hypertrophic phenotype depending on the filling pattern and the wall thickness. Patients with RCM and HCM can coexist in the same family and on occasions, in the same patient there may be a phenotypic overlap between them. Therefore, it is currently considered that RCM may represent a part of the phenotypic spectrum of HCM and not a different cardiomyopathy. In both entities, diastolic dysfunction predominates. In a low percentage of HCM/RCM patients with refractory HF, HT is the only therapeutic alternative. The restrictive biventricular physiology added to the small size of the LV chamber determines that patients with HCM/RCM are often less tolerant to inotropes and are not considered good candidates for mechanical circulatory support devices. In addition, CPET and/or echocardiography do not always reflect the severity of the disease, leading to an inadequate risk estimate and therefore higher waiting list mortality. For this reason, increasing the priority of HT in HCM/RCM has currently been established according to clinical parameters and without specific hemodynamic or pharmacological/mechanical support criteria.

In patients with HCM/RCM due to storage or infiltrative disease who have specific therapies, continuation of these treatments should be considered after HT, to prevent recurrence of heart disease and progression in other organs.

References

[1] Elliott P, Andersson B, Arbustini E, Bilinska Z, Cecchi F, Charron P, Dubourg O, Kühl U, Maisch B, McKenna WJ, Monserrat L, Pankuweit S, Rapezzi C, Seferovic P, Tavazzi L, Keren A. Classification of the cardiomyopathies: a position statement from the European Society Of Cardiology Working Group on Myocardial and Pericardial Diseases. *Eur Heart J*. 2008 Jan;29(2):270-6.

[2] Authors/Task Force members, Elliott PM, Anastasakis A, Borger MA, Borggrefe M, Cecchi F, Charron P, Hagege AA, Lafont A, Limongelli G, Mahrholdt H, McKenna WJ, Mogensen J, Nihoyannopoulos P, Nistri S, Pieper PG, Pieske B, Rapezzi C, Rutten FH, Tillmanns C, Watkins H. 2014 ESC Guidelines on diagnosis and management of hypertrophic cardiomyopathy: the Task Force for the Diagnosis and Management of Hypertrophic Cardiomyopathy of the European Society of Cardiology (ESC). *Eur Heart J.* 2014 Oct 14;35(39):2733-79.

[3] Fernández A, Acunzo RS, Avegliano G, Casabé JH,A, Dumont CA, Hita A, Ortiz M, Pérez de Arenaza D, Alday L, Antoni D, Baratta S, Cerdá M, Cianciulli TF, Costabel JP, Cura F, Darú V, Di Nunzio H, Elizari A, Favaloro R, Figal J, Galizio N, Ganum G, García D, González GE, González JL, Guerchicoff A, Guerchicoff M, Guevara E, Hershson A, Konopka IV, Labadet C, Lakowsky A, Lax J, Lev G, Lowenstein JA, Militello C, Morales C, Oberti P, Ochoa JP, Ontiveros G, Peidro

R, Quiroga A, Saccheri MC, Salmo F, Thierer J, Vigliano C, Vrancic JM. Argentine Consensus on the diagnosis and treatment of hypertrophic cardiomyopathy 2016. Argentine Society of Caridology. *Rev Argent Cardiol* 2017 May;85 (2):1-78.

[4] Ommen SR, Mital S, Burke MA, Day SM, Deswal A, Elliott P, Evanovich LL, Hung J, Joglar JA, Kantor P, Kimmelstiel C, Kittleson M, Link MS, Maron MS, Martinez MW, Miyake CY, Schaff HV, Semsarian C, Sorajja P. 2020 AHA/ACC Guideline for the Diagnosis and Treatment of Patients With Hypertrophic Cardiomyopathy: Executive Summary: A Report of the American College of Cardiology/American Heart Association Joint Committee on Clinical Practice Guidelines. *Circulation.* 2020 Dec 22;142(25):e533-e557.

[5] Harris KM, Spirito P, Maron MS, Zenovich AG, Formisano F, Lesser JR, Mackey-Bojack S, Manning WJ, Udelson JE, Maron BJ. Prevalence, clinical profile, and significance of left ventricular remodeling in the end-stage phase of hypertrophic cardiomyopathy. *Circulation.* 2006 Jul 18;114(3):216-25.

[6] Shirani J, Maron BJ, Cannon RO 3rd, Shahin S, Roberts WC. Clinicopathologic features of hypertrophic cardiomyopathy managed by cardiac transplantation. Am *J Cardiol.* 1993 Aug 15;72(5):434-40.

[7] Biagini E, Spirito P, Leone O, Picchio FM, Coccolo F, Ragni L, Lofiego C, Grigioni F, Potena L, Rocchi G, Bacchi-Reggiani L, Boriani G, Prandstraller D, Arbustini E, Branzi A, Rapezzi C. Heart transplantation in hypertrophic cardiomyopathy. *Am J Cardiol*. 2008 Feb 1;101(3):387-92.

[8] Fernández A, Vigliano CA, Casabé JH, Diez M, Favaloro LE, Guevara E, Favaloro RR, Laguens RP. Comparison of prevalence, clinical course, and pathological findings of left ventricular systolic impairment versus normal systolic function in patients with hypertrophic cardiomyopathy. *Am J Cardiol.* 2011 Aug 15;108(4):548-55.

[9] Cecchi F, Olivotto I, Gistri R, Lorenzoni R, Chiriatti G, Camici PG. Coronary microvascular dysfunction and prognosis in hypertrophic cardiomyopathy. *N Engl J Med.* 2003 Sep 11;349(11):1027-35.

[10] Thaman R, Gimeno JR, Murphy RT, Kubo T, Sachdev B, Mogensen J, Elliott PM, McKenna WJ. Prevalence and clinical significance of systolic impairment in hypertrophic cardiomyopathy. *Heart.* 2005 Jul;91(7):920-5.

[11] Olivotto I, Cecchi F, Gistri R, Lorenzoni R, Chiriatti G, Girolami F, Torricelli F, Camici PG. Relevance of coronary microvascular flow impairment to long-term remodeling and systolic dysfunction in hypertrophic cardiomyopathy. *J Am Coll Cardiol.* 2006 Mar 7;47(5):1043-8.

[12] Olivotto I, Maron BJ, Appelbaum E, Harrigan CJ, Salton C, Gibson CM, Udelson JE, O'Donnell C, Lesser JR, Manning WJ, Maron MS. Spectrum and clinical significance of systolic function and myocardial fibrosis assessed by cardiovascular magnetic resonance in hypertrophic cardiomyopathy. *Am J Cardiol.* 2010 Jul 15;106(2):261-7.

[13] Marstrand P, Han L, Day SM, Olivotto I, Ashley EA, Michels M, Pereira AC, Wittekind SG, Helms A, Saberi S, Jacoby D, Ware JS, Colan SD, Semsarian C, Ingles J, Lakdawala NK, Ho CY; SHaRe Investigators. Hypertrophic

Cardiomyopathy With Left Ventricular Systolic Dysfunction: Insights From the SHaRe Registry. *Circulation.* 2020 Apr 28;141(17):1371-1383.

[14] Melacini P, Basso C, Angelini A, Calore C, Bobbo F, Tokajuk B, Bellini N, Smaniotto G, Zucchetto M, Iliceto S, Thiene G, Maron BJ. Clinicopathological profiles of progressive heart failure in hypertrophic cardiomyopathy. *Eur Heart J.* 2010 Sep;31(17):2111-23.

[15] Rowin EJ, Maron MS, Chan RH, Hausvater A, Wang W, Rastegar H, Maron BJ. Interaction of Adverse Disease Related Pathways in Hypertrophic Cardiomyopathy. *Am J Cardiol.* 2017 Dec 15;120(12):2256-2264.

[16] Pasqualucci D, Fornaro A, Castelli G, Rossi A, Arretini A, Chiriatti C, Targetti M, Girolami F, Corda M, Orrù P, Matta G, Stefàno P, Cecchi F, Porcu M, Olivotto I. Clinical Spectrum, Therapeutic Options, and Outcome of Advanced Heart Failure in Hypertrophic Cardiomyopathy. *Circ Heart Fail.* 2015 Nov;8(6):1014-21.

[17] Fujino N, Shimizu M, Ino H, Yamaguchi M, Yasuda T, Nagata M, Konno T, Mabuchi H. A novel mutation Lys273Glu in the cardiac troponin T gene shows high degree of penetrance and transition from hypertrophic to dilated cardiomyopathy. *Am J Cardiol*. 2002 Jan 1;89(1):29-33.

[18] Mogensen J, Murphy RT, Kubo T, Bahl A, Moon JC, Klausen IC, Elliott PM, McKenna WJ. Frequency and clinical expression of cardiac troponin I mutations in 748 consecutive families with hypertrophic cardiomyopathy. *J Am Coll Cardiol.* 2004 Dec 21;44(12):2315-25.

[19] García-Giustiniani D, Arad M, Ortíz-Genga M, Barriales-Villa R, Fernández X, Rodríguez-García I, Mazzanti A, Veira E, Maneiro E, Rebolo P, Lesende I, Cazón L, Freimark D, Gimeno-Blanes JR, Seidman C, Seidman J, McKenna W, Monserrat L. Phenotype and prognostic correlations of the converter region mutations affecting the β myosin heavy chain. *Heart.* 2015 Jul;101(13):1047-53.

[20] Lopes LR, Garcia-Hernández S, Lorenzini M, Futema M, Chumakova O, Zateyshchikov D, Isidoro-Garcia M, Villacorta E, Escobar-Lopez L, Garcia-Pavia P, Bilbao R, Dobarro D, Sandin-Fuentes M, Catalli C, Gener Querol B, Mezcua A, Garcia Pinilla J, Bloch Rasmussen T, Ferreira-Aguar A, Revilla-Martí P, Basurte Elorz MT, Bautista Paves A, Ramon Gimeno J, Figueroa AV, Franco-Gutierrez R, Fuentes-Cañamero ME, Martinez Moreno M, Ortiz-Genga M, Piqueras-Flores J, Analia Ramos K, Rudzitis A, Ruiz-Guerrero L, Stein R, Triguero-Bocharán M, de la Higuera L, Ochoa JP, Abu-Bonsrah D, Kwok CYT, Smith JB, Porrello ER, Akhtar MM, Jager J, Ashworth M, Syrris P, Elliott DA, Monserrat L, Elliott PM. Alpha-protein kinase 3 (ALPK3) truncating variants are a cause of autosomal dominant hypertrophic cardiomyopathy. *Eur Heart J.* 2021 Aug 21;42(32):3063-3073.

[21] Spirito P, Maron BJ, Bonow RO, Epstein SE. Occurrence and significance of progressive left ventricular wall thinning and relative cavity dilatation in hypertrophic cardiomyopathy. *Am J Cardiol*. 1987 Jul 1;60(1):123-9.

[22] Shirani J, Pick R, Roberts WC, Maron BJ. Morphology and significance of the left ventricular collagen network in young patients with hypertrophic cardiomyopathy and sudden cardiac death. *J Am Coll Cardiol.* 2000 Jan;35(1):36-44.

[23] Kitamura M, Shimizu M, Ino H, Okeie K, Yamaguchi M, Funjno N, Mabuchi H, Nakanishi I. Collagen remodeling and cardiac dysfunction in patients with hypertrophic cardiomyopathy: the significance of type III and VI collagens. *Clin Cardiol.* 2001 Apr;24(4):325-9.

[24] Thaman R, Gimeno JR, Reith S, Esteban MT, Limongelli G, Murphy RT, Mist B, McKenna WJ, Elliott PM. Progressive left ventricular remodeling in patients with hypertrophic cardiomyopathy and severe left ventricular hypertrophy. *J Am Coll Cardiol.* 2004 Jul 21;44(2):398-405. doi: 10.1016/j.jacc.2004.01.054. PMID: 15261938.

[25] Maron BJ, Wolfson JK, Epstein SE, Roberts WC. Intramural ("small vessel") coronary artery disease in hypertrophic cardiomyopathy. *J Am Coll Cardiol.* 1986 Sep;8(3):545-57.

[26] Schwartzkopff B, Mundhenke M, Strauer BE. Alterations of the architecture of subendocardial arterioles in patients with hypertrophic cardiomyopathy and impaired coronary vasodilator reserve: a possible cause for myocardial ischemia. J Am Coll Cardiol. 1998 Apr;31(5):1089-96.

[27] Krams R, Ten Cate FJ, Carlier SG, Van Der Steen AF, Serruys PW. Diastolic coronary vascular reserve: a new index to detect changes in the coronary microcirculation in hypertrophic cardiomyopathy. *J Am Coll Cardiol.* 2004 Feb 18;43(4):670-7.

[28] Varnava AM, Elliott PM, Sharma S, McKenna WJ, Davies MJ. Hypertrophic cardiomyopathy: the interrelation of disarray, fibrosis, and small vessel disease. *Heart.* 2000 Nov;84(5):476-82.

[29] McDonagh TA, Metra M, Adamo M, Gardner RS, Baumbach A, Böhm M, Burri H, Butler J, Čelutkienė J, Chioncel O, Cleland JGF, Coats AJS, Crespo-Leiro MG, Farmakis D, Gilard M, Heymans S, Hoes AW, Jaarsma T, Jankowska EA, Lainscak M, Lam CSP, Lyon AR, McMurray JJV, Mebazaa A, Mindham R, Muneretto C, Francesco Piepoli M, Price S, Rosano GMC, Ruschitzka F, Kathrine Skibelund A; ESC Scientific Document Group. 2021 ESC Guidelines for the diagnosis and treatment of acute and chronic heart failure. *Eur Heart J.* 2021 Sep 21;42(36):3599-3726.

[30] Rogers DP, Marazia S, Chow AW, Lambiase PD, Lowe MD, Frenneaux M, McKenna WJ, Elliott PM. Effect of biventricular pacing on symptoms and cardiac remodelling in patients with end-stage hypertrophic cardiomyopathy. *Eur J Heart Fail.* 2008 May;10(5):507-13.

[31] Rowin EJ, Mohanty S, Madias C, Maron BJ, Maron MS. Benefit of Cardiac Resynchronization Therapy in End-Stage Nonobstructive Hypertrophic Cardiomyopathy. *JACC Clin Electrophysiol.* 2019 Jan;5(1):131-133.

[32] Glikson M, Nielsen JC, Kronborg MB, Michowitz Y, Auricchio A, Barbash IM, Barrabés JA, Boriani G, Braunschweig F, Brignole M, Burri H, Coats AJS, Deharo JC, Delgado V, Diller GP, Israel CW, Keren A, Knops RE, Kotecha D, Leclercq C, Merkely B, Starck C, Thylén I, Tolosana JM; ESC National Cardiac Societies; ESC Scientific Document Group. 2021 ESC Guidelines on cardiac pacing and cardiac resynchronization therapy. *Eur Heart J.* 2021 Sep 14;42(35):3427-3520.

[33] Cappelli F, Morini S, Pieragnoli P, Targetti M, Stefàno P, Marchionni N, Olivotto I. Cardiac Resynchronization Therapy for End-Stage Hypertrophic Cardiomyopathy: The Need for Disease-Specific Criteria. *J Am Coll Cardiol.* 2018 Jan 30;71(4):464-466.

[34] Hebl VB, Miranda WR, Ong KC, Hodge DO, Bos JM, Gentile F, Klarich KW, Nishimura RA, Ackerman MJ, Gersh BJ, Ommen SR, Geske JB. The Natural History of Nonobstructive Hypertrophic Cardiomyopathy. *Mayo Clin Proc.* 2016 Mar;91(3):279-87.

[35] Chan RH, Maron BJ, Olivotto I, Pencina MJ, Assenza GE, Haas T, Lesser JR, Gruner C, Crean AM, Rakowski H, Udelson JE, Rowin E, Lombardi M, Cecchi F, Tomberli B, Spirito P, Formisano F, Biagini E, Rapezzi C, De Cecco CN, Autore C, Cook EF, Hong SN, Gibson CM, Manning WJ, Appelbaum E, Maron MS. Prognostic value of quantitative contrast-enhanced cardiovascular magnetic resonance for the evaluation of sudden death risk in patients with hypertrophic cardiomyopathy. *Circulation.* 2014 Aug 5;130(6):484-95.

[36] Weng Z, Yao J, Chan RH, He J, Yang X, Zhou Y, He Y. Prognostic Value of LGE-CMR in HCM: A Meta-Analysis. *JACC Cardiovasc Imaging.* 2016 Dec;9(12):1392-1402.

[37] Braunwald E, Brockenbrough EC, Frye RL. Studies on digitalis. V. Comparison of the effects of ouabain on left ventricular dynamics in valvular aortic stenosis and hypertrophic subaortic stenosis. *Circulation.* 1962 Aug;26:166-73.

[38] Tafelmeier M, Baessler A, Wagner S, Unsoeld B, Preveden A, Barlocco F, Tomberli A, Popovic D, Brennan P, MacGowan GA, Ristic A, Velicki L, Olivotto I, Jakovljevic DG, Maier LS. Design of the SILICOFCM study: Effect of sacubitril/valsartan vs lifestyle intervention on functional capacity in patients with hypertrophic cardiomyopathy. *Clin Cardiol.* 2020 May;43(5):430-440.

[39] Nguyen A, Schaff HV, Nishimura RA, Geske JB, Dearani JA, King KS, Ommen SR. Apical myectomy for patients with hypertrophic cardiomyopathy and advanced heart failure. *J Thorac Cardiovasc Surg.* 2019 Apr 5:S0022-5223(19)30772-X.

[40] Cimiotti D, Budde H, Hassoun R, Jaquet K. Genetic Restrictive Cardiomyopathy: Causes and Consequences-An Integrative Approach. *Int J Mol Sci.* 2021 Jan 8;22(2):558.

[41] Kushwaha SS, Fallon JT, Fuster V. Restrictive cardiomyopathy. *N Engl J Med.* 1997 Jan 23;336(4):267-76.

[42] Vio R, Angelini A, Basso C, Cipriani A, Zorzi A, Melacini P, Thiene G, Rampazzo A, Corrado D, Calore C. Hypertrophic Cardiomyopathy and Primary Restrictive Cardiomyopathy: Similarities, Differences and Phenocopies. *J Clin Med.* 2021 May 1;10(9):1954.

[43] De Bortoli M, Vio R, Basso C, Calore M, Minervini G, Angelini A, Melacini P, Vitiello L, Vazza G, Thiene G, Tosatto S, Corrado D, Iliceto S, Rampazzo A, Calore C. Novel Missense Variant in MYL2 Gene Associated With Hypertrophic Cardiomyopathy Showing High Incidence of Restrictive Physiology. *Circ Genom Precis Med.* 2020 Apr;13(2):e002824.

[44] Repetti GG, Toepfer CN, Seidman JG, Seidman CE. Novel Therapies for Prevention and Early Treatment of Cardiomyopathies. *Circ Res*. 2019 May 24;124(11):1536-1550.

[45] Rapezzi C, Arbustini E, Caforio AL, Charron P, Gimeno-Blanes J, Heliö T, Linhart A, Mogensen J, Pinto Y, Ristic A, Seggewiss H, Sinagra G, Tavazzi L, Elliott PM. Diagnostic work-up in cardiomyopathies: bridging the gap between clinical phenotypes and final diagnosis. A position statement from the ESC Working Group on Myocardial and Pericardial Diseases. *Eur Heart J.* 2013 May;34(19):1448-58.

[46] Mogensen J, Kubo T, Duque M, Uribe W, Shaw A, Murphy R, Gimeno JR, Elliott P, McKenna WJ. Idiopathic restrictive cardiomyopathy is part of the clinical expression of cardiac troponin I mutations. *J Clin Invest*. 2003 Jan;111(2):209-16.

[47] Kaski JP, Syrris P, Burch M, Tomé-Esteban MT, Fenton M, Christiansen M, Andersen PS, Sebire N, Ashworth M, Deanfield JE, McKenna WJ, Elliott PM. Idiopathic restrictive cardiomyopathy in children is caused by mutations in cardiac sarcomere protein genes. *Heart.* 2008 Nov;94(11):1478-84.

[48] Gallego-Delgado M, Delgado JF, Brossa-Loidi V, Palomo J, Marzoa-Rivas R, Perez-Villa F, Salazar-Mendiguchía J, Ruiz-Cano MJ, Gonzalez-Lopez E, Padron-Barthe L, Bornstein B, Alonso-Pulpon L, Garcia-Pavia P. Idiopathic Restrictive Cardiomyopathy Is Primarily a Genetic Disease. *J Am Coll Cardiol.* 2016 Jun 28;67(25):3021-3.

[49] Fernández A, Politei J. Cardiac Manifestation of Fabry Disease: From hypertrophic cardiomyopathy to early diagnosis and treatment in patients without left ventricular hypertrophy. Journal of Inborn Errors of Metabolism & Screening 2016 Jan;4:1-9.

[50] Linhart A, Germain DP, Olivotto I, Akhtar MM, Anastasakis A, Hughes D, Namdar M, Pieroni M, Hagège A, Cecchi F, Gimeno JR, Limongelli G, Elliott P. An expert consensus document on the management of cardiovascular manifestations of Fabry disease. *Eur J Heart Fail.* 2020 Jul;22(7):1076-1096.

[51] Fernández A, Rodríguez MJ, Gómez JE. Fabry's disease. Rev Colomb Cardiol 2021 May;28(2):10-16.

[52] Aronow WS. Management of cardiac hemochromatosis. *Arch Med Sci*. 2018 Apr;14(3):560-568.

[53] Brodehl A, Pour Hakimi SA, Stanasiuk C, Ratnavadivel S, Hendig D, Gaertner A, Gerull B, Gummert J, Paluszkiewicz L, Milting H. Restrictive Cardiomyopathy is Caused by a Novel Homozygous Desmin (DES) Mutation p.Y122H Leading to a Severe Filament Assembly Defect. *Genes (Basel).* 2019 Nov 11;10(11):918.

[54] Lopez-Sainz A, Dominguez F, Lopes LR, Ochoa JP, Barriales-Villa R, Climent V, Linschoten M, Tiron C, Chiriatti C, Marques N, Rasmussen TB, Espinosa MÁ, Beinart R, Quarta G, Cesar S, Field E, Garcia-Pinilla JM, Bilinska Z, Muir AR, Roberts AM, Santas E, Zorio E, Peña-Peña ML, Navarro M, Fernandez A, Palomino-Doza J, Azevedo O, Lorenzini M, García-Álvarez MI, Bento D, Jensen MK, Méndez I, Pezzoli L, Sarquella-Brugada G, Campuzano O, Gonzalez-Lopez E, Mogensen J, Kaski JP, Arad M, Brugada R, Asselbergs FW, Monserrat L, Olivotto I, Elliott PM, Garcia-Pavia P; European Genetic Cardiomyopathies Initiative Investigators. Clinical Features and Natural History of PRKAG2 Variant Cardiac Glycogenosis. *J Am Coll Cardiol.* 2020 Jul 14;76(2):186-197.

[55] González-López E, Gagliardi C, Dominguez F, Quarta CC, de Haro-Del Moral FJ, Milandri A, Salas C, Cinelli M, Cobo-Marcos M, Lorenzini M, Lara-Pezzi E, Foffi S, Alonso-Pulpon L, Rapezzi C, Garcia-Pavia P. Clinical characteristics of wild-type transthyretin cardiac amyloidosis: disproving myths. *Eur Heart J.* 2017 Jun 21;38(24):1895-1904.

[56] Selcen D. Myofibrillar myopathies. *Neuromuscul Disord.* 2011 Mar;21(3):161-71.

[57] Reuser AJ, Verheijen FW, Bali D, van Diggelen OP, Germain DP, Hwu WL, Lukacs Z, Mühl A, Olivova P, Piraud M, Wuyts B, Zhang K, Keutzer J. The use of dried blood spot samples in the diagnosis of lysosomal storage disorders--current status and perspectives. Mol Genet Metab. 2011 Sep-Oct;104(1-2):144-8.

[58] Politei J, Frabasil J, Durand C, Di Pietrantonio S, Fernandez A, Albertón V, Velasquez Rivas D, Barriales-Villa R, Larrañaga-Moreira J, Schenone AB. Incidental finding of cornea verticillata or lamellar inclusions in kidney biopsy: measurement of lyso-Gb3 in plasma defines between Fabry disease and drug-induced phospholipidosis. *Biochim Biophys Acta Mol Basis Dis.* 2021 Jan 1;1867(1):165985.

[59] Palladini G, Sachchithanantham S, Milani P, Gillmore J, Foli A, Lachmann H, Basset M, Hawkins P, Merlini G, Wechalekar AD. A European collaborative study of cyclophosphamide, bortezomib, and dexamethasone in upfront treatment of systemic AL amyloidosis. *Blood.* 2015 Jul 30;126(5):612-5.

[60] Kastritis E, Palladini G, Minnema MC, Wechalekar AD, Jaccard A, Lee HC, Sanchorawala V, Gibbs S, Mollee P, Venner CP, Lu J, Schönland S, Gatt ME, Suzuki K, Kim K, Cibeira MT, Beksac M, Libby E, Valent J, Hungria V, Wong SW, Rosenzweig M, Bumma N, Huart A, Dimopoulos MA, Bhutani D, Waxman AJ, Goodman SA, Zonder JA, Lam S, Song K, Hansen T, Manier S, Roeloffzen W, Jamroziak K, Kwok F, Shimazaki C, Kim JS, Crusoe E, Ahmadi T, Tran N, Qin X, Vasey SY, Tromp B, Schecter JM, Weiss BM, Zhuang SH, Vermeulen J, Merlini G, Comenzo RL; ANDROMEDA Trial Investigators. Daratumumab-Based Treatment for Immunoglobulin Light-Chain Amyloidosis. *N Engl J Med.* 2021 Jul 1;385(1):46-58.

[61] Dubrey SW, Cha K, Anderson J, Chamarthi B, Reisinger J, Skinner M, Falk RH. The clinical features of immunoglobulin light-chain (AL) amyloidosis with heart involvement. *QJM.* 1998 Feb;91(2):141-57

[62] Lacy MQ, Dispenzieri A, Hayman SR, Kumar S, Kyle RA, Rajkumar SV, Edwards BS, Rodeheffer RJ, Frantz RP, Kushwaha SS, Clavell AL, Dearani JA, Sundt TM, Daly RC, McGregor CG, Gastineau DA, Litzow MR, Gertz MA. Autologous stem cell transplant after heart transplant for light chain (Al) amyloid cardiomyopathy. *J Heart Lung Transplant*. 2008 Aug;27(8):823-9.

[63] Dey BR, Chung SS, Spitzer TR, Zheng H, Macgillivray TE, Seldin DC, McAfee S, Ballen K, Attar E, Wang T, Shin J, Newton-Cheh C, Moore S, Sanchorawala V, Skinner M, Madsen JC, Semigran MJ. Cardiac transplantation followed by dose-intensive melphalan and autologous stem-cell transplantation for light chain amyloidosis and heart failure. *Transplantation.* 2010 Oct 27;90(8):905-11.

[64] Gillmore JD, Maurer MS, Falk RH, Merlini G, Damy T, Dispenzieri A, Wechalekar AD, Berk JL, Quarta CC, Grogan M, Lachmann HJ, Bokhari S, Castano A, Dorbala S, Johnson GB, Glaudemans AW, Rezk T, Fontana M, Palladini G, Milani P, Guidalotti PL, Flatman K, Lane T, Vonberg FW, Whelan CJ, Moon JC, Ruberg FL, Miller EJ, Hutt DF, Hazenberg BP, Rapezzi C, Hawkins PN. Nonbiopsy Diagnosis of Cardiac Transthyretin Amyloidosis. *Circulation.* 2016 Jun 14;133(24):2404-12.

[65] González-Moreno J, Losada-López I, Cisneros-Barroso E, Garcia-Pavia P, González-Costello J, Muñoz-Beamud F, Campistol JM, Fernandez-Torron R, Chapman D, Amass L. A Descriptive Analysis of ATTR Amyloidosis in Spain from the Transthyretin Amyloidosis Outcomes Survey. *Neurol Ther.* 2021 Dec;10(2):833-845.

[66] Etesami M, Gilkeson RC, Rajiah P. Utility of late gadolinium enhancement in pediatric cardiac MRI. *Pediatr Radiol.* 2016 Jul;46(8):1096-113.

[67] Senra T, Shiozaki AA, Salemi VM, Rochitte CE. Delayed enhancement by multidetector computed tomography in endomyocardial fibrosis. *Eur Heart J.* 2008 Feb;29(3):347.

[68] Charron P, Arad M, Arbustini E, Basso C, Bilinska Z, Elliott P, Helio T, Keren A, McKenna WJ, Monserrat L, Pankuweit S, Perrot A, Rapezzi C, Ristic A, Seggewiss H, van Langen I, Tavazzi L; European Society of Cardiology Working Group on Myocardial and Pericardial Diseases. Genetic counselling and testing in cardiomyopathies: a position statement of the European Society of Cardiology Working Group on Myocardial and Pericardial Diseases. *Eur Heart J.* 2010 Nov;31(22):2715-26.

[69] Cooper LT, Baughman KL, Feldman AM, Frustaci A, Jessup M, Kuhl U, Levine GN, Narula J, Starling RC, Towbin J, Virmani R. The role of endomyocardial biopsy in the management of cardiovascular disease: a scientific statement from the American Heart Association, the American College of Cardiology, and the European Society of Cardiology Endorsed by the Heart Failure Society of America and the Heart Failure Association of the European Society of Cardiology. *Eur Heart J.* 2007 Dec;28(24):3076-93.

[70] Rowin EJ, Maron BJ, Abt P, Kiernan MS, Vest A, Costantino F, Maron MS, DeNofrio D. Impact of Advanced Therapies for Improving Survival to Heart Transplant in Patients with Hypertrophic Cardiomyopathy. *Am J Cardiol.* 2018 Apr 15;121(8):986-996.

[71] Maron MS, Rowin EJ, Olivotto I, Casey SA, Arretini A, Tomberli B, Garberich RF, Link MS, Chan RHM, Lesser JR, Maron BJ. Contemporary Natural History and Management of Nonobstructive Hypertrophic Cardiomyopathy. *J Am Coll Cardiol.* 2016 Mar 29;67(12):1399-1409.

[72] Mehra MR, Canter CE, Hannan MM, Semigran MJ, Uber PA, Baran DA, Danziger-Isakov L, Kirklin JK, Kirk R, Kushwaha SS, Lund LH, Potena L, Ross HJ, Taylor DO, Verschuuren EAM, Zuckermann A; International Society for Heart Lung Transplantation (ISHLT) Infectious Diseases, Pediatric and Heart Failure and Transplantation Councils. The 2016 International Society for Heart Lung

Transplantation listing criteria for heart transplantation: A 10-year update. J *Heart Lung Transplant*. 2016 Jan;35(1):1-23.
[73] OPTN Review Board Guidance for Hypertrophic/Restrictive (HCM/RCM) Cardiomyopathy Exception Requests [online]. 2018 [cited 2021 October 24]. Available from: https://optn.transplant.hrsa.gov/media/2637/thoracic_guidance_review_board_hcm_rcm_201806.pdf.
[74] Organ Procurement and Transplantation Network: Policy 6: Allocation of Hearts and Hearts-Lungs [online]. 2021 [cited 2021 October 24]. Available from: http://optn.transplant.hrsa.gov/media/1200/optn_policies.pdf#nameddest=Policy_06.
[75] Coats CJ, Rantell K, Bartnik A, Patel A, Mist B, McKenna WJ, Elliott PM. Cardiopulmonary Exercise Testing and Prognosis in Hypertrophic Cardiomyopathy. *Circ Heart Fail.* 2015 Nov;8(6):1022-31.
[76] Magrì D, Re F, Limongelli G, Agostoni P, Zachara E, Correale M, Mastromarino V, Santolamazza C, Casenghi M, Pacileo G, Valente F, Morosin M, Musumeci B, Pagannone E, Maruotti A, Uguccioni M, Volpe M, Autore C. Heart Failure Progression in Hypertrophic Cardiomyopathy- Possible Insights From Cardiopulmonary Exercise Testing. *Circ J.* 2016 Sep 23;80(10):2204-11.
[77] Rowin EJ, Maron BJ, Kiernan MS, Casey SA, Feldman DS, Hryniewicz KM, Chan RH, Harris KM, Udelson JE, DeNofrio D, Roberts WC, Maron MS. Advanced heart failure with preserved systolic function in nonobstructive hypertrophic cardiomyopathy: under-recognized subset of candidates for heart transplant. *Circ Heart Fail*. 2014 Nov;7(6):967-75.
[78] Sridharan L, Wayda B, Truby LK, Latif F, Restaino S, Takeda K, Takayama H, Naka Y, Colombo PC, Maurer M, Farr MA, Topkara VK. Mechanical Circulatory Support Device Utilization and Heart Transplant Waitlist Outcomes in Patients with Restrictive and Hypertrophic Cardiomyopathy. *Circ Heart Fail*. 2018 Mar;11(3):e004665.
[79] Griffin JM, DeFilippis EM, Rosenblum H, Topkara VK, Fried JA, Uriel N, Takeda K, Farr MA, Maurer MS, Clerkin KJ. Comparing outcomes for infiltrative and restrictive cardiomyopathies under the new heart transplant allocation system. *Clin Transplant*. 2020 Dec;34(12):e14109.
[80] Uchmanowicz I, Łoboz-Rudnicka M, Szeląg P, Jankowska-Polańska B, Łoboz-Grudzień K. Frailty in heart failure. *Curr Heart Fail Rep*. 2014 Sep;11(3):266-73.
[81] Singh TP, Almond CS, Piercey G, Gauvreau K. Current outcomes in US children with cardiomyopathy listed for heart transplantation. *Circ Heart Fail*. 2012 Sep 1;5(5):594-601.
[82] Su JA, Menteer J. Outcomes of Berlin Heart EXCOR® pediatric ventricular assist device support in patients with restrictive and hypertrophic cardiomyopathy. *Pediatr Transplant*. 2017 Dec;21(8).
[83] Nordin S, Kozor R, Medina-Menacho K, Abdel-Gadir A, Baig S, Sado DM, Lobascio I, Murphy E, Lachmann RH, Mehta A, Edwards NC, Ramaswami U, Steeds RP, Hughes D, Moon JC. Proposed Stages of Myocardial Phenotype

Development in Fabry Disease. *JACC Cardiovasc Imaging*. 2019 Aug;12(8 Pt 2):1673-1683.

[84] Weidemann F, Reiser M. Fabry Disease: Cardiomyopathy Staging. *JACC Cardiovasc Imaging*. 2019 Aug;12(8 Pt 2):1684-1685.

[85] Karras A, De Lentdecker P, Delahousse M, Debauchez M, Tricot L, Pastural M, Bruneval P, Zemoura L, Duong Van Huyen JP, Lidove O. Combined heart and kidney transplantation in a patient with Fabry disease in the enzyme replacement therapy era. *Am J Transplant*. 2008 Jun;8(6):1345-8.

[86] Ortiz A, Germain DP, Desnick RJ, Politei J, Mauer M, Burlina A, Eng C, Hopkin RJ, Laney D, Linhart A, Waldek S, Wallace E, Weidemann F, Wilcox WR. Fabry disease revisited: Management and treatment recommendations for adult patients. *Mol Genet Metab*. 2018 Apr;123(4):416-427.

[87] Liao R, Ward JE. Amyloid Cardiomyopathy: Disease on the Rise. *Circ Res*. 2017 Jun 9;120(12):1865-1867.

[88] Maurer MS, Schwartz JH, Gundapaneni B, Elliott PM, Merlini G, Waddington-Cruz M, Kristen AV, Grogan M, Witteles R, Damy T, Drachman BM, Shah SJ, Hanna M, Judge DP, Barsdorf AI, Huber P, Patterson TA, Riley S, Schumacher J, Stewart M, Sultan MB, Rapezzi C; ATTR-ACT Study Investigators. Tafamidis Treatment for Patients with Transthyretin Amyloid Cardiomyopathy. *N Engl J Med*. 2018 Sep 13;379(11):1007-1016.

[89] Merlini G, Bellotti V. Molecular mechanisms of amyloidosis. *N Engl J Med.* 2003 Aug 7;349(6):583-96.

[90] Vranian MN, Sperry BW, Valent J, Hanna M. Emerging Advances in the Management of Cardiac Amyloidosis. *Curr Cardiol Rep*. 2015 Nov;17(11):100.

[91] Wechalekar AD, Gillmore JD, Hawkins PN. Systemic amyloidosis. *Lancet.* 2016 Jun 25;387(10038):2641-2654.

[92] Arruda-Olson AM, Zeldenrust SR, Dispenzieri A, Gertz MA, Miller FA, Bielinski SJ, Klarich KW, Scott CG, Grogan M. Genotype, echocardiography, and survival in familial transthyretin amyloidosis. *Amyloid.* 2013 Dec;20(4):263-8.

[93] Patel KS, Hawkins PN. Cardiac amyloidosis: where are we today? *J Intern Med.* 2015 Aug;278(2):126-44.

[94] Wechalekar AD, Schonland SO, Kastritis E, Gillmore JD, Dimopoulos MA, Lane T, Foli A, Foard D, Milani P, Rannigan L, Hegenbart U, Hawkins PN, Merlini G, Palladini G. A European collaborative study of treatment outcomes in 346 patients with cardiac stage III AL amyloidosis. *Blood.* 2013 Apr 25;121(17):3420-7.

[95] The Hereditary Amyloidosis mutations database. Mutations in Hereditary Amyloidosis [online]. 2021 [cited 2021 November 14]. Available from: http://amyloidosismutations.com/attr.html.

[96] Gillmore JD, Goodman HJ, Lachmann HJ, Offer M, Wechalekar AD, Joshi J, Pepys MB, Hawkins PN. Sequential heart and autologous stem cell transplantation for systemic AL amyloidosis. *Blood.* 2006 Feb 1;107(3):1227-9.

[97] Holmgren G, Ericzon BG, Groth CG, Steen L, Suhr O, Andersen O, Wallin BG, Seymour A, Richardson S, Hawkins PN. Clinical improvement and amyloid regression after liver transplantation in hereditary transthyretin amyloidosis. *Lancet.* 1993 May 1;341(8853):1113-6.

[98] Ericzon BG, Wilczek HE, Larsson M, Wijayatunga P, Stangou A, Pena JR, Furtado E, Barroso E, Daniel J, Samuel D, Adam R, Karam V, Poterucha J, Lewis D, Ferraz-Neto BH, Cruz MW, Munar-Ques M, Fabregat J, Ikeda S, Ando Y, Heaton N, Otto G, Suhr O. Liver Transplantation for Hereditary Transthyretin Amyloidosis: After 20 Years Still the Best Therapeutic Alternative? *Transplantation.* 2015 Sep;99(9):1847-54.

[99] Westermark P, Westermark GT. Seeding and Cross-seeding in Amyloid Diseases, In: Jucker M, Christen Y. Proteopathic Seeds and Neurodegenerative Diseases. Berlin: Springer;2016;47-60.

[100] Davis MK, Lee PH, Witteles RM. Changing outcomes after heart transplantation in patients with amyloid cardiomyopathy. *J Heart Lung Transplant.* 2015 May;34(5):658-66.

About the Editor

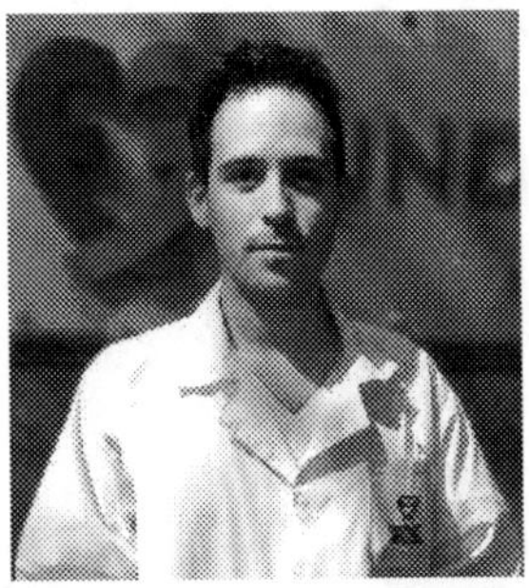

Elian Facundo Giordanino, MD
Cardiologist, Heart Failure and Heart Transplantation,
Favaloro Foundation University Hospital, Buenos Aires, Argentina
E-mail: elianfg@gmail.com
ORCID: 0000-0001-7380-4753

Elian Facundo Giordanino is a Cardiologist specialized in Heart Failure, Mechanical Circulatory Support and Heart Transplantation. He works in the Heart Failure and Heart Transplantation Division of the Favaloro Foundation University Hospital, Buenos Aires, Argentina.

In 2012, he graduated from Medical School University of Buenos Aires (UBA), Argentina and was awarded with the Gold Medal for the highest cumulative grade point average. After that, he was Coordinator and Editor in Chief of the *Journal of the Argentine Council of Cardiology Residents* and Coordinated the book, *Coronary Care Unit Manual CONAREC* (1st Edition, Buenos Aires, Argentina). In addition, he has published different research papers and chapters as well as peer reviewed several articles for the leading journals in the field such as the *Journal of Heart and Lung Transplantation* and *Transplant International Journal*.

Currently, he is Director of different courses in the field of Heart Failure and Heart Transplantation, as well as Principal Investigator in related clinical trials at his center. He is member of the International Society for Heart and Lung Transplantation (ISHLT), Heart Failure Association of the European Society of Cardiology (HFA-ESC) and the Argentinean Society of Cardiology (SAC).

List of Reviewers and Contributors

Reviewers

Absi, Daniel Oscar
Heart Failure and Heart Transplantation, Favaloro Foundation University Hospital, Buenos Aires, Argentina

Bertolotti, Mario Alejandro
Heart Failure and Heart Transplantation, Favaloro Foundation University Hospital, Buenos Aires, Argentina

Favaloro, Liliana Ethel
Heart Failure and Heart Transplantation, Favaloro Foundation University Hospital, Buenos Aires, Argentina

Favaloro, Roberto René
Heart Failure and Heart Transplantation, Favaloro Foundation University Hospital, Buenos Aires, Argentina

Renedo, María Florencia
Heart Failure and Heart Transplantation, Favaloro Foundation University Hospital, Buenos Aires, Argentina

Contributors

Absi, Daniel Oscar
Heart Failure and Heart Transplantation, Favaloro Foundation University Hospital, Buenos Aires, Argentina

Ahumada, Rosalía
Exercise Physiopathology Laboratory, Pneumonology Section, Department of Medicine, Favaloro Foundation University Hospital, Buenos Aires, Argentina

Andino Di Masi, Sergio Daniel
Infectious Diseases Department, Favaloro Foundation University Hospital, Buenos Aires, Argentina

Candioti Lehmann, Mariano Martin
Heart Failure and Heart Transplantation, Favaloro Foundation University Hospital, Buenos Aires, Argentina

Cáneva, Jorge Osvaldo
Exercise Physiopathology Laboratory, Pneumonology Section, Department of Medicine, Favaloro Foundation University Hospital, Buenos Aires, Argentina

Cicolini, Alejandro
Cardiovascular Intensive Care Unit, Favaloro Foundation University Hospital, Buenos Aires, Argentina

Favaloro, Liliana Ethel
Heart Failure and Heart Transplantation, Favaloro Foundation University Hospital, Buenos Aires, Argentina

Fernández, Adrián
Familial Cardiomyopathies Working Group, Clinical Cardiology Service, Favaloro Foundation University Hospital, Buenos Aires, Argentina

Gago, Rocío Emilia
Infectious Diseases Department, Austral University Hospital, Buenos Aires, Argentina

Ganum, Guillermo Eduardo
Echocardiography Department, Favaloro Foundation University Hospital, Buenos Aires, Argentina

Giordanino, Elian Facundo
Heart Failure and Heart Transplantation, Favaloro Foundation University Hospital, Buenos Aires, Argentina

Giorgio, Patricia Lourdes
Infectious Diseases Department, British Hospital, Buenos Aires, Argentina

Guevara, Eduardo
Echocardiography Department, Favaloro Foundation University Hospital, Buenos Aires, Argentina

Ibañez, Teresa Patricia
Heart Failure and Heart Transplantation, Favaloro Foundation University Hospital, Buenos Aires, Argentina

Martínez Rios, Melisa Belén
Infectious Diseases Department, Mendoza Central Hospital, Mendoza, Argentina

Martinez, Liliana
Heart Failure and Heart Transplantation, Favaloro Foundation University Hospital, Buenos Aires, Argentina

Moscoloni, Silvia Elsa
Heart Failure and Heart Transplantation, Favaloro Foundation University Hospital, Buenos Aires, Argentina

Moukarzel, Juan Alberto
Echocardiography Department, Favaloro Foundation University Hospital, Buenos Aires, Argentina

Ossés, Juan Manuel
Exercise Physiopathology Laboratory, Pneumonology Section, Department of Medicine, Favaloro Foundation University Hospital, Buenos Aires, Argentina

Padros, Karin
Histocompatibility, PRICAI-Favaloro Foundation University Hospital, Buenos Aires, Argentina

Pujato, Natalia Rosana
Infectious Diseases Department, ITAC Institute of Transplantation and High Complexity Buenos Aires, Argentina

Quiroga, Alejandro
Familial Cardiomyopathies Working Group, Clinical Cardiology Service, Favaloro Foundation University Hospital, Buenos Aires, Argentina

Ratto, Roxana Daniela
Heart Failure and Heart Transplantation, Favaloro Foundation University Hospital, Buenos Aires, Argentina

Renedo, María Florencia
Heart Failure and Heart Transplantation, Favaloro Foundation University Hospital, Buenos Aires, Argentina

Salmo, José Fabian
Echocardiography Department, Favaloro Foundation University Hospital, Buenos Aires, Argentina

Sánchez Luceros, Diego
Echocardiography Department, Favaloro Foundation University Hospital, Buenos Aires, Argentina

Scatularo, Cristhian Emmanuel
Heart Failure and Heart Transplantation, Favaloro Foundation University Hospital, Buenos Aires, Argentina

Seijo Behety, Milagros
Echocardiography Department, Favaloro Foundation University Hospital, Buenos Aires, Argentina

Trentadue, Julio Jorge
Department of Pediatrics, Favaloro Foundation University Hospital. Buenos Aires, Argentina

Vigliano, Carlos
Pathology Department, Favaloro Foundation University Hospital, Buenos Aires, Argentina

Villamandos. Silvina
Infectious Diseases Department, Juana F. Cabral. Corrientes Cardiology Institute

Yakobas, Norma Graciela
Heart Failure and Heart Transplantation, Favaloro Foundation University Hospital, Buenos Aires, Argentina

Zacarias, Orlando Omar
Heart Failure and Heart Transplantation, Favaloro Foundation University Hospital, Buenos Aires, Argentina

Zeppa, Federico Ignacio
Adult Congenital Heart Disease, Favaloro Foundation University Hospital, Buenos Aires, Argentina

Index

A

B

C

H

I

L

M

N

O

P

R

S

T

V

W